Histopathology

RECENT ADVANCES IN HISTOPATHOLOGY

Contents of Number 14

Edited by P. P. Anthony, R. N. M. MacSween

ISBN 0 443 039984

You can place your order by contacting your local medical bookseller or the Sales Promotion Department, Robert Stevenson House, 1–3 Baxter's Place, Leith Walk, Edinburgh EH1 3AF, UK

Tel: (031) 556 2424; Telex: 727511 LONGMN G; Fax: (031) 558 1278

Look out for *Recent Advances in Histopathology 16* in November 1993

RECENT ADVANCES IN

Histopathology

Edited by

Peter P. Anthony MBBS FRCPath
Consultant Pathologist and Professor of Clinical Histopathology, Royal Devon and Exeter
Hospitals and Postgraduate Medical School, University of Exeter, Exeter, UK

Roderick N. M. MacSween BSc MD FRCP(Glasg) FRCP(Edin)
FRCPath FRSE FIBiol
Professor of Pathology, University of Glasgow; Honorary Consultant in Pathology, Western
Infirmary, Glasgow, UK

NUMBER FIFTEEN

CHURCHILL LIVINGSTONE
EDINBURGH LONDON MADRID MELBOURNE NEW YORK AND TOKYO 1992

CHURCHILL LIVINGSTONE
Medical Division of Longman Group UK Limited

Distributed in the United States of America by Churchill
Livingstone Inc., 650 Avenue of the Americas, New York,
N.Y. 10011, and by associated companies, branches and
representatives throughout the world.

First published 1992

ISBN 0-443-04519-4
ISSN 0143-6953

British Library Cataloguing in Publication Data
A catalogue record for this book is available from the British
Library

Library of Congress Cataloging in Publication Data
is available

Printed in Great Britain by The Bath Press, Avon

Preface

Advances in histopathology continue and do so at a pace that shows no sign of slackening. Some relate to new developments in immunology and genetics but others, just as important, reflect a better understanding of the microscopic appearances of disease. Existing knowledge also needs re-appraisal from time to time so that its elements can be set in a more logical order. This volume, like its predecessors, attempts to cover a range of topics: basic sciences, new clinicopathological entities, improvements in laboratory technique and, both inevitably and necessarily, varying mixtures of these. Aspects of tumour pathology have received particular emphasis to reflect the many advances made in this area. Histopathology derives support from science and provides service to clinical practice: this represents a fundamental unifying characteristic of our discipline and in it lies our strength.

Exeter   P. P. Anthony
Glasgow   R. N. M. MacSween
1992

Contributors

Wladimir V. Bogomoletz MD FRCPath MIBiol
Head, Laboratoire d'Anatomie Pathologique, Institut Jean Godinot,
Reims, France

Margaret M. Esiri DM FRCPath
Clinical Reader in Neuropathology, Departments of Neuropathology and
Clinical Neurology, Radcliffe Infirmary, Oxford, UK

Christopher D. M. Fletcher MB BS MRCPath
Director, Soft Tissue Tumour Unit, and Senior Lecturer and Honorary
Consultant in Histopathology, St Thomas's Hospital (UMDS), London,
UK

Kenneth M. Grigor BSc MB ChB MD MRCPath
Senior Lecturer, Department of Pathology, University of Edinburgh,
Edinburgh, UK

Peter A. Hall BSc MD MRCPath
Professor of Pathology, Department of Histopathology, St Thomas's
Hospital (UMDS), London, UK

Sverre Heim MD PhD
Professor of Medical Genetics, Department of Clinical Genetics,
University Hospital, Lund, Sweden, and Department of Medical
Genetics, Odense University, Denmark

Peter Kirkpatrick MPhil DMS FIMLS
Head MLSO, Histopathology, Royal Cornwall Hospital, Treliske, Truro,
Cornwall, UK

Ian Lauder MB BS FRCPath
Professor of Pathology, University of Leicester; Honorary Consultant
Histopathologist, Leicestershire Health Authority, Leicester, UK

R. J. Marshall MA DM MRCPath
Consultant Histopathologist, Royal Cornwall Hospital, Truro, Cornwall,
UK

Peter R. Millard MD FRCPath
Consultant in Histopathology, John Radcliffe Hospital, Oxford, UK

F. Mitelman MD PhD
Professor and Chairman, Department of Clinical Genetics, University
Hospital, Lund, Sweden

Terence P. Rollason BSc MB ChB MRCPath
Senior Lecturer in Pathology, University of Birmingham; Honorary
Consultant Pathologist, South Health Authority, Birmingham, UK

Graham A. Russell BSc MB BS MRCPath
Honorary Lecturer, Bristol University; Senior Registrar in
Histopathology, Bristol Royal Hospital for Sick Children and Bristol
Maternity Hospital, Bristol, UK

J. C. E. Underwood MD FRCPath
Joseph Hunter Professor of Pathology, University of Sheffield, Sheffield,
UK

John N. Webb MA MD (Cantab) FRCP (Edin)
Honorary Senior Lecturer, University of Edinburgh; Consultant
Pathologist, and Head, Department of Pathology, Western General
Hospital, Edinburgh, UK

Contents

Differentiation, stem cells and tumour histogenesis

P. A. Hall

The practice of tumour histopathology is based upon the characterization of the phenotype or state of differentiation of cells in tissues using morphological assessment (*morphophenotype*), often supplemented by immunohistology (*immunophenotype*). We perceive that the various tissues, and cells within them, differ in their appearance because of their differing shapes, relationships and cytological detail and their abilities to interact with a range of tinctorial or other stains: properties that reflect the various patterns of cellular gene expression.

All somatic cells from an individual, with the exception of those that rearrange their antigen receptor genes (e.g. T and B lymphocytes) possess the same genome, comprising some 6×10^9 nucleotide bases encoding about 10^5 genes (Alberts et al 1989). While all the cells have the same *genotype* they differ in the expression of these genes: for example the set of genes expressed by a hepatocyte differs radically from that expressed by a neuron. The *phenotype* of a cell is thus determined by the set of genes chosen for expression by that cell: morphological and functional differences between cells represent the differences in these patterns. During development spatial and temporal expression of the genome is carefully regulated and in the adult this regulation persists as exquisitely controlled tissue-specific gene expression (Gilbert 1988). A fundamental problem in biology is to understand the cellular and molecular mechanisms involved in the processes of development and differentiation that give rise to numerous cellular phenotypes from the same genotype.

The tissues that make up both adult and developing organisms are composed of carefully integrated cell populations. Phenotypic variation within clonally derived progeny is a characteristic feature of normal tissues. This is particularly so in continually renewing populations such as epidermis, gut and bone marrow, in which stem cells give rise to differentiated, post-mitotic cells via transit amplifying populations (Hall & Watt 1989). In this review, the cell lineages that generate phenotypic diversity in tissues will be discussed, prefaced by an overview of the molecular mechanisms that regulate the state of cellular differentiation or phenotype. With this background, we will consider the nature of cell differentiation in neoplasia and the relationship of this to presumptive

1

histogenesis. A central theme of this essay is that those mechanisms that generate differing patterns of differentiation or phenotypic diversity in normal tissues persist in neoplasia (to greater or lesser degrees) and result in the phenotypic heterogeneity that is a characteristic feature of practically all tumours.

DIFFERENTIATION

Progression from simple to complex involves the spatially and temporally highly regulated process of selective gene expression in the cells that comprise an organism. Differentiation can thus be defined as the *process* of regulated gene expression that gives rise to different phenotypes from a common genotype. Differentiation can also refer to a *state* of regulated differential gene expression, or phenotype. Nuclear transplantation experiments have demonstrated that somatic cells differentiate by alterations in patterns of gene expression while retaining a complete genome (Gurdon 1962): differentiation occurs by regulation of gene expression by a composite of intrinsic and extrinsic factors (Grobstein 1964). There are many layers of control, and regulation is possible at every step in the pathway from DNA to protein via RNA intermediates (Fig. 1.1).

For most genes, control at the level of transcription of DNA into mRNA appears to be of primary significance. A general strategy in eukaryotes involves a *promoter* element. This is required for accurate and efficient transcription, located close upstream (5′) to the protein coding DNA sequence. The promoter acts together with more distantly located *enhancer* sequences. These are required to enhance the rate of transcription from the promoter, which may be either upstream (5′) or downstream (3′) and in either orientation. Most promoters and enhancers are modular in construction, being composed of a number of 8 to 20 base pair sequences, to which can bind sequence specific gene regulatory proteins, or transcription factors, which may act in a positive or negative manner. It is believed that a relatively small number of regulatory proteins can control transcription in a combinatorial manner, with input from several regulatory proteins determining gene activity. Regulation may be by inhibition of positive regulatory factors or by activation of negative factors. Interactions between different DNA binding proteins, between DNA binding proteins and other ligands, or their alteration by modification such as phosphorylation may alter the binding to DNA and the level of transcriptional activation or repression (Gierer 1973, Maniatis et al 1987, Alberts et al 1989).

A series of DNA binding proteins have been defined and their structures determined. Several generalizations can be made. They tend to have a modular design with separate DNA binding and modulating domains. However, there is remarkable evolutionary conservation of at least some parts of these molecules. It appears that the modulating domains can interact with other proteins and these interactions are essential for

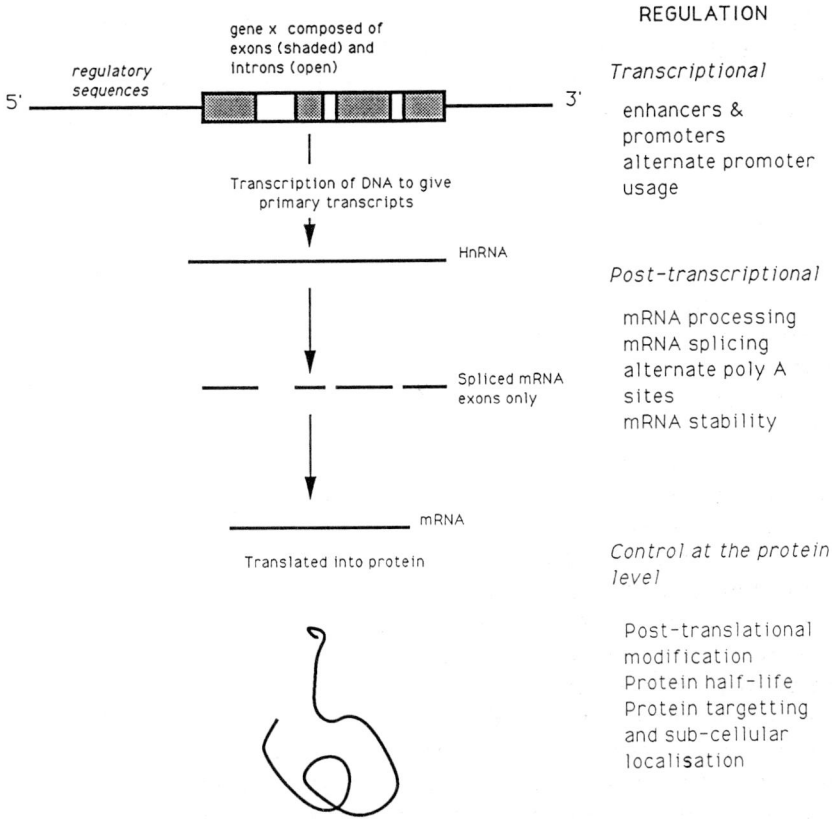

Fig. 1.1 The regulation of gene expression.

functioning of the transcriptional regulators. A nomenclature has arisen on transcriptional regulators including terms such as homeobox, zinc finger and leucine zipper. The 'homeobox' or homeodomain (Affolter et al 1990) is a highly conserved 60 amino acid sequence which appears to be part of the DNA binding domain and contains a 'helix-turn-helix' motif allowing binding to DNA by alignment of the helices with DNA coils. Some homeodomain containing transcriptional regulators also contain a second conserved region termed POU which also appears important in controlling gene expression, particularly in development (Kessel & Gruss 1990). The 'zinc finger' is a second form of DNA binding domain seen in transcriptional regulators where a single Zn^{2+} ion is co-ordinately bound to protein loops containing a pair of cysteines and a pair of histidines or two pairs of cysteines. The ability of a transcription factor to bind to a second protein (and thus to alter its properties) is sometimes a consequence of the presence of 'leucine zippers' i.e. regularly spaced leucine residues on both proteins. These leucines allow dimerization because of their hydrophobicity. The mechanisms of sequence specific transcriptional regulation based upon protein–DNA interactions are reviewed elsewhere (Whitelaw 1989).

It is now recognized that gene regulatory proteins may control (positively or negatively) their own transcription and that of other regulatory proteins forming cybernetic networks that determine the complex patterns of gene expression required in metazoan organisms (Johnson & McKnight 1989). Such networks may then generate stable states of gene expression as a consequence of the relative abundance of different transcription factors binding to enhancer and promoter elements. For example, in muscle it has been shown that a small number of DNA binding proteins (*myoD1*, *myd*, *myogenin*, etc) can regulate the myogenic phenotype (Olson 1990). The introduction into a fibroblast of *myoD1* in a suitable expression vector can induce a programme of muscle specific gene expression (Davis et al 1987) although other factors are also involved in the full expression of muscle differentiation (Hopwood & Gurdon 1990, Olson 1990). It seems probable that cascades of regulatory gene expression with mixtures of diffusible *trans* acting DNA binding proteins binding to *cis* regulatory sequences are central to the control of differentiation but other mechanisms also have a role. For example, the physical state of chromatin influences gene expression with heterochromatin being transcriptionally inactive, and methylation of cytosine residues may be an important means of inactivating certain genes (Alberts et al 1989, Holliday 1990).

Post-transcriptional modifications of RNA are a further important layer of control. The processing of mRNA and its export from the nucleus have been described and important structural alterations of mRNA can occur. For example, splicing events can give rise to a number of different mRNAs from the same gene by removal of exons, introns or use of internal splice sites. Such alternate splicing events can be important means of generating quite different proteins from the same gene in a manner related to development or differentiation (Andreadis et al 1987). The use of alternate promoter sequences may have a similar effect (Rathjen et al 1990). Another structural alteration involves the use of different 3' poly A addition sites which can give rise to proteins of different length. Control of translation of mRNA into protein may be effected by binding of regulatory proteins to the 5' mRNA leader sequence or by alterations in mRNA stability. For example, it has been found that regulatory proteins typically have mRNAs with very short half lives. Stability of mRNA is usually determined by intrinsic mRNA sequences, typically at the 3' end, and the half life may be extensively altered by extracellular signals including growth factors (Alberts et al 1989). Finally, the use of alternate translational start sites can give rise to quite different protein species from the same original mRNA.

The process of differentiation is associated with a progressive restriction in the potentiality of cells, so that in the adult, the cells of any given normal tissue have a very restricted capacity to express the whole genome. Furthermore, cells retain the memory of this restricted genotype, and they 'remember' their nature even when placed in a novel environment: patterns of gene expression are stable and heritable (Blau et al 1985). Although some modulation of differentiated phenotype can occur as a consequence of environmental stimuli such as growth factors, extracellular matrix molecules and contiguous cells (Bissell et al 1982, Gilbert 1988, Alberts et al 1989, Gerhart 1989), radical modifications are rarely observed: a keratinocyte does not spontaneously express a neural phenotype. The nature of the cell's memory of its state of differentiation is uncertain: it may in part reflect methlyation status and structural alterations of chromatin. However, it seems increasingly likely that transcriptional control by cascades of regulatory DNA binding proteins underpins this phenomenon (Schafer et al 1990). Whatever the mechanisms, it is clear that during development and differentiation external (epigenetic) influences induce heritable changes in gene expression (Holliday 1990).

CELL LINEAGES THAT GENERATE AND MAINTAIN CELLULAR DIVERSITY

In multicellular organisms the pattern of gene expression in a cell depends on its history (lineage) as well as on its environment. Cells become committed to certain fates prior to their differentiation, and this is associated with a progressive restriction in potential for genomic expression. The biochemical basis of commitment remains uncertain but it may involve activation of some signal transduction pathway that terminates in the alteration in the balance of competing hierarchies of transcriptional control. These then initiate a new programme of gene expression manifest as a new state of differentiation. Competence to respond to some inducing factor (presumably a growth factor) depends on the expression of appropriate receptors (Slack 1989).

Cell populations in adult tissues may be classified into three broad categories by the rate at which they renew themselves (Leblond 1963). *Static* populations such as in brain and peripheral nervous tissue are those where there is no cell division and where most of the cells formed during development persist in adult life. At the other extreme, in *continually renewing* populations such as in gut, skin and haemopoietic bone marrow there is continuous cell proliferation and a small population of stem cells gives rise to all terminally differentiated cells via a transit amplifying population. These stem cells have a high capacity for self-renewal and generate daughter cells committed to specific differentiation pathways (Hall & Watt 1989). The identity of stem cell populations and the mechanisms that regulate them in higher organisms have proved difficult to establish.

Intermediate between static and continually renewing cell populations are *conditional renewal* (or *slowly renewing*) populations such as in liver, breast and pancreas, where there is generally little cell division, but where proliferation can occur in response to certain stimuli. A question of considerable importance is whether the cell lineages in conditional renewal populations contain stem cells. The spatial arrangement of proliferative cells in conditional renewal populations is not in keeping with a stem cell hierarchy. However, in the endometrium an arrangement similar to gastro-intestinal crypts can be identified and in the adrenal gland proliferation is largely confined to the zona glomerulosa with subsequent migration into the other zones (Wright & Alison 1984). In the case of the liver there is considerable kinetic evidence suggesting that proliferative and differentiative heterogeneity does not exist (Wright & Alison 1984). In contrast, a range of in vivo and in vitro data supports the existence of liver stem cells (Sell 1990). In the rodent coagulating gland and prostate, there is evidence for interchange between proliferating and resting cell populations which argues against the existence of a defined stem cell compartment (Wright & Alison 1984). Thus in conditional renewal populations the case for the existence of stem cells remains unproven.

It is remarkable that despite many advances in biology we are still faced by fundamental problems in defining and understanding stem cells, lineages derived from them and how they are controlled. This is particularly so in the case of conditional renewal systems. However there have been advances in the analysis of cell lineages and of clonal architecture. In addition to the use of fluorescent dyes as cell markers, the introduction of retroviral vectors for lineage analysis in model systems has revolutionized the field (Price 1987). Other methods include the study of chimaeric animals and heterozygotes for X-linked genes and these have also been of great value (Ponder et al 1985, Griffiths et al 1988, Thompson et al 1990).

DIFFERENTIATION IN TUMOURS AND THE ORIGIN OF PHENOTYPIC HETEROGENEITY

Aberrant cellular differentiation is a common theme in neoplasia with the frequent abnormal expression of developmentally and/or spatially regulated genes. It is possible that this is a consequence of abnormal transcriptional control. However tumours are not anarchic: the patterns of differentiation observed are not random, and the dysregulation of gene expression is often intimately linked with their normal programme of differentiation. Indeed, the molecular events that occur in oncogenesis may exploit normal differentiation pathways (Harris 1990). Neoplastic cells may have impaired and altered differentiation programmes for a variety of reasons. For example, they may fail to receive environmental signals, misinterpret these signals, or possibly send abnormal signals to nearby cells (including other tumour cells and even themselves). The paradigms for this model are leukaemias and lymphomas (Greaves 1986) where detailed phenotypic analysis of tumours has revealed the existence of normal conterparts with similar features. This relationship has been observed in a wide range of neoplasms and tumour progression is frequently associated with progressive block to differentiation in a given lineage (Potter 1978, Greaves 1986, Pierce & Speers 1988). For example, in melanoma there are often phenotypically distinct subpopulations and detailed immunological analysis has shown that these reflect the phenotypes seen in the normal differentiation programme (Houghton et al 1987). Similar observations have recently been made in other tumours such as rhabdomyosarcomas (Carter et al 1990). The molecular basis of the abnormalities of differentiation observed remains obscure. They may reflect alterations in the many signal transduction pathways acting on the control of gene expression, including alterations in transcriptional control itself. It is possible that genes with regulatory roles in development and differentiation, including homeobox genes, represent a further class of potential 'oncogenes' (Perkins et al 1990).

Histopathologists are well aware that the patterns of differentiation in some tissues can change, a process termed metaplasia. Such phenomena are relatively stereotyped and only a small number of possibilities exist in any given tissue. The biological basis of metaplasia remains uncertain but Slack (1986) has argued that it represents a reprogramming of the differentiation pathways that stem cells and their progeny follow. An alternative mechanism would involve a differentiated cell type undergoing a process of de-differentiation followed by re-differentiation (Lugo & Putong 1983). The former hypothesis is attractive since it is consonant with the idea of homeotic transformations in other biological systems (Slack 1986) but it suffers from our lack of understanding of stem cell biology.

What evidence supports the concept of de-differentiation? In plants any differentiated cell can give rise to the whole organism (Steward et al 1964). Furthermore, in limb regeneration observed in amphibia de-differentiation to a primitive mesenchyme followed by re-differentiation is well described (Gilbert 1988). However, in mammalian systems direct evidence is scanty. Rao et al (1990) have reported differentiation of pancreatic exocrine tissue to hepatocytes but the lineage basis for this remains uncertain. This again raises the question of whether stem cells exist in conditional renewal systems. More persuasively, Barrandon et al (1989) have demonstrated that introduction of the adenovirus E1a gene into cultured keratinocytes can reverse the pattern of differentiation. The weight of evidence does not favour de-differentiation in most normal or pathological tissues, but rigorous experimental data are lacking in most instances.

We are well aware of the variation in appearance that is seen in different parts of the same tumour. While this is in part a consequence of mechanical factors, such as proximity to blood supply, the phenotypic variability is frequently an integral feature of a tumour. Indeed in many situations such heterogeneity represents a major diagnostic criterion and cellular heterogeneity may also be of therapeutic relevance (Mackillop et al 1983, Fidler & Poste 1985). What mechanisms generate this phenotypic heterogeneity in neoplasia?

The existence of heterogeneity within tumours could reflect an origin from more than one cell or the formation of cell hybrids by fusion (Woodruff 1990). It is generally accepted that tumours are clonally derived (Woodruff 1990, Wainscoat & Fey 1990) and cell fusion is probably a very unusual event in eukaryotic biology. It should also be noted, that the observation of monoclonal composition does not preclude polyclonal origin with subsequent clonal outgrowth (Bennett 1986), as has been observed in metastasis formation (Kerbel et al 1989).

An alternative hypothesis is that cellular heterogeneity reflects normal mechanisms of generating differentiated progeny including metaplasia (Buick & Pollack 1984, Heppner 1984, Nicholson 1987). Such a view is not inconsistent with the clonal origin of neoplasms (Nowell 1986, Woodruff 1989). Differentiation of cells within neoplastic clones with attendant switch from malignant to benign behaviour is well documented in a range of tumour types including squamous carcinomas, teratomas, neuroblastomas and leukaemia (Pierce & Speers 1988). These observations provide considerable support for the hypothesis that tumours are composed of cell lineages akin to those seen in the normal tissue (Potter 1978, Greaves 1986, Pierce & Speers 1988). In addition, the progressive acquisition of new molecular defects as a consequence of the genetic instability characteristic of tumour progression (Nowell 1986) is usually associated with progressive alterations in the differentiated state which may generate further evolutionary changes. We observe the features of tumour progression as altered patterns of differentiation: quantitative and qualitative alterations in gene expression occur, but we remain ignorant of the molecular basis of these changes.

STEM CELLS AND NEOPLASIA

The evidence for the existence of stem cells in neoplasia has been previously reviewed (Mackillop et al 1983, Buick & Pollack 1984, Hall 1989). At the simplest level, histological examination of many tumours show a spatial and phenotypic organization which resembles that of normal tissues, and there is, in general, an inverse relation between kinetic indices and phenotypic differentiation. Considerable clinical evidence points to the existence of a small fraction of the tumour population that must be eliminated by treatment in order to prevent regrowth (Steel 1977). This is supported by clonogenic assays in vitro which indicate that a small fraction of the cells within a tumour are clonogenic, and by a range of fractionation studies that suggest that self-renewal capacity and differentiation properties are restricted to subpopulations with differing physical properties (Mackillop et al 1983, Buick & Pollack 1984). Finally in some neoplasms, such as chronic granulocytic leukaemia or myelodysplasia, clonal markers have been found in multiple cell lineages which indicate neoplastic involvement of an early progenitor or stem cell (Fialkow et al 1987, Keinannen et al 1988, Janssen et al 1989). Stem cells may also exist in mesenchymal tissues with progenitor cells capable of multi-directional differentiation (Grigoriadis et al 1988), and this provides a conceptual framework for the existence of soft tissue tumours with multiple patterns of differentiation.

Neoplasia is recognized as being associated with the acquisition of multiple molecular abnormalities (Land et al 1983, Fearon & Vogelstein 1990) over prolonged periods of time (Cairns 1975). In continually renewing populations the only cells present for long periods and able to accrue the molecular events for oncogenesis are stem cells, and it has been argued that they are the targets of oncogenesis (Potten & Morris 1989). Certainly the observations from classical skin carcinogenesis models, with the capacity for prolonged intervals between initiation and promotion, support this notion as do recent observations of carcinogen adduct retaining cells in skin (Morris et al 1986).

The hypothesis that tumours recapitulate normal cell lineages accords well with cellular heterogeneity since tumours usually reflect either the phenotypic diversity present in the putative tissue of origin (e.g. the various phenotypes present in colorectal carcinoma are similar to those present in normal colorectal epithelium), or the potential phenotypic diversity seen in those forms of metaplasia that may occur in the putative tissue of origin (e.g. squamous metaplasia in bronchial epithelium and squamous carcinoma of the bronchus). There exist some rare tumours in which the patterns of differentiation do not reflect these two models. For example the combination of thyroid follicular neoplasms with parafollicular C cell (medullary) carcinoma does not reflect the generally accepted ontogenesis of these two lineages: the former from endoderm and the latter from neural crest (Wright 1990). Another example is 'metaplastic' carcinoma of the breast containing areas of frankly sarcomatous tumour with osseous or cartilaginous differentiation. These observations do not of themselves preclude stem cell lineages generating these tumours but suggest that the molecular regulation of differentiation in some tumours is radically deranged with expression of genes usually restricted to other lineages. However, these relatively rare circumstances are not completely random: certain patterns are seen suggesting that differentiation control mechanisms may have certain features in common.

DIFFERENTIATION, STEM CELLS AND HISTOGENESIS

In the context of neoplasia, histogenesis refers to the tissue of origin of tumours which are traditionally classified according to the extent to which they resemble their presumptive normal embryonic or adult counterpart. Given the preceding discussion of differentiation, cell lineage and phenotypic diversity in neoplasia, it is not unreasonable to propose that patterns of differentiation in neoplasia reflect potential patterns of differentiation in the corresponding normal tissue. It is a widely held premise that most tumours originate in stem cells or progenitor populations. Does the available evidence support this contention?

Consider, for example, chronic granulocytic leukaemia. It is clear that the tumour cells have a phenotype that resembles that of granulocytes. Does this mean that the tumour is derived from granulocytes? It does not, because this malignancy is a multilineage disorder in the majority of cases as evidenced by the presence of the Philadelphia chromosome in several haemopoietic lineages. The oncogenic events probably occur in an early progenitor or stem cell which has the potential for differentiation along several pathways. Similar arguments can be applied to a range of other haemopoietic neoplasms including acute myeloblastic and lymphoblastic leukaemias and the non-Hodgkin's lymphomas (Greaves 1986). Such arguments do not negate the value of conventional morphophenotypic or immunophenotypic classification of neoplasia. They do however caution against the uncritical acceptance of histogenetic statements based solely upon such observations.

The presence of multiple epithelial cell types in a clonally derived colorectal carcinoma cell line provides direct experimental support for the origin of these lineages from a single progenitor (Kirkland 1988). It has been shown that all non-endocrine epithelial cells are clonally derived in normal colonic epithelium of allophenic chimaeric mice and of mice heterozygous for X linked alleles (Ponder et al 1985, Griffiths et al 1988). Endocrine cells of gastric glands are similarly derived as demonstrated by in situ hybridization methods in XX/XY chimaeras (Thompson et al 1990).

Consequently, evidence exists in haemopoietic and colorectal tumours for a stem cell origin but not in other tumours. Pancreatic exocrine carcinomas show common morphological and immunohistochemical features with the epithelial cells of normal pancreatic ducts and there can be little doubt that they arise from the exocrine epithelium of the pancreas. However, a phenotypic similarity between the tumour and the normal ducts does not necessarily indicate an origin of one from the other. Recent observations point to a plasticity of pancreatic exocrine epithelium (Rao et al 1990). Furthermore, transgenic mice in which TGF alpha is expressed from an elastase promoter, derived from pancreatic acinar cells, develop ductal cell proliferations (Sandgren et al 1990). Also, in vitro culture studies have demonstrated that cells with acinar cell phenotype have the ability to differentiate into a ductal phenotype (Hall & Lemoine 1990 unpublished). Consequently it cannot be simply accepted that ductal pancreatic carcinomas arise in ductal cells: direct experimental evidence is required.

Phenotypic similarities between a tumour and a corresponding normal tissue are not incontrovertible evidence of histogenesis, simply because such data do not allow the discrimination between a series of alternative hypotheses as shown in Figure. 1.2. Bennett (1986) considered a hypothetical cell lineage composed of cells with phenotypes A, B and C and a tumour composed of cells with similar phenotypes B' and C'. What possible

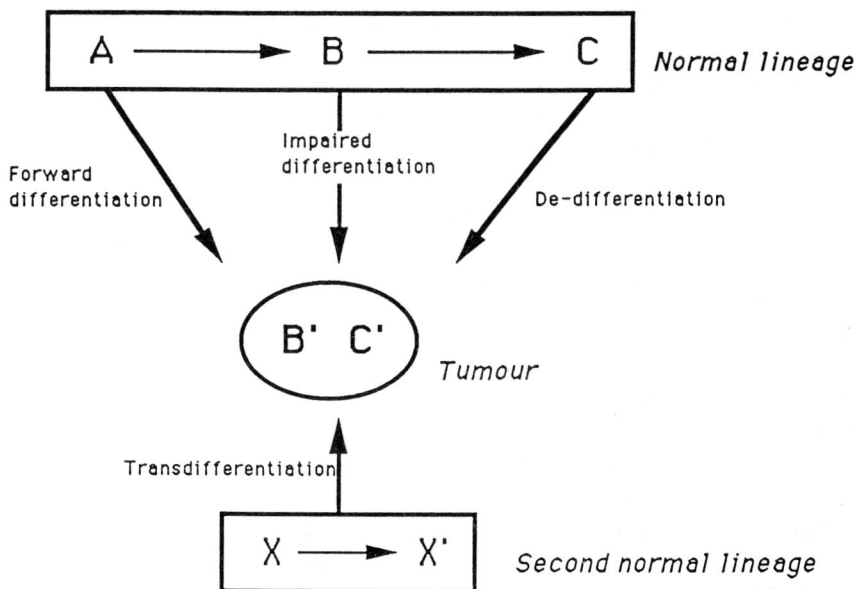

Fig. 1.2   Models of the possible cell of origin in neoplasia (after Bennett 1986).

targets exist for oncogenic change? The stem cell A may be a target giving rise to B′ and C′ by differentiation, as appears to occur in chronic granulocytic leukaemia, for example. Alternatively B may be the target. A third possibility is that the highly differentiated cell C is the target with an associated 'de-differentiation' to give phenotype B′ together with C′ as might occur in tumours arising from conditional renewal populations, such as breast and pancreas. A further point is that the various models are not mutually exclusive: tumours currently classified phenotypically as the same may be derived in different ways. For example, acute myeloid leukaemia appears to be heterogeneous with most cases showing multilineage involvement and thus presumptive stem cell or progenitor cell involvement, while other cases do not (Fialkow et al 1987, Keinannen et al 1988).

A further but remote possibility is that a cell in a separate lineage (say X) undergoes some transdifferentiation or metaplastic process in association with oncogenesis. This model may provide a clue to the occasional identification of neoplastic sarcomatous elements in epithelial tumours such as breast carcinoma. We can thus see that simple analysis of phenotype cannot allow definition of lineage inter-relationships. This will require much more complex analyses. These arguments are of particular relevance in the consideration of patterns of divergent differentiation so commonly observed by histopathologists in tumours at many sites (Mendelsohn & Maksem 1986).

It can be argued that tumours contain cells with stem cell properties (with the capacity for self-renewal and for giving rise to differentiated progeny), but this does not resolve the question of whether tumours arise from such cells. Many authorities accept, rather uncritically, the hypothesis that stem cells represent the target for oncogenic change (Steel 1977) but in the vast majority of neoplasms we cannot distinguish a stem cell origin from the acquisition of stem cell properties. Nor can we exclude the possibility of sequential molecular events within cell lineages, some early and some late (Fearon & Vogelstein 1990) which may make the question of cell of origin almost impossible to resolve.

It might be suggested that identification of cell lineage of origin is a more meaningful approach, not least because neoplasia represents altered patterns of differentiation in particular lineages. The notion is illustrated by the following example. Consider a hypothetical tumour that requires a series of seven molecular events (call them event 1, event 2 etc) for full neoplastic transformation. It may be that events 1 and 2 occur in a stem cell: but all its progeny will carry those molecular changes. Events 3 and 4 may occur in one daughter of the stem cell, an early transit amplifying cell, and events 5 and 6 in a daughter of this cell. Finally event 7, that ultimately leads to the formation of the tumour, occurs in one of the progeny of this cell. Can one really identify a cell of origin? Our lack of understanding of the lineage basis of many tissues and the sequential acquisition of molecular defects in neoplasia, particularly at early stages, makes further progress difficult at present.

PERSPECTIVE

Tumours are not anarchic: they, in general, behave according to rules. When new patterns of differentiation appear in a neoplasm they usually reflect those of the putative tissue of origin. However, it is not possible to make any statement regarding the cell of origin simply on the basis of phenotypic data. At present we define phenotype on the basis of morphology supplemented in some situations by immunophenotypic observations. This phenotype, or state of differentiation, is determined by the co-ordinated expression of a subset of the entire cellular genome. An understanding of how this is regulated, by transcriptional and post-transcriptional mechanisms, will increase the accuracy of our definitions and provide tools for investigating the altered patterns of differentiation seen in neoplasia. Furthermore, improved understanding of the cell lineages that make up normal tissues together with how these are regulated, will be central to our understanding of normal and abnormal differentiation, as will definition of the target cell for neoplastic transformation, whether it be a stem cell or not. With regard to the classification of tumours, as Gould (1986) has argued, it may be prudent to avoid questionable assumptions about the putative cell of origin, and restrict statements to objective characterization of cell lineage and phenotype, and perhaps as appropriate methods become available, the molecular mechanisms that regulate phenotype.

The arguments presented here in no way undermine the conventional practice of histopathology. On the contrary, they emphasize the importance of detailed morphological observations coupled with application of newer methods for the analysis of cellular phenotype. The study of the regulation of gene expression is the province of the histopathologist, and we need to be aware of the mechanisms by which normal tissues are regulated, including differentiation and the organization of cell lineages.

REFERENCES

Affolter M, Schier A, Gehring W J 1990 Homeodomains in proteins and the regulation of gene expression. Current Opinion in Cell Biology 2: 485–495
Alberts B, Bray D, Lewis J et al 1989 Molecular biology of the cell. Garland, New York
Andreadis A, Gallego M E, Nadal-Ginard B 1987 Generation of protein isoform diversity by alternative splicing: mechanistic and biological implications. Annual Review of Cell Biology 3: 207–242
Barrandon Y, Morgan J R, Mulligan R C et al 1989 Restoration of growth potential in paraclones of human keratinocytes by a viral oncogene. Proceedings of the National Academy of Sciences 86: 4102–4106
Bennett D C 1986 The cellular basis of carcinogenesis. In: Waring M J, Ponder B A J (eds) Biology of carcinogenesis. MTP Press, Lancaster, pp 65–81
Bissell M J, Hall H G, Parry G 1982 How does the extracellular matrix direct gene expression? Journal of Theoretical Biology 99: 31–68
Blau H M, Pavlath G K, Hardeman E C et al 1985 Plasticity of the differentiated state. Science 230: 758–766
Buick R N, Pollack M N 1984 Perspectives on clonogenic tumour cells, stem cells and oncogenes. Cancer Research 44: 4909–4918
Cairns J 1975 Mutation selection and the natural history of cancer. Nature 255: 197–200
Carter R L, Jameson C F, Philp E R et al 1990 Comparative phenotypes in rhabdomyosarcomas and developing muscle. Histopathology 17: 301–310
Davis R L, Weintraub H, Lassar A B 1987 Expression of a single transfected cDNA convert fibroblasts to myoblasts. Cell 51: 987–1000
Fearon E R, Vogelstein B 1990 A genetic model for colorectal carcinogenesis. Cell 61: 759–767
Fialkow P J, Singer J W, Raskind W et al 1987 Clonal development, stem cell differentiation and clinical remissions in acute nonlymphocytic leukaemia. New England Journal of Medicine 317: 468–473
Fidler I J, Poste G 1985 The cellular heterogeneity of malignant neoplasms: implications for adjuvant chemotherapy. Seminars in Oncology 12: 207–221
Gerhart J 1989 The primacy of cell interactions in development. Trends in Genetics 5: 233–237
Gierer A 1973 Molecular models and combinatorial principles in cellular differentiation and morphogenesis. CSH Symposia in Quantitative Biology 38: 951–961
Gilbert S F 1988 Developmental biology 2nd edn. Sinauer Associates Publ, Mass, Sunderland
Gould V E 1986 Histogenesis and differentiation: a re-evaluation of these concepts as criteria for the classification of tumours. Human Pathology 17: 212–214
Greaves M F 1986 Differentiation-linked leukaemogenesis. Science 236: 697–704
Griffiths D F R, Davies S J, Williams D et al 1988 Demonstration of somatic mutation and colonic crypt clonality by X-linked enzyme histochemistry. Nature 33: 461–463
Grigoriadis A E, Heersche J N M, Aubin J E 1988 Differentiation of muscle, fat, cartilage and bone from progenitor cells present in a bone-derived clonal cell population. Journal of Cell Biology 106: 2139–2151

14   RECENT ADVANCES IN HISTOPATHOLOGY

Grobstein C 1964 Cytodifferentiation and its controls. Science 143: 643–650
Gurdon J B 1962 Adult frogs derived from the nuclei of single somatic cells. Developmental
    Biology 4: 256–273
Hall P A 1989 Stem cells in neoplasia. Lancet i: 701–702
Hall P A, Watt F M 1989 Stem cells: the generation and maintenance of cellular diversity.
    Development 106: 619–633
Harris H 1990 The role of differentiation in the suppression of malignancy. Journal of Cell
    Science 97: 5–10
Heppner G H 1984 Tumour heterogeneity. Cancer Research 44: 2259–2265
Holliday R 1990 Paradoxes between genetics and development. Journal of Cell Science 97:
    395–398
Hopwood N D, Gurdon J B 1990 Activation of muscle genes without myogenesis by ectopic
    expression of MyoD in frog embryos. Nature 347: 197–200
Houghton A N, Real F X, Davis L J et al 1987 Phenotypic heterogeneity in melanoma.
    Relation to the differentiation program of melanoma cells. Experimental Cell Research 164:
    812–818
Janssen J W G, Buschle M, Layton M et al 1989 Clonal analysis of myelodysplastic
    syndrome: evidence of multipoint stem cell origin. Blood 73: 248–254
Johnson P F, McKnight S L 1989 Eukaryotic transcriptional regulation proteins. Annual
    Review Biochemistry 58: 799–839
Keinannen M, Griffin J D, Bloomfield C D et al 1988 Clonal chromosome abnormalities
    showing multiple-cell-lineage involvement in acute myeloid leukaemia. New England
    Journal of Medicine 318: 1153–1159
Kerbel R S, Cornil I, Korzak B 1989 New insights into evolutionary growth of tumours
    revealed by Southern gel analysis of tumours genetically tagged with plasmid or proviral
    DNA injections. Journal of Cell Science 94: 381–387
Kessel M, Gruss P 1990 Murine developmental control genes. Science 249: 374–379
Kirkland S C 1988 Clonal origin of columnar, mucous and endocrine cell lineages in human
    colorectal epithelium. Cancer 61: 1359–1363
Land H, Parada L, Weinberg R A 1983 Cellular oncogenes and multistep carcinogenesis.
    Science 222: 771–778
Leblond C P 1963 Classification of cell populations on the basis of their proliferative
    behaviour. NCI Monograph 14: 19–145
Lugo M, Putong P B 1983 Metaplasia: an overview. Archives of Pathology and Laboratory
    Medicine 108: 185–189
Mackillop W J, Ciampi A, Till J E et al 1983 A stem cell model of human tumour growth:
    implications for tumour clonogenic assays. Journal of the National Cancer Institute 70:
    9–16
Maniatis T, Goodbourne S, Fischer J A 1987 Regulation of inducible and tissue specific gene
    expression. Science 236: 1237–1245
Mendelsohn G, Maksem J A 1986 Divergent differentiation in neoplasms. Pathologic,
    biologic and clinical considerations. In: Sommers S C, Rosen P P, Fechner R E (eds)
    Pathology Annual, Volume 21, Appleton Century Crofts, Norwalk, pp 91–119
Morris R J, Fischer S M, Slaga T J 1986 Evidence that slowly cycling subpopulation of adult
    murine epidermal cells retains carcinogen. Cancer Research 46: 3061–3066
Nicholson G L 1987 Tumour cell instability, diversification and progression to the metastatic
    phenotype from oncogene to oncofetal expression. Cancer Research 47: 1473–1487
Nowell P C 1986 Mechanisms of tumour progression. Cancer Research 46: 2203–2207
Olson E N 1990 MyoD1 family: a paradigm for development. Genes & Development 4:
    1454–1461
Perkins A, Kongsuwan K, Visvader J et al 1990 Homeobox expression plus autocrine growth
    factor production elicits myeloid leukaemia. Proceedings of the National Academy of
    Sciences 87: 8398–8402
Pierce G B, Speers W C 1988 Tumours as caricatures of the process of tissue renewal:
    prospects for therapy by directing differentiation. Cancer Research 48: 1996–2004
Ponder B A J, Schmidt G H G, Wilkinson M M et al 1985 Derivation of mouse intestinal
    crypts from single progenitor cells. Nature 313: 689–691
Potten C S, Morris R J 1989 Epithelial stem cells. Journal of Cell Science (suppl) 10: 45–62
Potter V R 1978 Phenotypic diversity in experimental hepatomas: the concept of partially
    blocked ontogeny. British Journal of Cancer 38: 1–23

Price J 1987 Retroviruses and the study of cell lineage. Development 101: 409–420

Rao M S, Yeldandi A V, Reddy J K 1990 Differentiation and cell proliferation patterns in rat exocrine pancreas: role of type 1 and type 2 injury. Pathobiology 58: 37–43

Rathjen P D, Toth S, Willis A et al 1990 Differentiation inhibiting activity is produced in matrix-associated and diffusable forms that are generated by alternate promoter usage. Cell 62: 1105–1114

Sandgren E P, Luetteke N C, Palmiter R D 1990 Overexpression of TGF alpha in transgenic mice: induction of epithelial hyperplasia, pancreatic metaplasia and carcinoma of the breast. Cell 61: 1121–1135

Schafer B W, Blakely B T, Darlington G J et al 1990 The effect of cell history on response to helix-loop-helix family of myogenic regulators. Nature 344: 454–458

Sell S 1990 Is there a liver stem cell? Cancer Research 50: 3811–3815

Slack J M W 1986 Epithelial metaplasia and the second anatomy. Lancet ii: 268–270

Slack J M W 1989 Peptide regulatory factors in embryonic development. Lancet i: 1312–1315

Steel G G 1977 The kinetics of tumours. Oxford University Press, Oxford

Steward F C, Blakely L M, Kent A E et al 1964 Growth and organisation in cell free systems. Brookhaven Symposia in Biology 16: 73–88

Thompson E M, Fleming K A, Evans D J et al 1990 Gastric endocrine cells share a common origin with other gut cell lineages. Development 110: 477–481

Wainscoat J S, Fey M F 1990 Assessment of clonality in human tumours: a review. Cancer Research 50: 1355–1360

Whitelaw E 1989 The role of DNA-binding proteins in differentiation and transformation. Journal of Cell Science 94: 169–173

Woodruff M F A 1990 Cellular variation and adaption in cancer. Oxford University Press, Oxford

Wright N A, Alison M 1984 The biology of epithelial cell populations. Oxford University Press, Oxford

Wright N A 1990 Endocrine cells in non-endocrine tumours. Journal of Pathology 161: 85–87

2

Prognostic indices in epithelial neoplasms

J. C. E. Underwood

Accurate histopathological typing, grading and staging of tumours is of proven value in the clinical management of cancer patients by enabling selection of the most appropriate treatment.

Short-term survival is determined mainly by the grade and stage of a tumour, whereas long-term survival is more dependent on tumour type. In many cases, however, histopathological assessment correlates poorly with clinical outcome. Reasons for this include:

1. The criteria used for typing, grading and, to some extent, staging tumours involve subjective interpretation and are thus liable to observer error.
2. Routine histopathological techniques may not reveal all possible markers of prognostic importance.
3. Individual categories of type, grade and stage may overlap as regards clinical outcome.

These problems have motivated the development of new techniques to augment routine methods for assessing type, grade and stage, and thereby to improve the accuracy and reproducibility of prognostication. Recently, there has been a bewildering increase in the number and variety of these techniques, but their adoption in routine practice has been slow. Many laboratories may not have sufficient resources to implement them and the results do not necessarily influence clinical management of the individual patient. A critical appraisal is, therefore, appropriate.

The scope of this review is restricted to those techniques and reagents that are applicable to histological and cytological material and does not deal with, for example, biochemical assays of tumour homogenates. These techniques have intrinsic advantages: they are more widely available, they can often be applied to archival material, and the cellular location of the prognostic marker can be verified.

TISSUE SAMPLING FOR PROGNOSTIC INDICES

Whichever technique is to be used, it is essential that the tissue has been sampled adequately and that it is processed optimally. Malignant neoplasms

17

are commonly heterogeneous and some techniques perform best, or work only on tissue that has been processed according to strict protocols.

Sampling and sample size

Tumours are *typed* according to the features evident in the best differentiated areas and *graded* on the appearance of the least differentiated part. Several blocks should be taken from large neoplasms to ensure that the full range of appearances is seen. Further than this general statement, there is no basis on which to give a strict numerical ruling for the minimum number of blocks.

Having satisfied these basic requirements, for any quantitative assessment (e.g. mitotic index, AgNOR count) it is then necessary to determine the minimum number of histological sections and microscope fields to yield an acceptable estimate of the actual value (usually within $\pm 5\%$) of the feature being quantified. Few studies have been validated in this way (Quinn & Wright 1990) and the credibility of many must be questioned.

Tissue fixation and processing

Histopathologists feel most comfortable with techniques that work on paraffin sections from formalin-fixed tissue; the tissue requires no special handling, the sections are robust and of good quality, and the final preparations are permanent. However, even these routinely prepared tissue samples should be handled with care and fixed promptly, for any undue delay will have undesirable consequences, e.g.:
   diffusion artefacts in immunohistochemistry
   underestimate of mitotic rate
   autolysis.

Some techniques, for example Ki-67 immunostaining, require frozen sections of unfixed tissue, and others, like bromodeoxyuridine labelling, small samples of fresh viable tissue. Such restrictions usually limit the application of these techniques to prospective studies.

IDENTIFICATION OF TUMOUR SUBTYPES OF PROGNOSTIC IMPORTANCE

We are probably close to the limit of what can be deduced about tumour type from the histological growth pattern, ultrastructural features and the application of relatively simple tinctorial methods such as mucin stains. The future identification of tumour subtypes of prognostic importance is likely to be based on features rendered histologically visible only by immunohistochemistry, lectin binding and, molecular biological techniques (Ellis & Gown 1990).

Receptors for hormones and growth factors

Because hormones and growth factors have trophic effects on normal tissues, it is logical to determine their role in the behaviour of tumours. This is best done in tissue samples by seeking their receptors. Initially this could be done only by radioligand-binding assays on tumour homogenates, but this approach has severe limitations (Underwood 1983) and is being superseded by immunohistochemical methods. Although these methods lack the numerical precision of radioligand-binding assays, the results are more meaningful because they enable the cellular location (tumour cells versus stroma) of the receptors and permit assessment of cellular heterogeneity with respect to their expression.

Steroid receptors

The best-characterized steroid receptors with prognostic significance are oestrogen receptor (ER) and progesterone receptor (PR) in breast carcinomas. Androgen receptor (AR) determinations in prostatic carcinomas are also valuable, but immunohistochemical methods for this purpose are still awaited. The availability of ER and PR antibodies for immunohistochemistry has been a considerable advance. These highly specific reagents verify the cellular location of the receptors, assess tumour cell heterogeneity of their expression, and are applicable to small lesions derived from breast screening programmes.

ER and PR can be demonstrated in the nuclei of approximately 60% of female breast carcinomas by immunohistochemistry with specific monoclonal antibodies (Fig. 2.1). These antibodies recognize an epitope on the receptor that is impaired by routine formalin fixation and paraffin embedding. Several investigators have, however, successfully adapted the methodology so that these reagents can be used on paraffin sections; this can be achieved by using a cocktail of monoclonal antibodies (Giri et al 1989) or by enzymatic pretreatment of the sections with, for example, pronase. The assessment is carried out according to a strict protocol based on the proportion of stained tumour cell nuclei and the intensity of their staining; from these data, a staining index can be calculated.

Women whose tumours exhibit a high staining index for ER survive longer than those whose tumours are ER poor or negative. Treatment of the ER positive group with tamoxifen, which blocks the action of the receptor, confers a further clinical advantage (Coombes et al 1987).

The co-expression of ER and PR in a breast carcinoma is important. PR is induced by the action of oestrogens on ER positive breast epithelium; it is, therefore, a post-receptor marker of ER and, when present, signifies that the ER is functional (Giri et al 1988).

It has been argued that ER and PR assays are unnecessary since tamoxifen is a relatively safe drug, it can be administered to all breast cancer patients

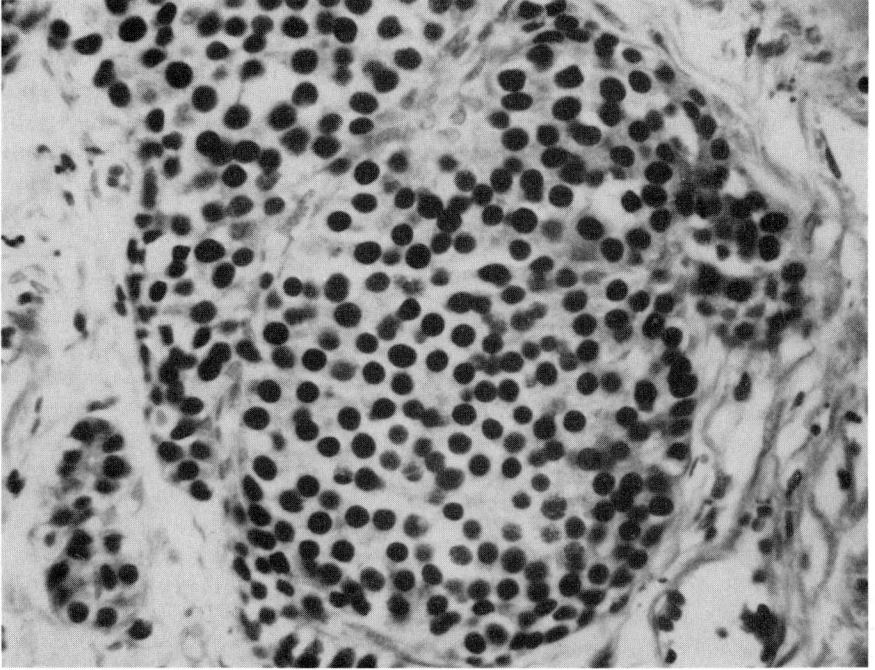

Fig. 2.1 Immunohistochemical demonstration of oestrogen receptor protein in breast carcinoma nuclei in paraffin sections. Such tumours are associated with a longer survival and a favourable response to tamoxifen therapy.

and the outcome reviewed after six months. However, by so doing, women with ER-negative tumours are denied 6 months of alternative treatment with cytotoxic chemotherapy.

Steroid-regulated proteins

Steroid hormones induce the synthesis of new proteins in receptor-positive cells. These 'post-receptor markers' are of importance in the prognostic assessment of tumours because their presence denotes a more favourable response to endocrine therapy.

Cathepsin D. Cathepsin D is a lysosomal protease which, like PR, is an oestrogen-regulated marker in ER-positive breast cancer cells; its presence verifies the functional integrity of the receptor pathway. Cathepsin D can be demonstrated readily by immunohistochemistry in routine paraffin sections. Its presence correlates with significantly prolonged survival in patients with ER-positive breast carcinomas, even in those with lymph node metastases (Henry et al 1990).

pS2. pS2 is a protein, the synthesis of which is oestrogen-regulated and it is rarely present in ER-negative breast cancers. pS2 is a marker of good prognosis and an indicator of a likely response to endocrine therapy (Foekens et al 1990). pS2 has, however, been reported to be present in normal gastric mucosa which is not known to be under the control of oestrogens (Rio et al 1988).

Epidermal growth factor receptor

Epidermal growth factor receptor (EGFR) can be demonstrated by immunohistochemistry in tissue sections.

In most tumours studied, EGFR expression is a marker for reduced disease-free interval and survival. It can be detected in approximately 50% of bladder carcinomas where it is associated with multiple tumours, recurrences and reduced survival (Neal et al 1990).

In breast carcinomas, EGFR expression correlates with poor prognosis and reciprocally with ER expression.

Oncogene and tumour-suppressor gene expression

Since the discovery of oncogenes and their expression in many human tumours, there has been considerable interest in their biological role and their use as markers of neoplastic behaviour (Bartow 1990).

Oncogenes can be studied at three molecular levels:

gene (DNA)

message (mRNA)

product (protein).

Unless the *gene* is amplified, i.e. into multiple copies in the genome, there is little point in simply determining its presence because it is found in the genome of all nuclei. However, some oncogenes become inappropriately active either because there has been a point mutation resulting in the synthesis of an abnormally active oncoprotein, or because there has been a chromosomal translocation or enhancer/promoter gene insertion causing the oncogene to be abnormally transcribed. These alterations at the DNA level can only be demonstrated by the techniques of molecular biology, but they are not easily adapted to provide morphological data of possible prognostic value.

In-situ hybridization can be used to demonstrate the *RNA message* for oncoprotein synthesis, but often the signal is weak and the methodology is not reliable for routine adoption. Nevertheless, the determination of oncogene expression at the level of the RNA message is potentially useful in view of the possible short half-life of the protein product which may make it difficult to detect immunohistochemically.

Most histological data on the prognostic significance of oncogene expression have been obtained from the immunohistochemical demonstration of the *oncoprotein* itself.

Immunohistochemistry reveals not only the presence or absence of the oncoprotein, but also abnormalities in its intracellular location. c-*erb*B-2, c-*myc*, *ras*, and the p53 tumour suppressor gene protein have been the most widely studied.

c-erbB-2/HER2/neu

c-*erb*B-2, HER2, and *neu* are synonymous; the different nomenclature reflects different routes to the discovery of this oncogene. In Europe, the gene is usually referred to as c-*erb*B-2; in the USA, HER2 or *neu* are the preferred designations. c-*erb*B-2 encodes for an oncoprotein located on the cell membrane. The location and molecular configuration are very suggestive of a receptor, the specific ligand for which is unknown.

In breast cancer, the tumour in which c-*erb*B-2 expression has been studied most extensively, there is a high incidence in intraduct carcinomas. Invasive breast carcinomas expressing c-*erb*B-2 are associated with a relatively poor survival (Wright et al 1989). Immunohistochemistry for c-*erb*B-2 is unusually easy to interpret in that tumours tend to be unequivocally positive or negative and dubious intermediate grades of staining are unusual.

c-myc

c-*myc* is the most widely studied nuclear oncoprotein. It interacts with nuclear DNA to stimulate DNA synthesis. Inappropriately increased expression may be associated with tumour development and progression. The p62 c-*myc* oncoprotein has been extensively studied by immuno-histochemistry. In general, increased expression is associated with more aggressive behaviour, a shorter disease-free interval and reduced survival time (Sowani et al 1989).

ras

The *ras* oncoprotein most extensively studied by immunohistochemistry is p21 (Ward et al 1989). Increased expression has been reported in hepato-cellular (Jagirdar et al 1989) and colorectal carcinomas (Salhab et al 1989), although in the latter study no correlation was found with differentiation grade, Dukes' stage or DNA ploidy. Similarly, no consistent differences in *ras* p21 expression were found between benign and malignant prostatic epithelium (Varma et al 1989). Although this oncoprotein has been found in ovarian carcinomas, there is no correlation with clinical outcome (Rodenberg et al 1988).

p53

p53 nuclear phosphoprotein is the subject of much current interest. First identified as a host cell protein binding to the transforming T-antigen of the

SV40 tumour-inducing virus, p53 behaves as a tumour suppressor gene in experimental models. However, it is converted from a recessive to a dominant oncogene by point mutations. Normal p53 protein resides in the nucleus; immunostaining often reveals the mutant form in both the cytoplasm and the nucleus.

In a recent immunohistochemical study of p53 in lung carcinomas (Iggo et al 1990), increased expression was observed in 28 of 40 cases contrasting with lack of staining in 7 pulmonary carcinoid tumours and 10 normal lung samples. In a small proportion of carcinomas further studied by the polymerase chain reaction, increased p53 expression corresponded to the presence of the mutant protein.

Lectin binding

Lectins bind to carbohydrate moieties and have proved to be useful probes for seeking diagnostic and prognostic changes in tumour cell-associated glycoproteins, notably in breast carcinomas. Peanut agglutinin (PNA) binding correlates positively with responsiveness to endocrine therapy (Remmele et al 1986), but it is less predictive than steroid receptor immunohistochemistry. *Helix pomatia* agglutinin (HPA) binding identifies a subgroup of breast cancer patients with an increased risk of nodal metastasis and decreased survival (Leathem & Brooks 1987).

Polymorphic epithelial mucins

Polymorphic epithelial mucins (PEM) are cell surface-associated glyco-proteins. The term is applied particularly to a family of glycoproteins which were initially found to be associated with breast epithelium, but are now known to be expressed more widely. PEMs include substances bearing epitopes recognized by the antibodies designated HMFG 1 and 2, NCRC 11 and B72.3.

HMFG 1 and 2 expression has no prognostic significance in breast cancer (Berry et al 1985). The diagnostic utility of B72.3 has been evaluated, but its prognostic value is uncertain.

NCRC 11 expression in breast cancer was shown initially to be associated with a lower incidence of nodal metastases and a prolonged survival (Ellis et al 1985), but other data are conflicting (Angus et al 1986).

NUCLEAR FEATURES AND TUMOUR GRADING

Nuclear features, such as size, staining intensity and mitotic activity, are invariably assessed in grading schemes for a wide variety of neoplasms (Underwood 1990). Because these features are usually assessed subjectively, there is ample scope for improving the reliability of grading by quantification.

Ploidy and prognosis

Abnormal chromosome numbers (triploid, aneuploid, etc.) can be determined by cytogenetic techniques, but these are inappropriate for routine
assessment of tumours because of sampling problems and the requirement
for viable tissue. The measurement of nuclear DNA content by flow or
static cytometric methods is regarded as an acceptable substitute for ploidy
analysis. However, abnormalities in *DNA content* ('DNA aneuploidy') do
not necessarily correspond to abnormalities in *chromosome number*. Cytometry requires that the nuclei are first stained with a dye that binds
stoichiometrically to DNA. Flow cytometry has the advantage that a large
number of nuclei can be analysed rapidly, but the disadvantage is that there
is no morphological check on the identity of the cells contributing to the
relevant peaks in the DNA histogram. Unless some separation technique is
employed, the cell suspension is likely to consist of possibly aneuploid
tumour cells and invariably diploid stromal cells in unknown proportions.
Static DNA cytometry uses image analysis of cytology preparations or
tissue sections. It takes longer, but it offers the advantage of selecting by
microscopy only tumour cells for measurement.

Many studies on several carcinoma types have shown a clear-cut tendency
for diploid tumours to have a better prognosis than tumours with abnormal
DNA ploidy (Quirke 1990).

Estimation of cell proliferation

Tumours are characterized by excessive cellular proliferation without
commensurate cell loss through apoptosis, necrosis or exfoliation and the
inevitable result is growth.

The proliferative fraction—the proportion of cells in S-phase—can be
computed mathematically from flow cytometric data. However, this method
suffers from the problem already alluded to, namely that the identity of the
cells in S-phase cannot be established. There are alternative methods
(Fig. 2.2) some of which require either in vivo labelling or in vitro
incubation of fresh tissue.

Mitotic activity

The *mitotic index* (the proportion of cells in mitosis) and the *mitotic count*
(the number of mitoses in a specified number of high-power fields) are well
established procedures in tumour grading. There are, however, important
limitations (Silverberg 1976, Donhuijsen 1986):

1. The histologically visible event of mitosis occupies only a short period
   in the cell cycle, so a large number of nuclei have to be counted to
   obtain statistically reliable estimates of the proportion of proliferating
   cells.

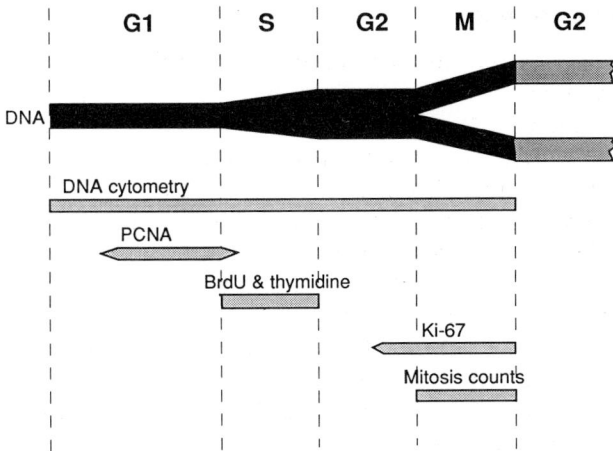

Fig. 2.2 Utility of different methods for assessing states in the proliferative cycle. DNA cytometry can distinguish between the G0 or G1 diploid states only from the accompanying S/G2/M peaks in the latter instance. ^{3}H-thymidine or BrdU labels incorporated during S-phase are carried onwards through the proliferative cycle where they can be detected by autoradiography or immunostaining respectively. PCNA and Ki-67 are expressed in the nuclei of proliferating cells; only the periods of synthesis and peak expression are shown. Mitoses are transient and may be difficult to identify.

2. The mitotic index or count may be exaggerated by mitoses arrested due to tumour chemotherapy (e.g. vincristine) or to an intracellular defect that blocks completion.
3. The recognition of mitotic figures is subject to observer error; some may be mistaken for pyknotic nuclei or lymphocytes and vice versa.
4. Criteria based on the number of mitoses per 'high-power field' are meaningless without specifying the size of the field; this varies between different makes of microscope.
5. The mitotic count per high-power field in epithelial neoplasms is influenced by variation in cellularity.
6. Any delay in fixation results in an underestimate of the number of mitoses, probably because those that have been initiated complete the process and no cells enter mitosis once the tissue has been deprived of its blood supply.

The effect of fixation can, however, be controlled. In one recent study (Cross et al 1990), a delay in fixation led to a 30% reduction at 2 h and a 50% reduction at 6 h in the mitotic frequency in colonic mucosal epithelium. Similarly, a fixation delay of 6 h led to a 43% reduction in the number of recognizable mitoses in a series of breast carcinomas (Start et al 1991). This has important implications for tumour grading based wholly or partly on mitotic indices.

These limitations have led to a search for alternative methods of estimating the cell proliferation rate in tumours.

^{3}H-thymidine uptake

Estimation of DNA synthesis by autoradiography of tissue sections incubated in tritiated thymidine is a well established method, but has found little use in clinical histopathology. This is due to the requirement for fresh viable tissue, tritiated thymidine, and autoradiographic skills. There have been few recent studies of the prognostic utility of this method (Meyer & Province 1988). However, it is encouraging to find a good correlation between the thymidine labelling index and some of the new methods, such as immunohistochemistry for proliferation antigens (Battersby & Anderson 1990).

Bromodeoxyuridine uptake

Bromodeoxyuridine (BrdU), a pyrimidine analogue, is incorporated into DNA during its synthesis. BrdU-labelled nuclei can be then demonstrated immunohistochemically using a specific monoclonal antibody or detected by flow cytometry. The main disadvantage of this technique is the necessity, shared with ^{3}H-thymidine uptake, for either the in vivo administration of BrdU (used therapeutically as a radiosensitiser) or the in vitro incubation of fresh viable tissue. This technique has been applied to clinical tumour kinetics (Wilson et al 1988) and the prognostic utility is likely to be similar to that of ^{3}H-thymidine uptake.

Proliferation antigens

Proliferation antigens are expressed in the nuclei of cells during specific stages of the cell cycle (Table 2.1). These include PAA (Dubey et al 1987), C_5F_{10} (Lloyd et al 1985), and DNA polymerase α (Namikawa et al 1987). However, the two most extensively studied are the Ki-67 epitope and PCNA.

Table 2.1   Characteristics of proliferation antigens

Proliferation antigen	Phase of cell cycle	Tissue processing	Cellular location
C_5F_{10}	M	Paraffin sections	Nucleus and cytoplasm
DNA polymerase α	G1 to G2	Frozen sections	Nucleus
Ki-67	Peak at G2/M	Frozen sections	Nucleus
PAA	G1 to M	Paraffin sections	Cell membrane and cytoplasm depending on cycle phase
PCNA/cyclin	Late G1/S	Paraffin sections	Nucleus

Ki-67. The monoclonal antibody Ki-67 identifies cells in the proliferative cycle, but reliably only in frozen sections. The applications have been comprehensively reviewed by Brown and Gatter (1990). There is no doubt about the reliability of Ki-67 immunostaining as a method for estimating proliferative activity in tissues, though its value as a prognostic marker is more strongly established in lymphomas than in other tumours such as carcinomas.

In breast carcinomas however, a high Ki-67 index (proportion of nuclei stained) correlates with the mitotic index and with parameters of tumour aggressiveness such as lymph node involvement (Charpin et al 1988). There is an inverse correlation with ER expression (Raymond & Leong 1989). There have been few studies correlating Ki-67 indices directly with prognosis, but a high Ki-67 index is associated with a tendency to early recurrence (Bouzubar et al 1989).

PCNA. PCNA (proliferating cell nuclear antigen/cyclin) was discovered independently from comparison of 2-dimensional gel electrophoresis patterns of proliferating and resting cells and from the specificity of a nuclear autoantibody occurring in patients with systemic lupus erythematosus.

Antibodies to PCNA may well supplant Ki-67 as the favoured reagent for immunohistochemical identification of cells in the proliferative cycle because they have the notable advantage of recognizing an epitope that survives formalin fixation and paraffin embedding of tissues (Garcia et al 1989) (Fig. 2.3). The PCNA immunostaining index correlates well with other measures of cellular proliferation in normal tissues and in lymphomas, but there may be deregulated increased or prolonged expression in some malignant epithelial neoplasms (Hall et al 1990).

Nucleolar organizer regions in interphase nuclei

Nucleolar organizer regions (NORs) are loops of DNA projecting into the nucleoli of interphase nuclei; they are thought to encode for ribosomal RNA. NORs are normally restricted to the five acrocentric chromosomes in the human karyotype. Some of the NOR-associated proteins (NORAPs) are argyrophilic and can be demonstrated as black dots by a silver-staining technique (Fig. 2.4). The structures thus demonstrated are known as AgNORs. Counts of AgNORs in interphase nuclei may assist in the distinction between benign and malignant neoplasms and in the grading of the latter (Crocker 1990).

The principal advantages of the AgNOR technique are the relative simplicity of the staining method and the ease of application to archival tissue. Disadvantages include the time-consuming and tedious counting of little dots, often tightly clustered, associated with the usual vagaries of observer error.

It must be emphasized that the number of dots revealed in interphase

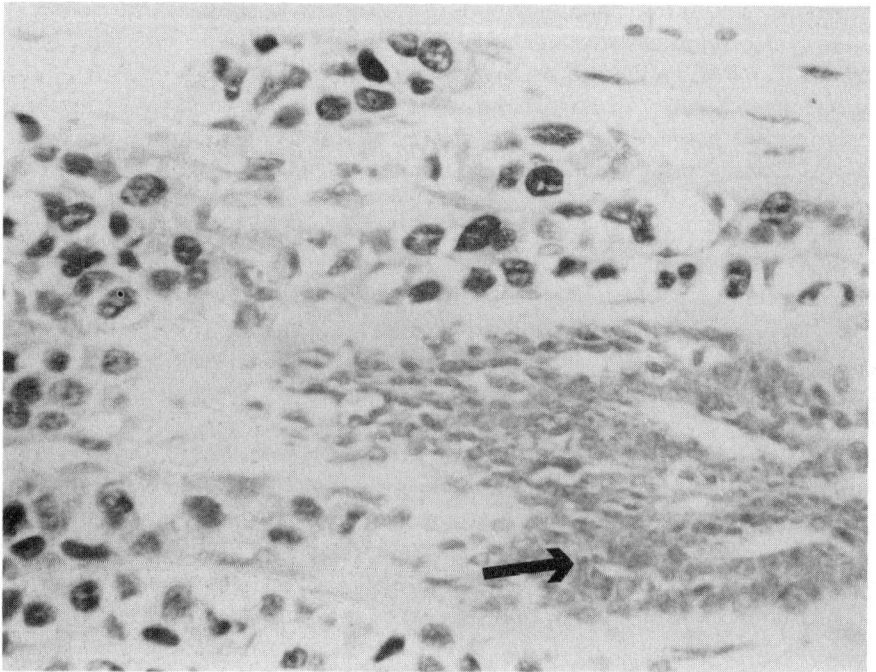

Fig. 2.3 Identification of breast carcinoma cells in the proliferative state by nuclear immunostaining with anti-PCNA. The non-neoplastic epithelium of a duct (arrowed) is PCNA-negative.

nuclei by the AgNOR technique does not necessarily correspond to the actual number of NORs in the karyotype (Underwood & Giri 1988). Because the AgNORs are often small, coalescent or overlapping, their apparent number is invariably less than the actual number present. Methods for counting AgNORs must be strictly consistent so that comparisons can be made between different studies (Crocker et al 1989).

Possible explanations for an *increased* number of countable AgNORs in interphase nuclei include:

increase in the number of NOR-bearing chromosomes in the karyotype

increased transcriptional activity producing more visible argyrophilic NORAPs

increased proliferation rate resulting in a larger proportion of cells showing pre- and post-mitotic NOR dispersion

defective nucleolar association.

In tumours, increased AgNOR counts in interphase nuclei are more likely to be attributable to cellular proliferation than to abnormal ploidy because:

1. Diploid cells in the proliferative cycle are transiently tetraploid in the G2 phase, thus resulting in a temporary doubling of the number of NOR-bearing acrocentric chromosomes.

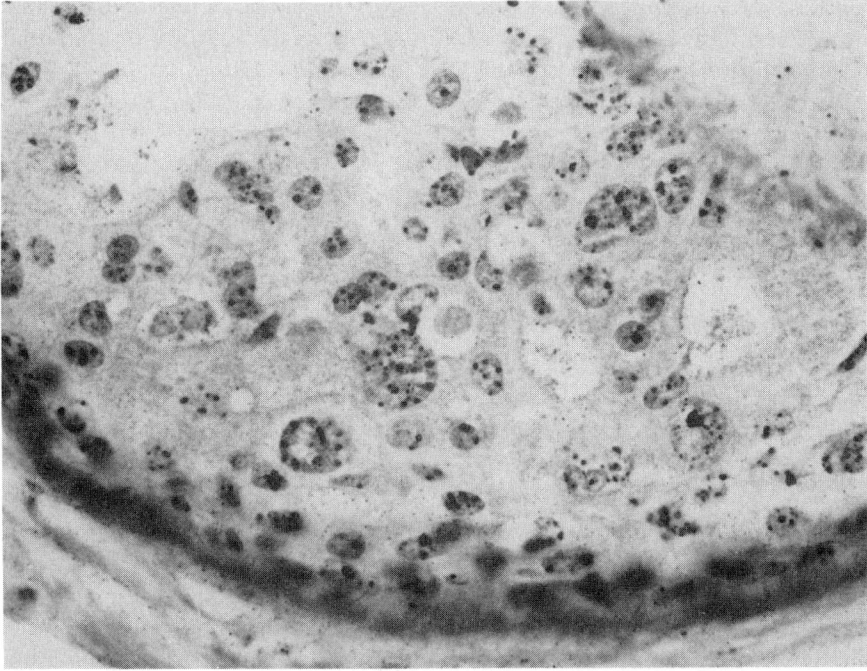

Fig. 2.4   AgNORs in the nuclei of invasive breast carcinoma cells. The larger numbers visible in malignant neoplastic cells is due not only to a possible increase in the absolute number of NORs in the karyotype, but also to their dispersion through the nucleoplasm of proliferating cells.

2. Immediately before and after mitotic division the NORs disperse and then reaggregate, thus leading to an increase in the number of *countable* AgNORs in nuclear profiles.

The number of countable AgNORs in interphase nuclei is probably related more to their dispersion through the nucleoplasm than to the actual number present; the AgNOR count may, therefore, be an index of AgNOR dispersion rather than the actual number present in the karyotype. Dispersion in itself may reflect the proliferative state: before mitotic division the nucleoli and the NORs within them disperse; after mitosis the NORs reaggregate and the nucleoli reform. Thus the AgNOR count rises before and after mitosis. Comparison with the Ki-67 immunostaining index shows a highly significant correlation in breast carcinomas (Dervan et al 1989).

Crocker, who has promulgated the AgNOR technique in tumour grading, recommends its use in non-Hodgkin's lymphomas, melanocytic tumours, mesothelial lesions, salivary gland tumours, gliomas and liver lesions and in the distinction between 'oat' cells and lymphocytes (Crocker 1990). It is reported to be of no diagnostic value in thyroid and prostatic carcinomas because of the overlap in AgNOR counts between different diagnostic categories. The technique has only limited diagnostic utility in epithelial lesions of the breast (Giri et al 1988), stomach and cervix.

As with all new techniques, the prognostic utility takes time to emerge. In a recent study of breast carcinomas (Sividris & Sims 1990), tumours associated with less than four involved lymph nodes possessed a mean AgNOR count of 2.81, whereas cases with more than four had a mean AgNOR count of 8.57; this was a highly significant difference. In endometrial curettings, an AgNOR count of greater than 9 is reported to be suggestive of the presence of invasive carcinoma (Wilkinson et al 1990). Recent work suggests that AgNOR size may be just as important as the number of AgNOR dots per nucleus, for example in assessing grades of cervical intraepithelial neoplasia (Egan et al 1990).

Nuclear morphometry

The nuclei of malignant cells are characteristically larger, less regular in outline, more densely staining, and have larger and more numerous nucleoli than those in benign or normal cells. These features are often assessed subjectively in grading systems for carcinomas and other neoplasms. These characteristics, not all of which have any known intrinsic functional significance, are quantifiable and have been shown to be *prognostically* relevant in a variety of neoplasms. The application of nuclear morphometry to tumour grading overcomes the limitations of observer error in subjective assessments.

The prognostic utility of nuclear morphometry has been reviewed recently by Stephenson (1990). In breast carcinomas, for example, nuclear density and area correlate with mitotic activity and tumour recurrence rates (Stenkvist et al 1982). A high mean nucleolar area ($>6\,\mu m^2$) and pleomorphic nucleoli (standard deviation $>2.49\,\mu m^2$) are associated with a markedly reduced survival (Baak 1985). By selecting areas of the section containing the largest and most atypical nuclei, nuclear area correlates strongly with tumour grade and stage in bladder carcinomas (Blomjous et al 1990).

REFINEMENTS IN TUMOUR STAGING

The stage of a malignant neoplasm at the time of presentation is one of the most important prognostic factors, a fact well illustrated by the Dukes' staging scheme for colorectal carcinomas. Staging often relies on fairly obvious features—depth of invasion, presence of lymph node metastases— which can be determined by careful gross inspection of specimens and routine histology. New reagents for immunohistochemistry have refined these long-established staging criteria.

Basement membrane integrity

Basement membranes are complex extracellular laminar structures formed at the interface between epithelial or endothelial and connective tissues (Abrahamson 1986).

They have been the subject of considerable research in the context of tumour invasion and metastasis (Liotta 1984). Experimental evidence suggests an important role for laminin, a basement membrane constituent, and for laminin, receptors in preventing tumour cell invasion and metastasis. Enzymes such as type IV collagenase and proteinases degrade basement membranes and thus facilitate the progression of malignancy. The integrity of basement membranes in carcinomas is often regarded as a criterion of great importance in the distinction between in-situ and invasive neoplasia. The microanatomical barrier of the subepithelial basement membrane is crucial in this demarcation, but the idea that its *loss* is fundamental to invasion may be an oversimplification (van den Hooff 1989). Moreover, invasive carcinoma cells may retain the ability to synthesize some basement membrane constituents.

Using immunohistochemistry for laminin and type IV collagen, basement membrane material has been found around the invasive groups of tumour cells in basal cell and squamous cell carcinomas (van Cauwenberge et al 1983; Gusterson et al 1984) and even within lymph node metastases of the latter (Carter et al 1985).

The possible prognostic significance of finding basement membrane materials in invasive tumours is illustrated by a study on bladder cancer in which the presence of intact or only partially fragmented membranes, identified by type IV collagen immunohistochemistry, was associated with a more favourable prognosis (Daher et al 1987).

Type VII collagen appears to be a better marker for epithelial basement membranes in carcinomas. Unlike type IV collagen which is present in all basement membranes, including those around vascular endothelial cells, type VII collagen is restricted to the epithelial:stromal interface. However, in a study of breast carcinomas type VII collagen was detected immunohistochemically in 11% of invasive tumours (Wetzels et al 1989).

Vascular and lymphatic invasion

Vascular and/or lymphatic invasion is a marker of tumour aggressiveness, but it rarely features in staging systems because of the difficulty in recognizing it with certainty in routinely stained sections; conversely, retraction artefact around groups of tumour cells often mimics vascular invasion.

Good markers for vascular invasion in tumours are:
factor-VIII-related antigen (Factor VIIIrAg)
Ulex europeaus lectin
α-actin.

Factor VIIIrAg is synthesized by mature vascular endothelium. There is doubt, however, about its reliability as a vascular marker in tumours. This is probably because the blood vessels in tumours are relatively young and the endothelial cells are immature. This has led to a search for more reliable markers in this situation.

Ulex europeaus lectin binds to sugar moieties associated with blood group glycoproteins expressed on endothelial cells. It has proved to be a good marker of intratumoural vessels. In one recent study of bladder carcinomas (Larsen et al 1990), *Ulex* lectin staining confirmed vascular invasion in only five out of 36 cases suspected on routine histology; the rest were attributed to retraction artefact. This lectin, however, also binds to red blood cells and epithelia of ABH blood group secretors.

α-actin is present in the smooth muscle cell cytoplasm of blood vessel walls. This is a more robust structure than the vascular endothelium itself, so it enables the recognition of relatively advanced vascular involvement.

The relative diagnostic and prognostic utility of lectin or immuno-histochemical vascular staining in tumours has been shown for carcinomas of the breast (Lee et al 1986), thyroid (Stephenson et al 1986) and large bowel (Lapertosa et al 1989).

Micrometastases

A large proportion of patients with carcinomas, but without overt metastases, eventually relapse sometime after resection of the primary lesion. This is because, at the time of excision of the primary tumour, minute metastases were already present but were too small to be detected by clinical examination, imaging techniques or routine biopsy histology. Regional lymph nodes and the bone marrow are common sites for micrometastases.

It has been suggested that a rigorous search for micrometastases is worthwhile, especially in breast cancer (Neville 1990). Lymph node micrometastases can only be detected reliably by examining multiple sections; the search is assisted by immunohistochemistry using epithelial cytokeratin antibodies. A similar approach reveals occult metastatic carcinoma cells in bone marrow aspirates and trephine biopsies.

A recent study (International [Ludwig] Breast Cancer Study Group 1990) revealed nodal micrometastases in 9% of breast cancer cases previously deemed to be node-negative after routine histological examination. These patients had a shorter disease-free interval and a decreased survival than patients who were genuinely node negative. The authors of this report recommend cutting each axillary lymph node into 2 mm slices, processing each slice for histology, and performing immunohistochemistry for breast epithelial markers as previously advocated by Wells et al (1984).

A similar meticulous search for tumour cells in bone marrow aspirates, using immunohistochemical epithelial markers, may enable the identification of patients with occult bone metastases (Cote et al 1988). Such patients may benefit from early systemic chemotherapy.

CONCLUSIONS

New diagnostic techniques are often received with uninhibited enthusiasm, followed by a period of scepticism as the original expectations are not fulfilled, then finally adopted for selective use.

Most of the techniques and markers cited above have been evaluated in retrospective studies; a few have been used prospectively; hardly any have yet been adopted in routine practice.

Tumour typing has been refined by the immunohistological detection of markers associated with subtypes of different clinical behaviour. Some of these markers, such as steroid receptors, are of immediate clinical utility because they identify patients who are more likely to benefit from particular therapies.

Tumour grading can be made more objective by the quantification of nuclear features (e.g. DNA ploidy, nuclear shape and size, AgNOR counts) and estimation of the proliferative state. Mitosis counting seems simple, but there are major caveats. Reagents such as anti-PCNA are likely to prove increasingly popular for the assessment of the proliferative state of tumour cells in fixed and paraffin-embedded tissue.

Tumour staging can be made more precise by developing techniques for the earlier recognition of the steps in the progression of an invasive carcinoma, e.g. transgression of the basement membrane, vascular invasion, micrometastases.

These improved methods have undeniable research potential and they continue to illuminate our knowledge of cancer biology.

REFERENCES

Abrahamson D R 1986 Recent studies on the structure and pathology of basement membrane. Journal of Pathology 149: 257–278

Angus B, Napier J, Purvis J et al 1986 Survival in breast cancer related to tumour oestrogen receptor status and immunohistochemical staining for NCRC 11. Journal of Pathology 149: 301–306

Baak J P A 1985 The relative prognostic significance of nucleolar morphometry in invasive ductal breast cancer. Histopathology 9: 437–444

Bartow S A 1990 Diagnostic and prognostic applications of oncogenes in surgical pathology. American Journal of Surgical Pathology 14 (Suppl 1): 5–15

Battersby S, Anderson T J 1990 Correlation of proliferative activity in breast tissue using PCNA/cyclin. Human Pathology 21: 781

Berry N, Jones D B, Smallwood J et al 1985 The prognostic value of the monoclonal antibodies HMFG1 and HMFG2 in breast cancer. British Journal of Cancer 51: 179–186

Bouzubar N, Walker K J, Griffiths K et al 1989 Ki-67 immunostaining in primary breast cancer: pathological and clinical associations. British Journal of Cancer 59: 943–947

Blomjous C E, Vos W, Schipper N W 1990 The prognostic significance of selective nuclear morphometry in human urinary bladder carcinoma. Human Pathology 21: 409–413

Brown D C, Gatter K C 1990 Monoclonal antibody Ki-67: its use in histopathology. Histopathology 17: 489–503

Carter R L, Burman J F, Barr L et al 1985 Immunohistochemical localization of basement membrane type IV collagen in invasive and metastatic squamous carcinomas of the head and neck. Journal of Pathology 147: 159–164

van Cauwenberge D, Pierard G E, Foidart J M et al 1983 Immunohistochemical localisation of laminin, type IV and type V collagen in basal cell carcinomas. British Journal of Dermatology 108: 163–170

Charpin C, Andrac L, Vacheret H et al 1988 Multiparametric evaluation (SAMBA) of growth fraction (monoclonal antibody Ki-67) in breast carcinoma tissue sections. Cancer Research 48: 4368–4374

Coombes R C, Berger U, McClelland R A et al 1987 Prediction of endocrine response in breast cancer by immunocytochemical detection of oestrogen receptor in fine-needle aspirates. Lancet ii: 701–703

Cote R J, Rosen P P, Hakes T B et al 1988 Monoclonal antibodies detect occult breast carcinoma metastases in the bone marrow of patients with early stage disease. American Journal of Surgical Pathology 12: 333–340

Crocker J 1990 Nucleolar organiser regions. In: Underwood J C E (ed) Pathology of the nucleus. Springer Verlag, Berlin, pp 91–149

Crocker J, Boldy D A R, Egan M J et al 1989 How should we count AgNORs? Proposals for a standardised nomenclature. Journal of Pathology 158: 189–194

Cross S S, Start R D, Smith J H F 1990 Does delay in fixation affect the number of mitotic figures in processed tissue? Journal of Clinical Pathology 43: 597–599

Daher N, Abourachid H, Bove N et al 1987 Collagen type IV staining pattern in bladder carcinomas: relationship to prognosis. British Journal of Cancer 55: 665–671

Dervan P A, Gilmartin L G, Loftus B M et al 1989 Breast carcinoma kinetics: argyrophilic nucleolar organizer region counts correlate with Ki67 scores. American Journal of Clinical Pathology 92: 401–407

Donhuijsen K 1986 Mitosis counts: reproducibility and significance in grading of malignancy. Human Pathology 17: 122–125

Dubey D P, Staunton D E, Parekh A C et al 1987 Unique proliferation-associated marker expressed on activated and transformed human cells defined by monoclonal antibody. Journal of the National Cancer Institute 78: 203–212

Egan M, Freeth M, Crocker J 1990 Relationship between intraepithelial neoplasia of the cervix and the size and number of nucleolar organiser regions. Gynecologic Oncology 36: 30–33

Ellis G K, Gown A M 1990 New applications of monoclonal antibodies to the diagnosis and prognosis of breast cancer. Pathology Annual (Part 2) 193–235

Ellis I O, Hinton C P, McNay J et al 1985 Immunocytochemical staining of breast carcinoma with the monoclonal antibody NCRC 11: a new prognostic indicator. British Medical Journal 290: 881–883

Foekens J A, Rio M C, Seguin P et al 1990 Prediction of relapse and survival in breast cancer patients by pS2 protein status. Cancer Research 50: 3832–3837

Garcia R L, Coltrera M D, Gown A M 1989 Analysis of proliferative grade using anti-PCNA/cyclin monoclonal antibodies in fixed, embedded tissues. American Journal of Pathology 134: 733–739

Giri D D, Goepel J R, Rogers K et al 1988 Immunohistochemical demonstration of progesterone receptor in breast carcinoma: correlation with radioligand binding assays and oestrogen receptor immunohistology. Journal of Clinical Pathology 41: 444–447

Giri D D, Dundas S A C, Nottingham J F 1989 Oestrogen receptors in benign epithelial lesions and intraduct carcinoma of the breast: an immunohistochemical study. Histopathology 15: 575–584

Gusterson B A, Warburton M J, Mitchell D et al 1984 Invading squamous cell carcinoma can retain a basal lamina. Laboratory Investigation 51: 82–87

Hall P A, Levison D A 1990 Assessment of cell proliferation in histological material. Journal of Clinical Pathology 43: 184–192

Hall P A, Levison D A, Woods A L et al 1990 Proliferating cell nuclear antigen (PCNA) immunolocalisation in paraffin sections: an index of cell proliferation with evidence of deregulated expression in some neoplasms. Journal of Pathology 162: 285–294

Henry J A, McCarthy A L, Angus B et al 1990 Prognostic significance of the oestrogen-regulated protein, cathepsin D, in breast cancer: an immunohistochemical study. Cancer 65: 265–271

van den Hooff A 1989 An essay on basement membranes and their involvement in cancer. Perspectives in Biology and Medicine 32: 401–413

Iggo R, Gatter K, Bartek J et al 1990 Increased expression of mutant forms of p53 oncogene in primary lung cancer. Lancet 335: 675–679

International (Ludwig) Breast Cancer Study Group 1990 Prognostic importance of occult axillary lymph node micrometastases from breast cancers. Lancet 335: 1565–1568

Jagirdar J, Nonomura A, Patil J et al 1989 ras oncogene p21 expression in hepatocellular carcinoma. Journal of Experimental Pathology 4: 37–46

Lapertosa G, Baracchini P, Fulcheri E et al 1989 Prognostic value of the immunocytochemical detection of extramural venous invasion in Dukes' C colorectal adenocarcinomas: a preliminary study. American Journal of Pathology 135: 939–945

Larsen M P, Steinberg G D, Brendler C B et al 1990 Use of *Ulex europaeus* agglutinin I (UEAI) to distinguish vascular and "pseudovascular" invasion in transitional cell carcinoma of bladder with lamina propria invasion. Modern Pathology 3: 83–88

Leathem A J, Brooks S A 1987 Predictive value of lectin binding on breast cancer recurrence and survival. Lancet i: 1054–1056

Lee A K C, DeLellis R A, Silverman M L et al 1986 Lymphatic and blood vessel invasion in breast carcinoma: a useful prognostic indicator. Human Pathology 17: 984–987

Liotta L A 1984 Tumour invasion and metastasis: role of the basement membrane. American Journal of Pathology 117: 339–348

Lloyd R V, Wilson B S, Vaarani J et al 1985 Immunocytochemical characterization of a monoclonal antibody that recognises mitosing cells. American Journal of Pathology 121: 274–283

Meyer J S, Province M 1988 Proliferative index of breast carcinoma by thymidine labeling: prognostic power independent of stage, oestrogen and progesterone receptors. Breast Cancer Research and Treatment 12: 191–204

Namikawa R, Ueda R, Suchi T et al 1987 Double immunoenzymatic detection of surface phenotype of proliferating lymphocytes in situ with monoclonal antibodies against DNA polymerase α and lymphocyte membrane antigens. American Journal of Clinical Pathology 87: 725–731

Neal D E, Sharples L, Smith K et al 1990 The epidermal growth factor receptor and the prognosis of bladder cancer. Cancer 65: 1619–1625

Neville A M 1990 Are breast cancer axillary node micrometastases worth detecting? Journal of Pathology 161: 283–284

Quinn C M, Wright N A 1990 The clinical assessment of proliferation and growth in human tumours: evaluation of methods and applications as prognostic variables. Journal of Pathology 160: 93–102

Quirke P 1990 Flow cytometry in the quantitation of DNA aneuploidy and cell proliferation in human disease. In: Underwood J C E (ed) Pathology of the nucleus. Springer Verlag, Berlin, pp 216–256

Raymond W A, Leong A S-Y 1989 The relationship between growth fractions and oestrogen receptors in human breast carcinoma, as determined by immunohistochemical staining. Journal of Pathology 158: 203–211

Remmele W, Hildebrand U, Hienz H A et al 1986 Comparative histological, histochemical, immunohistochemical and biochemical studies on oestrogen receptors, lectin receptors, and Barr bodies in human breast cancer. Virchow's Archiv A 409: 127–147

Rio M C, Bellocq J P, Daniel J Y et al 1988 Breast-cancer associated pS2 protein: synthesis and secretion by normal stomach mucosa. Science 251: 705–708

Rodenberg C J, Koelma I A, Nap M et al 1988 Immunohistochemical detection of the *ras* oncogene product p21 in advanced ovarian cancer: lack of correlation with clinical outcome. Archives of Pathology and Laboratory Medicine 112: 151–154

Salhab N, Jones D J, Bos J L et al 1989 Detection of ras gene alterations and ras proteins in colorectal cancer. Diseases of the Colon and Rectum 32: 659–664

Silverberg S G 1976 Reproducibility of the mitosis count in the histologic diagnosis of smooth muscle tumours of the uterus. Human Pathology 7: 451–454

Sividris E, Sims B 1990 Nuclear organiser regions: new prognostic variable in breast carcinomas. Journal of Clinical Pathology 43: 390–392

Sowani A, Ong G, Dische S et al 1989 c-*myc* oncogene expression and clinical outcome in carcinoma of the cervix. Molecular Cell Probes 3: 117–123

Start R D, Flynn M S, Roger K et al 1991 Delayed fixation significantly decreases observed mitotic figures in breast carcinoma. Journal of Pathology 163: 154A

Stenkvist B, Bengtsson E, Dahlqvist B et al 1982 Predicting breast cancer recurrence. Cancer 50: 2884–2893

Stephenson T J 1990 Quantitation of the nucleus. In: Underwood J C E (ed) Pathology of the nucleus. Springer Verlag, Berlin, pp 151–213

Stephenson T J, Griffiths D W R, Mills P M 1986 Comparison of *Ulex europaeus* I lectin binding and factor-VIII related antigen as markers of vascular endothelium in follicular carcinoma of the thyroid. Histopathology 10: 251–260

Underwood J C E 1983 Oestrogen receptors in human breast cancer: review of histopathological correlations and critique of histochemical methods. Diagnostic Histopathology 6: 1–22

Underwood J C E 1990 Nuclear morphology and grading in tumours. In: Underwood J C E (ed) Pathology of the nucleus. Springer Verlag, Berlin, pp 1–5

Underwood J C E, Giri D D 1988 Nucleolar organizer regions as diagnostic discriminants for malignancy. Journal of Pathology 155: 95–96

Varma V A, Austin G E, O'Connell A C 1989 Antibodies to ras oncogene p21 proteins lack immunohistochemical specificity for neoplastic epithelium in human prostate tissue. Archives of Pathology and Laboratory Medicine 113: 16–19

Ward J M, Perantoni A O, Santos E 1989 Comparative immunohistochemical reactivity of monoclonal and polyclonal antibodies to H-ras p21 in normal and neoplastic tissues of rodents and humans. Oncogene 4: 203–213

Wells C A, Heryet A, Brochier J et al 1984 The immunocytochemical detection of axillary micrometastases in breast cancer. British Journal of Cancer 50: 193–197

Wetzels R H, Holland R, van Haelst U J et al 1989 Detection of basement membrane components and basal cell keratin 14 in noninvasive and invasive carcinomas of the breast. American Journal of Pathology 134: 571–579

Wilkinson N, Buckley C H, Chawner L et al 1990 Nucleolar organiser regions in normal, hyperplastic and neoplastic endometria. International Journal of Gynecology and Oncology 9: 55–59

Wilson G D, McNally N J, Dische S et al 1988 Measurement of cell kinetics in human tumours in vivo using bromodeoxyuridine incorporation and flow cytometry. British Journal of Cancer 58: 423–431

Wright C, Nicholson S, Angus B et al 1989 Expression of C-erbB-2 oncoprotein: a prognostic indicator in human breast cancer. Cancer Research 49: 2087–2090

3

Cytogenetics of solid tumours

S. Heim F. Mitelman

Attempts to explain neoplastic growth have historically been dominated by two partly opposing lines of reasoning: one, with its roots in humoral theories of disease, maintains that tumours are the result of a general process in which a disturbed balance of positive and negative growth-regulatory influences is the dominating pathogenetic factor; the other views neoplasia as an essentially local phenomenon that only secondarily affects total-body homeostasis. The latter view has prevailed and since the advent of modern pathology towards the end of the last century, cancer, and indeed all neoplasms, are considered to be cellular disorders. The tumour cells are at fault, not the host organism.

One mechanism whereby a propensity for unrestricted growth could be retained in generation after generation of dividing cells would be through stable rearrangements—mutations—of the cells' genetic make up. This somatic mutation theory of cancer was first clearly espoused by Theodor Boveri (1914) in *Zur Frage der Entstehung maligner Tumoren*, which also stated his conviction that tumours originate from a single cell, and that they must hence be monoclonal. Boveri's seminal insights drew heavily on experimental evidence reached also by others, in particular David von Hansemann (1890), who described the occurrence of aberrant mitoses in carcinomas. The direct cause of the transformation of a cell from normal to neoplastic was seen as an acquired genetic change and, in Boveri's opinion, mostly a chromosomal change. Thus, the cellular theory of carcinogenesis was restated in genetic terms, and the resulting somatic mutation theory has remained the paradigmatic view of tumour pathogenesis to this day.

NEOPLASTIC CELLS HAVE CLONAL CHROMOSOMAL ABNORMALITIES

Several technical innovations—including the introduction of improved tissue culture methods, the use of colchicin to arrest cell division in metaphase by inhibition of the mitotic spindle, and spreading of metaphase chromosomes by exposing the cells to a hypotonic solution—ushered in an era of intense progress in human cytogenetics in the middle of this century. Four years after the correct chromosome number of man had been established, Nowell & Hungerford (1960) described the first specific cancer-associated karyotypic abnormality, the Philadelphia chromosome (Ph[1]) that characterizes chronic myeloid leukaemia (CML).

Although the stage thus seemed set for quick and relatively effortless discoveries of tumour-specific chromosomal aberrations, progress in cancer cytogenetics was slow during the 1960s. Malignancies other than CML did not seem to have consistent chromosomal changes; instead, variable aberrations were detected even in what, by all conventional criteria, appeared to be identical neoplasms. Furthermore, the karyotypes would vary from normal to exceedingly complex, containing numerous unidentifiable rearrangements and with no apparent order in their distribution. The arguments for a primary role of chromosome abnormalities in the causation of human neoplasia seemed unconvincing, and many researchers were reluctant to accept that chromosome abnormalities in most solid tumours and leukaemias could be anything but randomly occurring epiphenomena without any direct pathogenetic importance.

These doubts were overcome when, after the introduction of banding techniques around 1970, analyses of haematological malignancies finally established that clonal chromosome aberrations are the rule rather than the exception in these neoplasms, that the pattern of abnormalities is non-random, and that some haematologic-cytogenetic correlations are so specific as to make the respective aberrations practically pathognomonic (Heim & Mitelman 1987, 1989, Whang-Peng & Knutsen 1989, Heim 1990, Mitelman et al 1990, Sandberg 1990). In solid tumour cytogenetics, on the other hand, corresponding breakthroughs were achieved only during the 1980s (Sandberg et al 1988, Mitelman et al 1989). The principal reason for this delay was the difficulty in bringing the neoplastic cells of many solid tumour types to divide in vitro and the technical quality of chromosome preparations was also generally poor. These methodological difficulties have now been at least partially overcome (Limon et al 1986, Mandahl 1991), and with the expansion of the data base, the fundamental conclusions reached in haematological malignancies have been shown to apply also for solid tumours. In most neoplasms that have been studied, the tumour cells were shown to have acquired clonal chromosomal abnormalities that are non-randomly distributed throughout the genome, and sometimes they are remarkably specific for the tumour type in question. Contrary to what was once believed, clonal aberrations are not restricted to malignant tumours but are also found, albeit in a lesser degree, in benign neoplasms. From the cytogenetic point of view, the qualitative borderline is between non-neoplastic and neoplastic cells and not between benign and malignant tumours. For practical purposes, the finding of clonal, acquired chromosome abnormalities means that the sampled disease process is of a neoplastic nature. Some reservations that apply specifically to solid tumours will be discussed below.

The fact that not all individual tumours of any given histological type have clonal abnormalities may, upon superficial consideration, seem to contradict the implications of the somatic mutation theory of cancer. There are two principal reasons why this is not so. First, in many cases with an apparently normal karyotype, the majority or perhaps all the cells that divide belong to the tumour stroma rather than to the parenchyma and the results may be misleading. This illustrates one of the dilemmas inherent in cytogenetics: after the cells have been processed for chromosome analysis, they no longer retain those phenotypic characteristics that enable their unequivocal, individual identification. Second, the absence of chromosomal abnormalities does not rule out the existence of submicroscopic genetic changes. The haploid chromosome complement contains approximately 300 bands, each harbouring, on average, 10^7 base pairs or maybe 100 genes. Since rearrangements involving chromatin pieces smaller than one band are extremely difficult to detect microscopically, extensive genetic changes may be hidden in what appears to be a normal karyotype. Nevertheless, it is surprising that the reshuffling of genetic material in cancer cells usually involves such large segments that more than 50% of all tumours have karyotypic changes.

The karyotypic complexity of solid tumours in general surpasses that of haematological neoplasms. Sometimes the aberrations are truly massive, rendering the identification of the various abnormalities well-nigh impossible. In order to assess the nature and importance of tumour-associated chromosomal abnormalities, and thereby to generate some conceptual order out of what may seem like a confusing chaos of aberrations, it is useful to classify the changes into three main categories:

1. *Primary abnormalities*. These are essential in establishing the neoplasm and presumably represent rate-limiting steps in tumorigenesis. They may be found as the sole karyotypic change and are as a rule strongly correlated with tumour type.

2. *Secondary abnormalities*. The often pronounced genomic instability of tumour cells predisposes to new aberrations, probably of a wholly random nature, but perhaps so that the nature of the primary change facilitates some additional aberrations more than others. The ensuing genetic diversity provides a fertile soil for Darwinian selection within the tumour cell population. Cells harbouring additional changes that give them an evolutionary edge, i.e. they proliferate more vigorously or have longer lifetimes, will outgrow their neighbours and gradually dominate the karyotype (Nowell 1976, Heim et al 1988a). Although secondary changes, too, are non-random in distribution, they are usually less specific than primary changes.

3. *Cytogenetic noise*. Sometimes the karyotypic picture of solid tumours is so chaotic that, although a core number of shared aberrations is found in all metaphases, no two cells have exactly the same chromosome complement. It is reasonable to believe that many of the non-clonal abnormalities seen are evolutionarily neutral or even deleterious; they generate diversity but possess no selective advantage, which is indeed why they show up as 'one

cell only' aberrations. Their presence however, signals the existence of massive genetic instability, a characteristic that is bound to facilitate clonal evolution and, consequently, rapid tumour progression.

In spite of much recent progress in the chromosomal analysis of solid tumours, this area of cancer cytogenetics still accounts for only 21% of the total data base of 14 000 neoplasms with reported clonal abnormalities (Mitelman 1991); the remainder are haematological malignancies. Thus the most common human tumours, those responsible for the largest morbidity and mortality from neoplastic disease, are also the ones about which the least information is available. This notwithstanding, a rough picture at least is now emerging of the characteristic changes in several major human neoplasms, and for some, our understanding approaches that of leukaemia subgroups. The following summary will focus on chromosomal morphology and on what are at present understood to be the characteristic karyotypic profiles in different tumour types. Only occasionally are the karyotypic data detailed enough to allow a separate discussion of primary and secondary abnormalities. The molecular genetic findings in solid tumours are outside the scope of this review and will be alluded to only when the data can be directly correlated with well-established cytogenetic features. Suffice it to emphasize that genes with a negative regulatory growth influence (tumour suppressor genes or anti-oncogenes) and genes which stimulate cell division (oncogenes) have both been detected in the human genome. Although some of the changes that alter the function of these two classes of gene are too small to be microscopically detectable, many are visible as cytogenetic rearrangements. Chromosome aberrations may activate oncogenes quantitatively through interference with regulatory structures or qualitatively through the generation of hybrid genes. Loss of anti-oncogene function may occur through cytogenetically detectable loss of chromatin material. The molecular genetics of cancer has been reviewed by, amongst others, Klein (1988) and Weinberg (1989).

CYTOGENETIC NOMENCLATURE

Before going on to describe the characteristic chromosome abnormalities of different tumour types, a brief description of cytogenetic terminology may be appropriate. For a complete and authoritative summary of the current language of cytogenetics the reader is referred to ISCN (1985).

After staining metaphase cells with a banding technique, the chromosomes are seen as a continuous series of transverse dark and light bands (Fig. 3.1). Each band can be designated individually by listing (a) the chromosome number (1–22 for the autosomes and X or Y for the sex chromosomes); (b) the chromosome arm (the centromere divides the chromosome into a short 'p' and a long 'q' arm); (c) the region (a region is an area delimited by specific landmarks, i.e. constant, distinct morphological features) and (d) the band number (bands are counted from the centromere

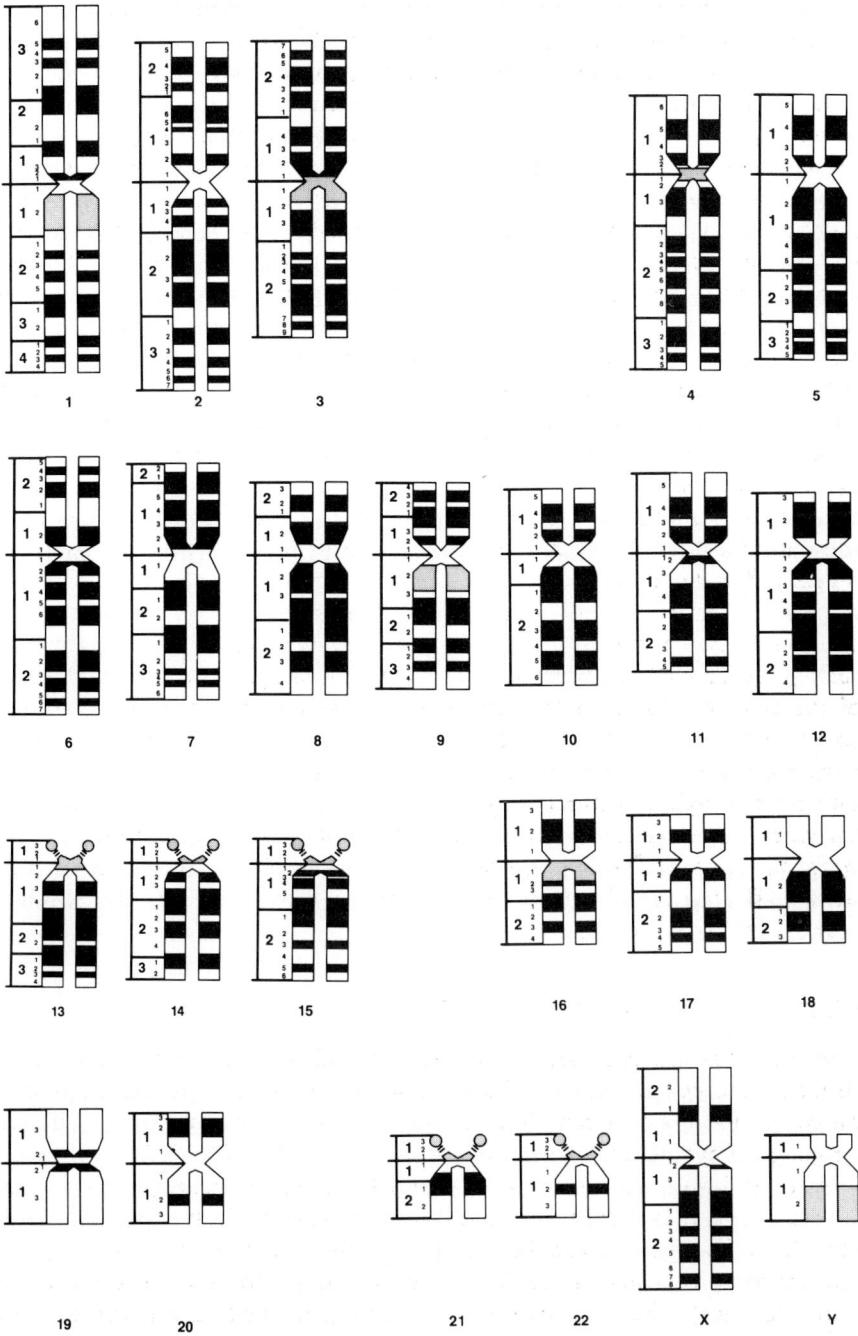

Fig. 3.1 Idiogram of the 22 autosomes and two sex chromosomes of man. Any band can be described by four items of information: the chromosome number, the arm, the region, and the band number within that region.

outward towards the telomere) within the region. Thus 12q13 means chromosome 12, long arm, region 1, band 3. If sub-bands are discernible, these are marked with additional numbers separated from the conventional band number by a full stop.

The normal human karyotypes are 46,XX for women and 46,XY for men. Karyotypic abnormalities may be numerical, meaning the loss or gain of whole chromosomes (written by placing a − or + sign before the chromosome in question), or structural. The most common structural aberrations are translocations (abbreviated t; chromatin material is exchanged between chromosomes) and deletions (del; chromosome material is lost). Loss of material can also be indicated by writing a − sign after the chromosome arm, e.g. 6q− means that material has been lost, whether by deletion or unbalanced translocation is unknown, from the long arm of chromosome 6. Isochromosomes (abbreviated i) are mirror images around their centromeres; they are symmetrical with two long or two short arms instead of one of each. 47,XX,del(3)(p13),+i(17q) therefore means a female karyotype in which the short arm of one chromosome 3 distal to 3p13 has been lost, but also where an isochromosome for the long arm of chromosome 17 has been gained.

KARYOTYPIC PROFILES IN DIFFERENT TUMOUR TYPES

Respiratory tract

Upper airways

Only about 30 karyotypically abnormal *squamous cell carcinomas* (SCC) of the head and neck region (mouth, pharynx, paranasal sinuses, larynx) have been reported. A recurring feature has been the presence of cytogenetically unrelated clones (Jin et al 1990a,b). This could mean that the primary genetic alteration is submicroscopic and that the visible aberrations are only secondary, or the findings could indicate multiclonal carcinogenesis within a cancer-prone epithelial field (Slaughter et al 1953). However, it is also possible that the clonal aberrations, which are mostly balanced translocations, are not representative of the tumour parenchyma but occur in stromal fibroblasts or other subepithelial cells. The iconoclastic implication of the latter explanation would of course be that non-neoplastic cells can carry acquired, clonal chromosomal abnormalities, at least when they are present in mucosa or skin subjected to long-term carcinogenic exposure.

The distribution of breakpoints in the chromosomal rearrangements in head and neck SCC seems to be non-random; bands 1p22 and 11q13 are preferentially involved (Jin et al 1990c). Cytogenetic signs of gene amplification, i.e. double minute chromosomes (dmin) and homogeneously staining regions (hsr), are also detected, something that may be consonant with reports of amplification of oncogenes whose normal location is in these bands (Zhou et al 1988, Berenson et al 1989, Tsuda et al 1989).

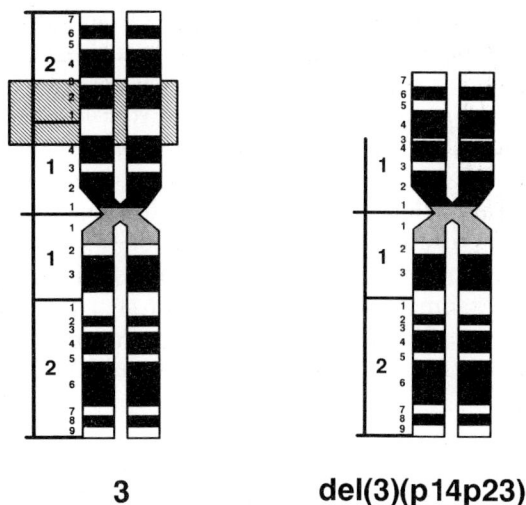

3   **del(3)(p14p23)**

Fig. 3.2   A deletion of the short arm of chromosome 3, here illustrated as a del(3) (p14p23), is the most consistent cytogenetic rearrangement in lung carcinomas. 3p − is also common in other carcinomas, especially of the kidney.

Lung

Early analyses established that many *small cell lung carcinomas* (SCLC) were characterized by loss of chromosome material from the short arm of chromosome 3 (Fig. 3.2), often as a del(3)(p14p23) (Whang-Peng et al 1982, Whang-Peng & Lee 1985). Zech et al (1985) detected comparable 3p deletions also in *non-small cell lung carcinomas* (NSCLC), albeit at lower frequencies. Molecular genetic investigations indicate that loss of genetic material from 3p band 3p21 may constitute a least common deleted segment in which a tentative tumour suppressor gene is located and this may be a central event in the development of lung cancer. A variety of oncogene activation changes have also been identified at various stages of tumour progression (Birrer & Minna 1989).

NSCLC, like SCLC, generally have complex karyotypes (Campbell et al 1989, Lukeis et al 1990, Miura et al 1990b, Viegas-Péquignot et al 1990). The small number of cases analysed does not allow a detailed picture to emerge; the breakpoints seem to be non-randomly distributed, but no other highly characteristic changes than 3p − have been detected. An isochromosome for 8q has been repeatedly described in adenocarcinomas (Jin et al 1988, Miura et al 1990a).

Pleura

About 70 *mesotheliomas* with clonal abnormalities have been reported. The karyotypes are complex and no specific aberrations are known. Tiainen et al

(1989) found that -22, $+7$, -1, -3, -9, $+11$, and -14 were common numerical aberrations and that deletions or translocations of 1p11–p22 were the most common structural rearrangements. Flejter et al (1989) detected a pattern of recurring chromatin loss from 1p, 3p, and 22q, which led them to suggest that these regions harbour loci for tumour suppressor genes of importance in mesothelioma tumorigenesis. In the series of 30 karyotypically abnormal malignant mesotheliomas analysed by Hagemeijer et al (1990), two main patterns of non-random abnormalities were observed. Most tumours had a hypodiploid and/or hypotetraploid modal chromosome number, loss of chromosomes 4 and 22, and structural rearrangements leading to loss of material from 9p and 3p. A minority had a hyperdiploid chromosome number, gain of chromosomes 7, 5, and 20, and deletion of 3p.

Digestive tract

Salivary glands

Adenomas of the salivary gland are among the cytogenetically best characterized epithelial tumours; more than 150 cases with clonal chromosome abnormalities are known. Large series and recent reviews were published by Bullerdiek et al (1987, 1988), Mark et al (1988), and Sandros et al (1990). The bands or regions 3p21, 8q12, and 12q13–15 are frequently rearranged and the first two often are recombined in t(3;8)(p21;q12) (Fig. 3.3).

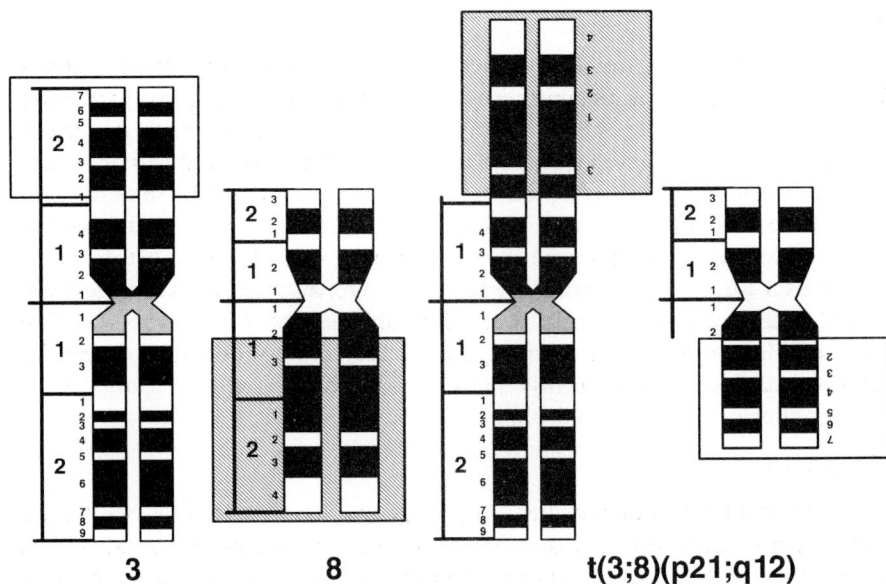

Fig. 3.3   The reciprocal translocation t(3;8) (p21;q12) characterizes a subgroup of salivary gland adenomas.

Sometimes more complex three-way rearrangements occur, and occasional variant translocations may involve either 3p21 or 8q12 without visible involvement of the other. The subset with 12q-rearrangements—repeated recombinations with 9p12–22, but a score of other translocation partners have also been recorded—usually has no structural changes of chromosomes 3 and 8 and so appears to be a pathogenetically distinct group.

Deletions of 6q seem to be the most common structural aberrations in *adenocarcinomas* and other malignant salivary gland tumours; the most common numerical changes have been loss of the Y chromosome and trisomy 8 (Sandros et al 1988, 1990). Analysis of two respiratory tract adenoid cystic carcinomas showed rearrangement of 9p to be the first cytogenetic change (Higashi et al 1991), which suggests that the 6q− aberrations here, and by inference also in other salivary gland carcinomas, are secondary phenomena despite their frequent presence.

Liver

The only *hepatocellular carcinoma* with chromosome aberrations that has been reported had a pseudodiploid karyotype with several rearrangements that included a 6q− (Simon et al 1990). Trisomy 20 and dmin were detected in two *hepatoblastomas* investigated by Mascarello et al (1990). Fletcher et al (1991) analysed four hepatoblastomas and found trisomy 20 and partial trisomy 2 (2q23–2q35 was the shortest region of overlap) in all cases.

Pancreas

For pancreatic tumours the data are scarce indeed. The largest series hitherto analysed included nine *carcinomas* with clonal aberrations (Johansson et al 1991). The − Y found as the sole anomaly in three tumours is probably not tumour specific (see below). The most common structural rearrangements affected 6q, 1p, 17, 3p, and 8p and the most common numerical changes were + 2, + 10, + 11, + 14, and + 20. The findings suggest that loss of genetic material from the short arms of 3, 8, and 17 and from the long arm of chromosome 6 might be important. Similar patterns of loss have been found in several other settings, and it is probable that we are witnessing the cytogenetic contours of a common tumorigenic pathway that is shared by adenocarcinomas of several organs and cell types.

Oesophagus

Except for three tumours at the oesophago-gastric junction (see below), no oesophageal squamous cell carcinomas with chromosome aberrations have been reported. Garewal et al (1989) analysed short-term cultures from 15 cases of *Barrett's oesophagus* and found a balanced t(3;6) in one, trisomy for chromosomes 5 and 7 in another, and clonal loss of the Y chromosome in seven. It is highly questionable whether these changes should be taken to mean that a neoplastic process had already begun in the premalignant epithelium.

Stomach

Only about 30 *carcinomas* with clonal karyotypic abnormalities have been reported. Ferti-Passantonopoulou et al (1987) described five tumours and found that the most common aberrations involved chromosomes 9 and 8, including trisomy 9, i(9q), 9p+, +8, and i(8q). Misawa et al (1990) examined seven cases and found complex numerical and structural changes in six but no characteristic karyotypic feature was discernible. Rodriguez et al (1990) analysed nine carcinomas, and found that the region 11p13–15 was rearranged in eight. Other aberrations repeatedly encountered were i(5p) and rearrangements of 3p21. Cytogenetic signs of gene amplification (hsr and dmin) were also present.

Small intestine

No information is available on adenocarcinomas of the small bowel. Mark (1976) and Dal Cin et al (1988a) reported two *leiomyosarcomas*, both of which had a hypodiploid chromosome number, deletions of the short arm of chromosome 1, and monosomy for chromosomes 14, 15, 18, and 22.

Large intestine

Although some 150 tumours with clonal chromosome aberrations have been described, the changes are complex and the technical difficulties in getting well-banded preparations are great. Mitelman et al (1974) and Reichmann et al (1985) reported numerical aberrations in *adenomas*, a feature that may turn out to be common in other nonmalignant glandular neoplasms (see also under thyroid and ovaries).

Adenocarcinomas usually have much more complex changes (Muleris et al 1987a, Ferti et al 1988, Yaseen et al 1990). Based on a review of 93 karyotypically abnormal cases, Muleris et al (1990) recently reiterated the group's previous conclusions that the most common changes are rearrangements of chromosome 17 (leading to loss of the short arm) and loss of one chromosome 18. They favour a subdivision of karyotypically abnormal colorectal adenocarcinomas into at least three groups. First, there is a subset of tumours that are near diploid, monosomic for 17p and chromosome 18, and which also have a range of other less constant aberrations usually leading to monosomy for given genomic segments. Second are the mono-somic polyploid tumours which, apart from their higher chromosome number, have a pattern of chromosomal imbalances similar to that of the first group. The third subset are the trisomic-type tumours, which may have lost either 17p or chromosome 18, and whose other anomalies mostly consist of gains of entire chromosomes.

Molecular genetic studies have significantly added to our knowledge of the genetic changes that characterize colorectal tumorigenesis. Based on allelic deletion analysis, Fearon & Vogelstein (1990) deduced that alterations on at least four to six loci, presumably inactivation mutations of tumour suppressor genes or anti-oncogenes, are required for carcinoma formation. Two of the genes that are most consistently inactivated are *p53* in 17p and *DCC* in 18q. It seems likely, therefore, that cytogenetic aberrations involving these regions are pathogenetically important as they may affect the same genes whose inactivation have been detected at the molecular level.

Information on *squamous cell carcinomas* of the anal canal is restricted to a single series of seven chromosomally abnormal tumours (Muleris et al 1987b). The most consistent aberrations were rearrangements leading to loss of genetic material from 11q and 3p.

Urinary tract

Kidney

The examination of more than 250 cytogenetically abnormal *renal cell carcinomas* (RCC) has revealed several karyotype characteristics. The primary cytogenetic abnormality in this tumour type involves loss of genetic material from the short arm of chromosome 3, mostly as the result of a simple deletion that may or may not be the sole aberration (Kovacs et al 1987, Dal Cin et al 1988b, Kovacs & Frisch 1989, Walter et al 1989). The extent of the common minimal deleted segment (if indeed one exists) is uncertain and it has hitherto not been possible to distinguish it from that found in lung tumours or from the less frequent 3p deletions encountered in mesotheliomas and carcinomas of the breast, salivary glands, and ovaries. On the other hand, Kovacs et al (1989) demonstrated that loss of 3p material may be restricted to nonpapillary RCCs, where it was found in more than 90% of cases. Few of the rare renal *oncocytomas* have been examined and they seem to be similar to papillary RCC in that they lack 3p— changes. Welter et al (1989) reported mitochondrial DNA mutations in oncocytomas; similar changes have not been detected in other renal tumours.

Most RCC with 3p— also have non-random secondary changes (Kovacs & Frisch 1989, Walter et al 1989). Frequent among these are aberrations of chromosome 5 resulting in trisomy for distal 5q, and of chromosome 14 resulting in loss of distal 14q. Trisomy 7, monosomy 8 and 9, loss of a sex chromosome, and structural or numerical aberrations involving chromosome 6 have also been found. Sex chromosome loss and small clones with trisomy 7 have now been detected in short-term cultures of non-neoplastic renal tissue, and their relevance in RCC is therefore questionable (Elfving et al 1990, Limon et al 1990).

The karyotypic profile of *nephroblastoma* differs from that of RCC (Douglass et al 1985, Slater et al 1985, Solis et al 1988, Hohenfellner et al 1989). Rearrangements of 3p are uncommon. The most frequent changes affect chromosome 1, often resulting in partial trisomy for the long arm. Some tumours have deletions of 11p13, where a locus for the aniridia-Wilms' tumour syndrome is located. The importance of chromosome 11 (probably gene(s) in 11p) is also testified to by the finding that when a normal chromosome 11 was introduced into a Wilms' tumour cell line, this resulted in suppression of tumorigenic capacity (Weissman et al 1987). However, these are unlikely to be the only loci that are important. Most Wilms' tumours do not have 11p changes, and it is reasonable to interpret the cytogenetic heterogeneity as a reflection of the pathogenetic complexity now known to characterize the development of these tumours (Francke 1990).

Bladder

Most of the nearly 100 known *transitional cell carcinomas* (TCC) with karyotypic aberrations were reported in the early or mid 1980s and the findings have been reviewed by Perucca et al (1990). Chromosome 1 shows the highest number of aberrations, but they vary widely in nature, and the impression is that most, if not all, are secondary and nonspecific. Also frequently involved are chromosomes 3 (especially the short arm), 5 (often an isochromosome for 5p), 7 (trisomy), 9 (mostly loss of one copy), and 10 (deletions of the long arm). Somewhat less common are various changes affecting chromosomes 6, 8, 11, 13, and 17. Combinations of abnormalities are the rule rather than the exception. The most frequent solitary changes, and thus the automatic candidates for a primary pathogenetic role, have been monosomy 9, trisomy 7, and del(10q). Except for trisomy 7, most karyotypic abnormalities in TCC involve loss of genetic material, which is taken to imply that anti-oncogene loss or inactivation is an essential element in tumorigenesis.

Breast

Close to 150 breast *carcinomas* with clonal chromosome aberrations have been reported. Large consecutive series were described by Rodgers et al (1984), Gebhart et al (1986), and Hill et al (1987). More recent reports include Dutrillaux et al (1990), Geleick et al (1990), and Mitchell & Santibanez-Koref (1990); the field was reviewed by Hainsworth & Garson (1990). The chromosome that is most commonly rearranged is chromosome 1, 1p seemingly more than 1q, and perhaps with a breakpoint cluster in 1p13. Other genomic regions that are frequently rearranged, often so that loss of genetic material occurs, are 3p, 6q, 11p and 11q, 16q, and 17p. Several molecular genetic analyses have demonstrated loss of heterozygosity on chromosomes 1 and 3, 13q, and 17p (references in Mitchell & Santibanez-Koref 1990).

Reproductive organs

These include both male and female sex organs.

Ovary

Roughly 200 ovarian tumours with clonal chromosome abnormalities are known; recent reports include those by Pejovic et al (1989) and Bello & Rey (1990). No consistent differences have been detected between the major *carcinoma* subtypes, but it is apparent that highly differentiated tumours are on average less karyotypically complex than their poorly differentiated counterparts (Pejovic et al 1990b). The aberrations often include structural rearrangements of 6q and 11p, mostly leading to loss of genetic material, as well as 19p + markers in which the material added to 19p13 is unknown. Even more common are aberrations of chromosome 1, but these are scattered along both the long and short arms and seem likely to be secondary, late changes. As deletions of 6q and 19p + markers are recurrent abnormalities in cancers other than those of the ovary, they too most likely reflect general cytogenetic pathways in carcinogenesis.

Simple but characteristic karyotypic changes have been detected in *benign tumours* of the ovary. Leung et al (1990), Mrozek et al (1990) and Pejovic et al (1990a) described trisomy 12—mostly as the sole chromosome abnormality—in one serous cystadenoma, one mucinous cystadenoma, one granulosa cell tumour, four fibromas, one fibrothecoma, and one thecoma. Trisomy 12 is otherwise found as the only change in uterine leiomyomas (see below) and in chronic lymphatic leukaemias (references in Sandberg, 1990).

Uterus

Most *cervical carcinomas* with chromosome aberrations have been reported by Atkin et al (1990). No consistent pattern of abnormalities has emerged, but chromosomes 1, 2, 3, 6, 9, 11, and 17 seem to be non-randomly involved. Isochromosomes—including i(1q), i(4p) or i(5p), and small metacentric markers—are common.

Only about 50 *endometrial carcinomas* with chromosome abnormalities have been reported. Couturier et al (1988) described frequent involvement of chromosome 1, often leading to partial trisomy or tetrasomy for 1q. Other imbalances included trisomy for chromosomes 2, 7, 10, and 12. Milatovich et al (1990) also reported gain of 1q material, but found no other consistent abnormality. They also described clonal aberrations in three endometrial *mixed Müllerian tumours* of the homologous; all had massive abnormalities that included changes of chromosomes 1, 3, and 5.

Leiomyomas of the uterus have been extensively studied and more than 200 tumours with clonal aberrations are known (Mark et al 1990, Nilbert & Heim 1990, Pandis et al 1991a). Several cytogenetic subgroups have emerged, characterized by the presence of the abnormalities t(12;14) (q14–15;q23–24), del(7)(q21q31), trisomy 12, and rearrangements of 6p. The breakpoints of the t(12;14) have been mapped at high resolution level to 12q15 and 14q24.1 (Pandis et al 1990a). A surprising finding has been that macroscopically discrete uterine leiomyomas may share the same clonal abnormalities (references in Nilbert & Heim 1990); this could be explained if intramyometrial spread of tumour cells is the underlying cause of some multiple leiomyomas. Sometimes clonal evolution is evident, often as chromosome 1 aberrations or the formation of ring chromosomes; among the strongly tumour-associated aberrations, del(7q) may occur secondarily to t(12;14) or +12 (Pandis et al 1990b). When multiple aberrations are found, the leiomyomas tend to be of the cellular type, to show more mitotic activity, and to contain atypical cells (Pandis et al 1991b).

Testis

Less than 100 testicular *germ cell tumours* (TGCT) with cytogenetic abnormalities have been reported; among the larger series are those of Delozier-Blanchet et al (1987), Bosl et al (1989), and Castedo et al (1989a,b); the topic was recently reviewed by de Jong et al (1990). The most common chromosomal aberration is an i(12p) which is present, sometimes in more than one copy, in TGCT of all histological subtypes. Numerous additional structural rearrangements are the rule rather than the exception. Most frequently involved in these secondary changes is chromosome 1, but otherwise no clear-cut pattern has emerged. The chromosome number in TGCT is usually in the hyperdiploid to hypotetraploid range, with higher modal numbers in seminomas. de Jong et al (1990) have used the cytogenetic information to assess existing theories for the pathogenetic relationship between *nonseminomatous germ cell tumours* and *seminomas*. They concluded that the karyotype data best fit a model in which both have a common origin and also a common tumorigenic pathway, but where the seminomas represent an intermediate stage in nonseminomatous germ cell tumour development.

Prostate

Most prostatic *adenocarcinomas* that have been cytogenetically analysed had normal karyotypes; only some 20 tumours with clonal chromosome aberrations have been reported. No consistent abnormalities are known. Brothman et al (1990) reported loss of chromosomes 1, 2, 5, and Y, gain of chromosomes 7, 14, 20, and 22, and structural rearrangements of chromosome arms 2p, 7q, and 10q to be the commonest changes. Lundgren et al

(1991) found breakpoint cluster regions in, or non-random loss of, 7q, 8p, and 10q and suggested that these regions harbour loci of importance in prostatic carcinogenesis.

Endocrine glands

Data are limited to the thyroid.

Thyroid

Some 20 *carcinomas* of the thyroid have been found to have cytogenetic abnormalities. Jenkins et al (1990) described clonal aberrations in a series which included three follicular, two anaplastic, and four papillary cancers. They concluded that rearrangements of 10q characterize nonmedullary carcinomas, especially when the growth pattern is papillary. Whereas the papillary carcinomas had relatively simple karyotypic aberrations, the karyotypes of the follicular and anaplastic tumours were complex and included changes seen in several other malignancies, e.g. 3p rearrangements.

From the equally limited data on thyroid *adenomas*, two different karyotypic profiles have been identified. In the series of Teyssier & Ferre (1989), simple structural aberrations were the most common. On the other hand, Bondeson et al (1989) and van den Berg et al (1990) found that gain of several whole chromosomes (often +4 or +5, +7, +9, +12, and +16) constituted a characteristic aberration pattern.

Nervous system

Characteristic karyotypic abnormalities, monosomy 22 but sometimes only del(22q), were demonstrated in *meningiomas* more than a decade ago (Mark 1977, Zang 1982). Later research has emphasized that the secondary aberrations of meningiomas are non-random; chromosome 14 and chromosome arms 1p and 11p have been implicated in the clonal evolution of these tumours (Rey et al 1988). The consistent loss of 22q material has led to the hypothesis that a tumour suppressor gene exists in this region and analyses of loss of polymorphic loci along the long arm of chromosome 22 have narrowed the likely position of this tentative locus to somewhere in 22q12.3 – qter (Dumanski et al 1990).

Nearly 200 karyotypically abnormal malignant *gliomas* have been reported. A characteristic feature has been the high frequency of double minutes (dmin), but other aberrations—in particular trisomy 7, loss of a sex chromosome, loss of one chromosome 10 or 22, and loss of material from chromosome arms 9p and 17p—also occur (Bigner et al 1988, 1990, Jenkins et al 1989). A conundrum in glioma cytogenetics has been that, whereas some tumours have complex karyotypes with several structural rearrangements, other equally malignant examples seem to have only simple numerical aberrations, in particular trisomy 7, monosomy 10, monosomy 22, and −X or −Y. This led to the suggestion that the primary genetic change in gliomas is a simple gain or loss of a whole chromosome (Bigner et al 1986). However, recent evidence indicates that a solitary +7 and/or sex chromosome loss do not represent tumour parenchyma cells in gliomas (Lindström et al 1991), and so their significance is doubtful.

Primitive neuroectodermal tumours (PNET) of the central nervous system are the most common malignant brain tumours in children. Biegel et al (1989a) described 19 cytogenetically abnormal PNETs and drew the conclusion that chromosomes 5, 6, 11, 16, 17, and X or Y were non-randomly involved in aberrations; dmin were also repeatedly observed. Particularly striking, however, was the frequent finding of an i(17q), which was the sole aberration in three tumours.

More than 100 *neuroblastomas* with abnormal karyotypes have been described (Brodeur & Fong 1989). The characteristic profile in this tumour type includes deletions towards the tip of the short arm of chromosome 1 and signs of gene amplification in the form of hsr and dmin (Kaneko et al 1987, Hayashi et al 1989). The hsr and dmin are more frequent in advanced tumours and are especially common in established cell lines. Although the amplicon may vary, it often includes the *MYCN* locus and amplification of this oncogene thus seems to be particularly characteristic of neuroblastoma, especially of advanced and rapidly progressive disease.

Approximately 70% of human neuroblastomas have cytogenetically visible deletions in 1p, and attempts have been made to delineate more precisely the area that contains the tentative tumour suppressor gene or antioncogene. Weith et al (1989) used a panel of polymorphic DNA probes to map a consensus deletion to 1p36.1−2. They found no evidence that the 1p deletion was directly correlated with *MYCN* amplification and so these two neuroblastoma-associated genetic alterations seem to result from different molecular mechanisms.

Retinoblastoma is found as both an autosomal dominant and a sporadic, non-hereditary tumour. Among the seminal contributions that have sprung from the study of these two modes of disease is Knudson's two-hit model, which explains how cancers that are autosomal dominant at the organism level may nevertheless be autosomal recessive at the level of individual target cells (Knudson 1989). A retinoblastoma susceptibility locus (RB) exists in 13q14, and both alleles must be inactivated before the cell becomes neoplastic. Patients with bilateral tumours have one allele inactivated in the germ line. The importance of the 13q14 locus has been demonstrated directly by introducing a cloned, intact RB gene into retinoblastoma or osteosarcoma cells (Huang et al 1988). This resulted in suppression of the tumour phenotype. The lessons learned from retinoblastoma genetics are being extended to more common neoplasms and so retinoblastoma continues to play a paradigmatic role in our conception of how homozygous inactivation or loss of anti-oncogenes is essential in carcinogenesis (Scrable et al 1990).

Among the roughly 100 retinoblastomas with aberrant karyotypes that have been reported, the most common change, found in one third of cases, has been i(6p) (Kusnetsova et al 1982, Benedict et al 1983, Squire et al 1985). The relative scarcity of acquired cytogenetic aberrations affecting 13q14 might at first glance seem puzzling in the light of the pathogenetic knowledge referred to above. The reason for this is probably that deletions in and around 13q14 are likely to jeopardize cellular fitness if they are so big as to be microscopically visible. Nevertheless, direct cytogenetic evidence of a homozygous deletion in 13q13.3–14.2, i.e. loss of the retinoblastoma locus in 13q14.1, was described by Lemieux et al (1989). Both the molecular genetic and the cytogenetic evidence thus support the notion that loss of both antioncogene alleles is necessary before a tumour develops (Scrable et al 1990).

Skin

Only ten *squamous cell carcinomas* with chromosome abnormalities have been reported. Aledo et al (1989) described cytogenetically independent clones and emphasized the non-random involvement of telomeric and centromeric regions to form what they call 'jumping translocations' in lesions from xeroderma pigmentosum patients. Heim et al (1989) found multiple clones in three invasive carcinomas. Doubt remains as to whether the multiple, apparently unrelated clones repeatedly detected in skin and upper airway tumours really represent genomic rearrangements in tumour cells.

Mertens et al (1991) analysed 33 *basal cell carcinomas*, eight of which had clonal chromosome aberrations. Cytogenetically unrelated clones were detected in two cases and short-term cultures yielded non-clonal, structural rearrangements. Again, it is premature to pass judgment as to whether the cytogenetic findings really signify multiclonal tumorigenesis, or whether the acquired clonal aberrations occurred in stromal cells.

Clonal chromosome abnormalities have been reported in about ten *Merkel cell carcinomas* (Sozzi et al 1988, Koduru et al 1989). The most consistent karyotypic feature has been aberrations of chromosome 1, often resulting in partial trisomy for the distal part of the long arm (1q22 — qter).

Less than 100 *malignant melanomas* with cytogenetic abnormalities are known. Chromosomes 1, 6, and 7 are clearly non-randomly involved (Parmiter & Nowell 1988). Other chromosomes that seem likely to harbour loci of importance in these tumours are 9 and 11 (loss of material from the short arm has been described), and 10 (loss of 10q material). The breakpoints in chromosome 1 are mostly in the region 1p11–22. The chromosome 7 involvement is mostly in the form of trisomy. The non-random involvement of chromosome 6 is due to numerous translocations and deletions of the long arm, with clustering to 6q12–25. Trent et al (1989) have called attention to the repeated occurrence of a t(1;6) in which the proximal part of 6q (6q11–13) is recombined with either 1p22 or 1q12–21. The importance of 6q loci in melanoma tumorigenesis is further underlined by the findings of Trent et al (1990b), who introduced a normal chromosome 6 into a melanoma cell line: this caused the cell line to revert to a non-neoplastic phenotype.

A particularly characteristic karyotypic pattern is emerging for *uveal melanomas*. Horsman et al (1990) reported −3 and i(8q) in one locally invasive tumour and Sisley et al (1990) described another five cases with abnormal karyotypes. In three of them, monosomy 3 and i(8q) were found. Finally, Prescher et al (1990) found additional 8q material (the smallest multiplied area was mapped to 8q21–8qter) in eight and monosomy 3 in six of 14 uveal melanomas. The two findings coexisted in five cases.

Bone and connective tissue

Ten *osteosarcomas* with clonal chromosome abnormalities have been reported; the largest series, six cases with aberrations, was that of Biegel et al (1989b). The aberrations were complex and no consistent changes were detected.

The characteristic chromosomal rearrangement of *Ewing's sarcoma* is the reciprocal translocation t(11;22)(q24;q12) (Fig. 3.4). Turc-Carel et al (1988) reviewed more than 80 tumours and found the t(11;22), or less often a variant rearrangement, in 90%. The t(11;22) may be the sole change, but other aberrations are usually present. Mugneret et al (1988) and Douglass et al (1990) found that the most common secondary changes of these were trisomy 8 and a der(16)t(1;16) (q21;q13).

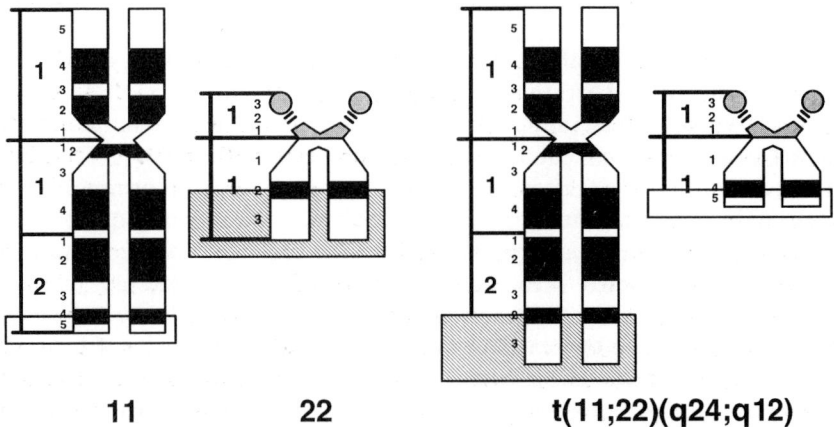

11   22   t(11;22)(q24;q12)

Fig. 3.4   The reciprocal translocation t(11;22)(q24;q12) characterizes Ewing's sarcoma as well as the rare variants peripheral neuroepithelioma, Askin tumour, and aesthesioneuroblastoma.

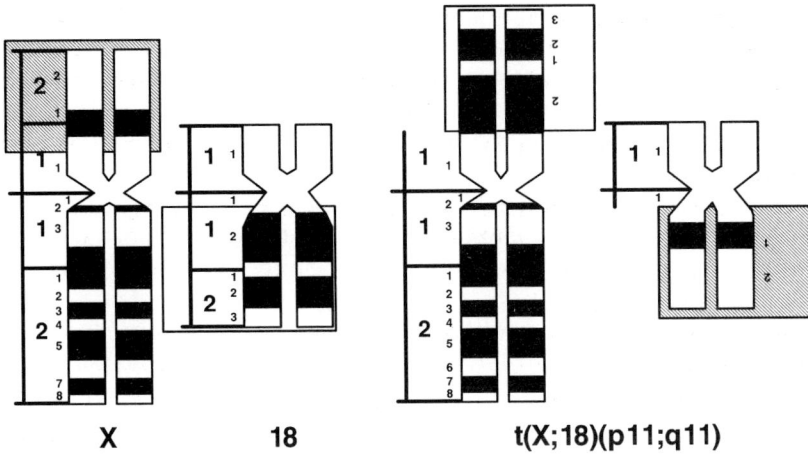

X   18   t(X;18)(p11;q11)

Fig. 3.5   The reciprocal translocation t(X;18)(p11;q11) is specific for synovial sarcoma.

A cytogenetically indistinguishable t(11;22) to that found in Ewing's sarcoma has been repeatedly demonstrated in *peripheral neuroepithelioma, Askin tumour,* and *aesthesioneuroblastoma* (Turc-Carel et al 1988, Douglass et al 1990). This has strengthened speculations that all four tumours may actually be variations on the same theme and that they share the same pathogenesis. Whether the breakpoints differ or are identical at the molecular level, is still unknown.

Mandahl et al (1990) described clonal abnormalities in one of six *chondromas* and in seven of ten *chondrosarcomas*. The most common numerical aberrations were monosomies for chromosomes 6, 10, 11, 13, 18, and 22. Structural rearrangements involved chromosome 1 in five tumours, chromosomes 6, 12, and 15 in three. No specific karyotypic abnormalities were detectable.

A new addition to the list of specific chromosomal abnormalities in mesenchymal tumours may be t(9;22)(q22;q12) in *extraskeletal myxoid chondrosarcoma*. The data are still limited, but of the four such tumours that have been reported, three had a 9;22-translocation with the 9q22 and 22q12 breakpoints, an aberration that has not been seen in any other tumour type (Örndal et al 1991a).

Synovial sarcomas are characterized by the only specific rearrangement known to involve one of the sex chromosomes (Fig. 3.5), a t(X;18)(p11;q11) (Turc-Carel et al 1987a). Limon et al (1991) reported tumour karyotypes that were mostly pseudodiploid or neardiploid. Whereas half of the primary tumours had t(X;18) as the sole change, most metastases had additional, secondary changes, involving chromosomes 1 and 12 particularly often. No cytogenetic differences were discernible between the karyotypic profiles of monophasic and biphasic synovial sarcomas.

Malignant fibrous histiocytoma is the most common soft tissue sarcoma, but the number of cases with known karyotypic abnormalities is still less than 30. The aberrations reported by Mandahl et al (1989b) included a high number of telomeric associations, rings, and dicentric chromosomes, and in several tumours hsr and dmin. The structural rearrangements often affected 19p13 (giving rise to 19p+ markers), 11p (mostly deletions), 1q (mostly deletions), and 3p (again mostly leading to loss of material). Molenaar et al (1989) found deletions of 1q to be recurrent changes.

The only two *infantile fibrosarcomas* that have been reported showed addition of several whole chromosomes as the only change (Speleman et al 1989, Mandahl et al 1989a).

Large series of cytogenetically well characterized *lipomas* have been published by Mandahl et al (1988) and Sreekantaiah et al (1991). The most specific rearrangement appears to be a reciprocal translocation between chromosomes 3 and 12, a t(3;12)(q27–28;q14–15). The same region of chromosome 12 may also recombine with a host of other chromosomes or undergo intrachromosomal rearrangements. Some typical lipomas have no visible 12q changes; among them, rearrangements of 6p and 13q seem to be the most common. Many lipomas appear to be cytogenetically normal. These are often multiple rather than solitary which may reflect pathogenetic differences.

A subgroup of lipogenic tumours demonstrate histological features and biological behaviour that place them in between the overtly malignant and the undoubtedly benign: they are variously termed *atypical lipomas* or *highly differentiated liposarcomas*. Regardless of what they are called, these tumours tend to be characterized by supernumerary ring chromosomes of unknown origin (Turc-Carel et al 1987b, Heim et al 1988b, Mandahl et al 1988). Such ring markers are also common in malignant fibrous histiocytomas (Mandahl et al 1989b), in dermatofibrosarcoma protuberans (Mandahl et al 1989c), and as secondary aberrations in uterine leiomyomas (Nilbert & Heim 1990). In general, supernumerary rings seem to be a feature of highly differentiated mesenchymal tumours of low or questionable malignancy (Örndal et al 1991b).

A specific chromosomal rearrangement, t(12;16)(q13;p11) (Fig. 3.6), has been detected in almost all of 20 karyotypically abnormal *myxoid* and *mixed liposarcomas* (Turc-Carel et al 1986, Molenaar et al 1989). Most of the karyotypes were pseudodiploid or neardiploid. Secondary aberrations were sometimes present. The t(12;16) has not been found in *round cell* or *poorly differentiated liposarcomas* and these tumours are so far without any characterizing karyotypic features.

The breakpoints of t(12;16) have recently been mapped to sub-bands 12q13.3 and 16p11.2 (Eneroth et al 1990). It is unclear whether the 12q breakpoint of liposarcomas is identical to that of lipomas or pleomorphic adenomas of the salivary gland, where all three bands within 12q13–15 have been implicated. On the other hand, the cytogenetic evidence now suggests that the liposarcoma breakpoint on 12q is proximal to the 12q breakpoint in

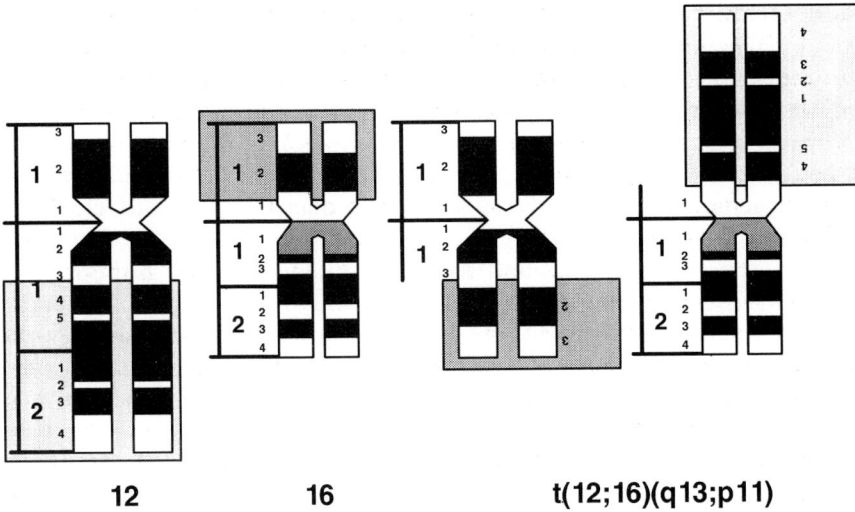

12   **16**   **t(12;16)(q13;p11)**

Fig. 3.6   The reciprocal translocation t(12;16)(q13;p11) is specific for myxoid liposarcoma. The breakpoints have now been mapped at high resolution level to sub-bands 12q13.3 and 16p11.2.

leiomyomas, which appears to be in 12q15 (Pandis et al 1990a). The molecular nature of the various 12q rearrangements in benign and malignant tumours has not been elucidated.

All our knowledge about *leiomyomas* is derived from the study of uterine tumours. Information about *leiomyosarcoma* is restricted to some 20 tumours with karyotypic abnormalities but no characteristic pattern has emerged. Something akin to the lipoma–myxoid liposarcoma relationship, is detectable, and at least two leiomyosarcomas have had rearrangements that mapped to 12q13 and 14q23 (Nilbert et al 1990).

No *rhabdomyoma* has been cytogenetically characterized. Some 40 *rhabdomyosarcomas* with karyotypic abnormalities have been reported. Douglass et al (1987) detected the specific t(2;13)(q35;q14) in five rhabdomyosarcomas amongst which the alveolar, embryonal, and undifferentiated subtypes were all represented. The tumours also had numerous secondary aberrations. Wang-Wuu et al (1988) found t(2;13) in four of seven alveolar rhabdomyosarcomas but in none of eight tumours of the embryonal subtype. Their data also indicated that +2 might be another non-random aberration, particularly among embryonal rhabdomyosarcomas.

CLINICAL IMPORTANCE OF SOLID TUMOUR CYTOGENETICS

In haematological neoplasms, where the knowledge of chromosome abnormalities is much more complete than is the case with solid tumours, cytogenetic analysis now plays an integral part in the diagnostic work-up of individual patients (Heim 1990, Sandberg 1990). The karyotypic findings in peripheral blood, bone marrow, or lymph node cells may unequivocally confirm that the disease process is neoplastic, disclose what type of neoplasm it is, and they may also give information of prognostic value. In practice, cytogenetic and other diagnostic modalities complement each other to achieve a picture of any given case that is as accurate, clear and detailed as it can be.

The technical difficulties and the still limited data have hitherto precluded the introduction of cytogenetics into the routine diagnostic practice of solid tumours. The indications are that this situation may now be changing. The major clinical usefulness of chromosome analysis will often lie in the digital nature of the result: either clonal chromosome aberrations are present, which means that the disease is neoplastic, or the karyotype is normal, in which case the information is of no value. This categorical statement may have to be modified somewhat, as has been alluded to repeatedly above: simple numerical but still clonal aberrations (especially $-X$ or $-Y$ and $+7$) may occur in non-neoplastic cells, and the same may be true for solitary reciprocal translocations encountered in short-term mucosa and skin cultures. However, when massive, acquired, clonal chromosomal abnormalities are detected, this means that the cells come from a neoplasm. When that sample has been taken from say, a pleural effusion of unknown cause, a situation where classical cytological or other diagnostic methods sometimes fail, cytogenetic methods may establish the correct diagnosis.

Another difficulty arises in the differential diagnosis of tumour types. We have pointed out the karyotypic characteristics corresponding to various nosological entities and emphasized that some aberrations are as good as specific for a given tumour, e.g. t(11;22) for Ewing's sarcoma and the related neural crest tumours, t(2;13) for rhabdomyosarcoma, t(X;18) for synovial sarcoma and t(12;16) for myxoid liposarcoma. Thus, cytogenetics may offer significant help in one of the most difficult differential diagnostic situations in oncology, the evaluation of small round-cell tumours in children. Because Ewing's sarcoma, metastatic neuroblastoma, rhabdomyosarcoma, and non-Hodgkin lymphoma all have distinguishing karyotypic features, chromosome analysis may, with obvious therapeutic benefit for the patient, differentiate unequivocally between these diagnostic possibilities. The cytogenetic diagnosis can even be made on fine needle aspirates, obviating the need for an open biopsy (Åkerman et al 1988).

Whether karyotype features will turn out to be an independent prognostic parameter in solid tumour cytogenetics, as they have done in haematological malignancies, remains largely untested. We shall confine ourselves to four situations in which prognostic correlations have been made and which therefore serve as a pointer to the future.

1. Sandberg (1986) summarized the then existing cytogenetic information on bladder tumours for the purpose of determining its clinical

importance. He found that noninvasive tumours of grades I and II tended to have near-diploid karyotypes with only occasional markers, whereas grade III tumours were often grossly abnormal with numerous markers. Superficially invasive grade II tumours had more aberrations than noninvasive lesions but without the massive abnormalities of the more aggressive carcinomas. Among the noninvasive papillary tumours, the presence of cytogenetic markers appeared to have predictive value: recurrence occurred in 90% of cases with markers compared with less than 5% in which no abnormal chromosomes were found.

2. The karyotype seems to be prognostically important in neuroblastoma also. Kaneko et al (1987) reported that whereas a near-triploid chromosome number was associated with excellent prognosis, the outcome for patients with near-diploid or pseudodiploid tumours was dismal. Hypotetraploid tumours seemed to have karyotypic and clinical features in common with the near- or pseudodiploid. The conclusion was that, at least from a clinical point of view, the near-triploid tumours constitute a distinct subentity. Christiansen & Lampert (1988) analysed 28 patients with neuroblastomas of different stage. Their life table analyses showed a 90% probability of surviving in patients lacking a 1p rearrangement, as compared to less than 10% in patients with an abnormal 1p. They concluded that the tumour karyotype, in particular whether or not a visible rearrangement of the short arm of chromosome 1 was present, was the most important factor in determining the outcome.

3. Trent et al (1990a) correlated clinical outcome with cytogenetic features in 62 patients with metastatic malignant melanoma. They found that patients with structural rearrangements of chromosome 7 or 11 had significantly shorter survival than patients without such abnormalities.

4. Finally, Rydholm et al (1990) compared clinical and pathological features in nine patients with malignant fibrous histiocytoma and a 19p+ marker with the same parameters in 13 patients with malignant fibrous histiocytoma but without 19p+. After a median follow-up time of 18 months, distant metastases and/or local recurrence occurred in eight of the nine patients with 19p+ but in only four of 13 without 19p+. On the other hand, patients with supernumerary ring markers appeared to have a reduced relapse risk.

Many of the correlation analyses outlined above are preliminary. It is in the nature of tentative conclusions that they may have to be modified as research progresses and further knowledge is gained. They all illustrate the important point, however, that the practical usefulness of investigating the acquired genetic abnormalities of tumour cells does not come into its own only after the pathogenetic mechanisms of tumourigenesis have been laid bare in all their intricacies. Even before any such fundamental understanding is achieved, the chromosomal abnormalities may serve as disease markers. When these are statistically compared with other parameters, the associations that emerge may help improve diagnostic and prognostic precision. This development has already taken place in haematological cytogenetics, and solid tumour cytogenetics is now quickly heading in the same direction.

REFERENCES

Åkerman M, Alvegård T, Eliasson J et al 1988 A case of Ewing's sarcoma diagnosed by fine needle aspiration. Light microscopy, electron microscopy and chromosomal analysis. Acta Orthopaedica Scandinavica 59: 589–592

Aledo R, Dutrillaux B, Lombard M et al 1989 Cytogenetic study on eleven cutaneous neoplasms and two pre-tumoral lesions from xeroderma pigmentosum patients. International Journal of Cancer 44: 79–83

Atkin N B, Baker M C, Fox M F 1990 Chromosome changes in 43 carcinomas of the cervix uteri. Cancer Genetics and Cytogenetics 44: 229–241

Bello M J, Rey J A 1990 Chromosome aberrations in metastatic ovarian cancer: relationship with abnormalities in primary tumors. International Journal of Cancer 45: 50–54

Benedict W F, Banerjee A, Mark C et al 1983 Nonrandom chromosomal changes in untreated retinoblastomas. Cancer Genetics and Cytogenetics 10: 311–333

Berenson J R, Yang J, Mickel R A 1989 Frequent amplification of the bcl-1 locus in head and neck squamous cell carcinomas. Oncogene 4: 1111–1116

Biegel J A, Rorke L B, Packer R J et al 1989a Isochromosome 17q in primitive neuroectodermal tumors of the central nervous system. Genes, Chromosomes & Cancer 1: 139–147

Biegel J A, Womer R B, Emanuel B S 1989b Complex karyotypes in a series of pediatric osteosarcomas. Cancer Genetics and Cytogenetics 38: 89–100

Bigner S H, Mark J, Bullard D E et al 1986 Chromosomal evolution in malignant human gliomas starts with specific and usually numerical deviations. Cancer Genetics and Cytogenetics 22: 121–135

Bigner S H, Mark J, Burger P C et al 1988 Specific chromosomal abnormalities in malignant human gliomas. Cancer Research 88: 405–411

Bigner S H, Mark J, Bigner D D 1990 Cytogenetics of human brain tumors. Cancer Genetics and Cytogenetics 47: 141–154

Birrer M J, Minna J D 1989 Genetic changes in the pathogenesis of lung cancer. Annual Review of Medicine 40: 305–317

Bondeson L, Bengtsson A, Bondeson A-G et al 1989 Chromosome studies in thyroid neoplasia. Cancer 64: 680–685

Bosl G J, Dmitrovsky E, Reuter V E et al 1989 Isochromosome of chromosome 12: clinical useful marker for male germ cell tumors. Journal of the National Cancer Institute 81: 1874–1878

Boveri T 1914 Zur Frage der Entstehung maligner Tumoren. Gustav Fischer, Jena

Brodeur G M, Fong C 1989 Molecular biology and genetics of human neuroblastoma. Cancer Genetics and Cytogenetics 41: 153–174

Brothman A R, Peehl D M, Patel A M et al 1990 Frequency and pattern of karyotypic abnormalities in human prostate cancer. Cancer Research 50: 3795–3803

Bullerdiek J, Bartnitzke S, Weinberg M et al 1987 Rearrangements of chromosome region 12q13-q15 in pleomorphic adenomas of the human salivary gland (PSA). Cytogenetics and Cell Genetics 45: 187–190

Bullerdiek J, Chilla R, Haubrich J et al 1988 A causal relationship between chromosomal rearrangements and the genesis of salivary gland pleomorphic adenomas. Archives of Otorhinolaryngology 245: 244–249

Campbell L, Brown J, Garson O M et al 1989 Cytogenetic abnormalities in lung cancer. In: Hansen H H (ed) Basic and clinical concepts of lung cancer. Kluwer Academic Publishers, Boston, pp 123–136

Castedo S M M J, de Jong B, Oosterhuis J W et al 1989a Chromosomal changes in human primary testicular nonseminomatous germ cell tumors. Cancer Research 49: 5696–5701

Castedo S M M J, de Jong B, Oosterhuis J W et al 1989b Cytogenetic analysis of ten human seminomas. Cancer Research 49: 439–443

Christiansen H, Lampert F 1988 Tumour karyotype discriminates between good and bad
prognostic outcome in neuroblastoma. British Journal of Cancer 57: 121–126
Couturier J, Vielh P, Salmon R J et al 1988 Chromosome imbalance in endometrial
adenocarcinoma. Cancer Genetics and Cytogenetics 33: 67–76
Dal Cin P, Boghosian L, Sandberg A A 1988a Cytogenetic findings in leiomyosarcoma of the
small bowel. Cancer Genetics and Cytogenetics 30: 285–288
Dal Cin P, Li F P, Prout Jr G R et al 1988b Involvement of chromosomes 3 and 5 in renal cell
carcinoma. Cancer Genetics and Cytogenetics 35: 41–46
de Jong B, Oosterhuis J W, Castedo S M M J et al 1990 Pathogenesis of adult testicular germ
cell tumors. A cytogenetic model. Cancer Genetics and Cytogenetics 48: 143–167
Delozier-Blanchet C D, Walt H, Engel E et al 1987 Cytogenetic studies of human testicular
germ cell tumours. International Journal of Andrology 10: 69–77
Douglass E C, Wilimas J A, Green A A et al 1985 Abnormalities of chromosomes 1 and 11 in
Wilms' tumor. Cancer Genetics and Cytogenetics 14: 331–338
Douglass E C, Valentine M, Etcubanas E et al 1987 A specific chromosomal abnormality in
rhabdomyosarcoma. Cytogenetics and Cell Genetics 45: 148–155
Douglass E C, Rowe S T, Valentine M et al 1990 A second nonrandom translocation,
der(16)t(1;16)(q21;q13), in Ewing sarcoma and peripheral neuroectodermal tumor.
Cytogenetics and Cell Genetics 53: 87–90
Dumanski J P, Rouleau G A, Nordenskjöld M et al 1990 Molecular genetic analysis of
chromosome 22 in 81 cases of meningioma. Cancer Research 50: 5863–5867
Dutrillaux B, Gerbault-Seureau M, Zafrani B 1990 Characterization of chromosomal
anomalies in human breast cancer. A comparison of 30 paradiploid cases with few
chromosome changes. Cancer Genetics and Cytogenetics 49: 203–217
Elfving P, Cigudosa J C, Lundgren R et al 1990 Trisomy 7, trisomy 10, and loss of the Y
chromosome in short-term cultures of normal kidney tissue. Cytogenetics and Cell
Genetics 53: 123–125
Eneroth M, Mandahl N, Heim S et al 1990 Localization of the chromosomal breakpoints of
the t(12;16) in liposarcoma to subbands 12q13.3 and 16p11.2. Cancer Genetics and
Cytogenetics 48: 101–107
Fearon E R, Vogelstein B 1990 A genetic model for colorectal tumorigenesis. Cell 61:
759–767
Ferti A D, Panani A D, Raptis S 1988 Cytogenetic study of rectosigmoidal adenocarcinomas.
Cancer Genetics and Cytogenetics 34: 101–109
Ferti-Passantonopoulou A D, Panani A D, Vlachos J D et al 1987 Common cytogenetic
findings in gastric cancer. Cancer Genetics and Cytogenetics 24: 63–73
Flejter W L, Li F P, Antman K H et al 1989 Recurring loss involving chromosomes 1, 3, and
22 in malignant mesothelioma: possible sites of tumor suppressor genes. Genes,
Chromosomes & Cancer 1: 148–154
Fletcher J A, Kozakewich H P, Pavelka K et al 1991 Consistent cytogenetic aberrations in
hepatoblastoma: a common pathway of genetic alterations in embryonal liver and skeletal
muscle malignancies? Genes, Chromosomes & Cancer 3: 37–43
Francke U 1990 A gene for Wilms tumour? Nature 343: 692–694
Garewal H S, Sampliner R, Liu Y et al 1989 Chromosomal rearrangements in Barrett's
esophagus. A premalignant lesion of esophageal adenocarcinoma. Cancer Genetics and
Cytogenetics 42: 281–286
Gebhart E, Brüderlein S, Augustus M et al 1986 Cytogenetic studies on human breast
carcinomas. Breast Cancer Research and Treatment 8: 125–138
Geleick D, Müller H, Matter A et al 1990 Cytogenetics of breast cancer. Cancer Genetics and
Cytogenetics 46: 217–229
Hagemeijer A, Versnel M A, Van Drunen E et al 1990 Cytogenetic analysis of malignant
mesothelioma. Cancer Genetics and Cytogenetics 47: 1–28
Hainsworth P J, Garson O M 1990 Breast cancer cytogenetics and beyond. Australian and
New Zealand Journal of Surgery 60: 327–336
Hayashi Y, Kanda N, Inaba T et al 1989 Cytogenetic findings and prognosis in
neuroblastoma with emphasis on marker chromosome 1. Cancer 63: 126–132
Heim S 1990 Cytogenetics in the investigation of haematological disorders. In: Cavill I (ed)
Baillière's Clinical Haematology vol 3, number 4. Baillière Tindall, London, pp 921–948
Heim S, Mitelman F 1987 Cancer cytogenetics. Alan R Liss, New York

Heim S, Mitelman F 1989 Primary chromosome abnormalities in human neoplasia. Advances in Cancer Research 52: 1–43

Heim S, Mandahl N, Mitelman F 1988a Genetic convergence and divergence in tumor progression. Cancer Research 48: 5911–5916

Heim S, Mandahl N, Rydholm A et al 1988b Different karyotypic features characterize different clinico-pathologic subgroups of benign lipogenic tumors. International Journal of Cancer 42: 863–867

Heim S, Mertens F, Jin Y et al 1989 Diverse chromosome abnormalities in squamous cell carcinomas of the skin. Cancer Genetics and Cytogenetics 39: 69–76

Higashi K, Jin Y, Johansson M et al 1991 Rearrangement of 9p13 as the primary chromosomal aberration in adenoid cystic carcinoma of the respiratory tract. Genes, Chromosomes & Cancer 3: 21–23

Hill S M, Rodgers C S, Hultén M A 1987 Cytogenetic analysis in human breast carcinoma. II. Seven cases in the triploid/tetraploid range investigated using direct preparations. Cancer Genetics and Cytogenetics 24: 45–62

Hohenfellner K, Holl M, Gutjahr P et al 1989 Cytogenetische befunde bei Wilmstumor. Klinische Pädiatrie 201: 293–298

Horsman D E, Sroka H, Rootman J et al 1990 Monosomy 3 and isochromosome 8q in a uveal melanoma. Cancer Genetics and Cytogenetics 45: 249–253

Huang H-J S, Yee J-K, Shew J-Y et al 1988 Suppression of the neoplastic phenotype of the RB gene in human cancer cells. Science 242: 1563–1566

ISCN 1985 An international system for human cytogenetic nomenclature. Birth Defects: Original Article Series, Vol. 21, No. 1, National Foundation—March of Dimes, New York

Jenkins R B, Kimmel D W, Moertel C A et al 1989 A cytogenetic study of 53 human gliomas. Cancer Genetics and Cytogenetics 39: 253–279

Jenkins R B, Hay I D, Herath J F et al 1990 Frequent occurrence of cytogenetic abnormalities in sporadic nonmedullary thyroid carcinoma. Cancer 66: 1213–1220

Jin Y, Mandahl N, Heim S et al 1988 Isochromosomes i(8q) or i(9q) in three adenocarcinomas of the lung. Cancer Genetics and Cytogenetics 33: 11–17

Jin Y, Heim S, Mandahl N et al 1990a Multiple clonal chromosome aberrations in squamous cell carcinomas of the larynx. Cancer Genetics and Cytogenetics 44: 209–216

Jin Y, Heim S, Mandahl N et al 1990b Unrelated clonal chromosomal aberrations in carcinomas of the oral cavity. Genes, Chromosomes & Cancer 1: 209–215

Jin Y, Higashi K, Mandahl N et al 1990c Frequent rearrangement of chromosomal bands 1p22 and 11q13 in squamous cell carcinomas of the head and neck. Genes, Chromosomes & Cancer 2: 198–204

Johansson B, Bardi G, Heim S et al 1991 Nonrandom chromosomal rearrangements in pancreatic carcinomas. Cancer (in press)

Kaneko Y, Kanda N, Maseki N et al 1987 Different karyotypic patterns in early and advanced stage neuroblastomas. Cancer Research 47: 311–318

Klein G 1988 Oncogenes and tumor suppressor genes. Acta Oncologica 27: 427–437

Knudson A G 1989 Hereditary cancers disclose a class of cancer genes. Cancer 63: 1888–1891

Koduru P R, Dicostanzo D P, Jhanwar S C 1989 Non random cytogenetic changes characterize Merkel cell carcinoma. Disease Markers 7: 153–161

Kovacs G, Frisch S 1989 Clonal chromosome abnormalities in tumor cells from patients with sporadic renal cell carcinomas. Cancer Research 49: 651–659

Kovacs G, Szücs S, De Riese W et al 1987 Specific chromosome aberrations in human renal cell carcinoma. International Journal of Cancer 40: 171–178

Kovacs G, Wilkens L, Tapp T et al 1989 Differentiation between papillary and nonpapillary renal cell carcinomas by DNA analysis. Journal of the National Cancer Institute 81: 527–530

Kusnetsova L E, Prigogina E L, Pogosianz H E et al 1982 Similar chromosomal abnormalities in several retinoblastomas. Human Genetics 61: 201–204

Lemieux N, Milot J, Barsoum-Homsy M et al 1989 First cytogenetic evidence of homozygosity for the retinoblastoma deletion in chromosome 13. Cancer Genetics and Cytogenetics 43: 73–78

Leung W-Y, Schwartz P E, Ng H-T et al 1990 Trisomy 12 in benign fibroma and granulosa cell tumor of the ovary. Gynecologic Oncology 38: 28–31

Limon J, Dal Cin P, Sandberg A A 1986 Application of long-term collagenase disaggregation for the cytogenetic analysis of human solid tumors. Cancer Genetics and Cytogenetics 23: 305–313

Limon J, Mrozek K, Heim S et al 1990 On the significance of trisomy 7 and sex chromosome loss in renal cell carcinoma. Cancer Genetics and Cytogenetics 49: 259–263

Limon J, Mrozek K, Mandahl N et al 1991 Cytogenetics of synovial sarcoma: presentation of ten new cases and review of the literature. Genes, Chromosomes & Cancer (in press)

Lindström E, Salford L G, Heim S et al 1991 Trisomy 7 and sex chromosome loss are not representative of tumor parenchyma cells in malignant glioma. Genes, Chromosomes & Cancer (in press)

Lukeis R, Irving L, Garson M et al 1990 Cytogenetics of non-small cell lung cancer: analysis of consistent non-random abnormalities. Genes, Chromosomes & Cancer 2: 116–124

Lundgren R, Mandahl N, Heim S et al 1991 Cytogenetic analysis of 57 primary prostatic adenocarcinomas. Genes, Chromosomes & Cancer (in press)

Mandahl N 1991 Methods in solid tumor cytogenetics. In: Rooney D E, Czepulkowski B H (eds) Human cytogenetics: a practical approach, Vol 2: Malignancy and acquired chromosome abnormalities. IRL Press (in press)

Mandahl N, Heim S, Arheden K et al 1988 Three major cytogenetic subgroups can be identified among chromosomally abnormal solitary lipomas. Human Genetics 79: 203–208

Mandahl N, Heim S, Rydholm A et al 1989a Nonrandom numerical chromosome aberrations (+8, +11, +17, +20) in infantile fibrosarcoma. Cancer Genetics and Cytogenetics 40: 137–139

Mandahl N, Heim S, Willén H et al 1989b Characteristic karyotype anomalies identify subtypes of malignant fibrous histiocytoma. Genes, Chromosomes & Cancer 1: 9–14

Mandahl N, Heim S, Willén H et al 1989c Supernumerary ring chromosome as the sole cytogenetic abnormality in a dermatofibrosarcoma protuberans. Cancer Genetics and Cytogenetics 49: 273–275

Mandahl N, Heim S, Arheden K et al 1990 Chromosomal rearrangements in chondromatous tumors. Cancer 65: 242–248

Mark J 1976 G-band analyses of a human intestinal leiomyosarcoma. Acta Pathologica Microbiologica Scandinavica Section A 84: 538–540

Mark J 1977 Chromosomal abnormalities and their specificity in human neoplasms: an assessment of recent observations by banding techniques. Advances in Cancer Research 24: 165–222

Mark J, Sandros J, Wedell B et al 1988 Significance of the choice of tissue culture technique on the chromosomal patterns in human mixed salivary gland tumors. Cancer Genetics and Cytogenetics 33: 229–244

Mark J, Havel G, Grepp C et al 1990 Chromosomal patterns in human benign uterine leiomyomas. Cancer Genetics and Cytogenetics 44: 1–13

Mascarello J T, Jones M C, Kadota R P et al 1990 Hepatoblastoma characterized by trisomy 20 and double minutes. Cancer Genetics and Cytogenetics 47: 243–247

Mertens F, Heim S, Mandahl N et al 1991 Cytogenetic analysis of 33 basal cell carcinomas. Cancer Research 51: 954–957

Milatovich A, Heerema N A, Palmer C G 1990 Cytogenetic studies of endometrial malignancies. Cancer Genetics and Cytogenetics 46: 41–54

Misawa S, Horiike S, Taniwaki M et al 1990 Chromosome abnormalities of gastric cancer detected in cancerous effusions. Japanese Journal of Cancer Research 81: 148–152

Mitchell E L D, Santibanez-Koref M F 1990 1p13 is the most frequently involved band in structural chromosomal rearrangements in human breast cancer. Genes, Chromosomes & Cancer 2: 279–289

Mitelman F 1991 Catalog of chromosome aberrations in cancer. 4th edn Wiley-Liss, New York

Mitelman F, Mark J, Nilsson P G et al 1974 Chromosome banding pattern in human colonic polyps. Hereditas 78: 63–68

Mitelman F, Heim S, Mandahl N 1989 Chromosome abnormalities in solid tumors. In: Ting S W, Chen J S, Schwartz M K (eds) Human tumor markers. Elsevier, Amsterdam, pp 75–88

Mitelman F, Kaneko Y, Trent J M 1990 Report of the committee on chromosome changes in neoplasia. Cytogenetics and Cell Genetics 55: 358–386

Miura I, Resau J, Tomiyasu T et al 1990a Isochromosome (8q) in four patients with
  adenocarcinoma of the lung. Cancer Genetics and Cytogenetics 48: 203–207
Miura I, Siegfried J M, Resau J et al 1990b Chromosome alterations in 21 non-small cell lung
  carcinomas. Genes, Chromosomes & Cancer 2: 328–338
Molenaar W M, DeJong B, Buist J et al 1989 Chromosomal analysis and the classification of
  soft tissue sarcomas. Laboratory Investigation 60: 266–274
Mrozek K, Nedoszytko B, Babinska M et al 1990 Trisomy of chromosome 12 in a case of
  thecoma of the ovary. Gynecologic Oncology 36: 413–416
Mugneret F, Lizard S, Aurias A et al 1988 Chromosomes in Ewing's sarcoma. II.
  Nonrandom additional changes, trisomy 8 and der(16)t(1;16). Cancer Genetics and
  Cytogenetics 32: 239–245
Muleris M, Salmon R-J, Dutrillaux A-M et al 1987a Characteristic chromosomal imbalances
  in 18 near-diploid colorectal tumors. Cancer Genetics and Cytogenetics 29: 289–301
Muleris M, Salmon R-J, Girodet J et al 1987b Recurrent deletions of chromosomes 11q and
  3p in anal canal carcinoma. International Journal of Cancer 39: 595–598
Muleris M, Salmon R-J, Dutrillaux B 1990 Cytogenetics of colorectal adenocarcinomas.
  Cancer Genetics and Cytogenetics 46: 143–156
Nilbert M, Heim S 1990 Uterine leiomyoma cytogenetics. Genes, Chromosomes & Cancer 2:
  3–13
Nilbert M, Mandahl N, Heim S et al 1990 Complex karyotypic changes, including
  rearrangements of 12q13 and 14q24, in two leiomyosarcomas. Cancer Genetics and
  Cytogenetics 48: 217–223
Nowell P C 1976 The clonal evolution of tumor cell populations. Acquired genetic lability
  permits stepwise selection of variant sublines and underlies tumor progression. Science
  194: 23–28
Nowell P C, Hungerford D A 1960 A minute chromosome in human granulocytic leukemia.
  Science 132: 1497
Örndal C, Mandahl N, Rydholm A et al 1991a Chromosomal abnormality t(9;22) (q22;q12)
  in an extraskeletal myxoid chondrosarcoma characterized by fine needle aspiration
  cytology, electron microscopy, immunohistochemistry and DNA flow cytometry.
  Cytopathology (in press)
Örndal C, Mandahl N, Rydholm A et al 1991b Supernumerary ring chromosomes in five
  bone and soft tissue tumors of low or borderline grade malignancy. Genes, Chromosomes
  & Cancer (Submitted)
Pandis N, Heim S, Bardi G et al 1990a High resolution mapping of consistent leiomyoma
  breakpoints in chromosomes 12 and 14 to 12q15 and 14q24.1. Genes, Chromosomes &
  Cancer 2: 227–230
Pandis N, Heim S, Bardi G et al 1990b Parallel karyotypic evolution and tumor progression
  in uterine leiomyoma. Genes, Chromosomes & Cancer 2: 310–317
Pandis N, Heim S, Bardi G et al 1991a Chromosome analysis of 96 uterine leiomyomas.
  Cancer Genetics and Cytogenetics (in press)
Pandis N, Heim S, Willén H et al 1991b Histologic-cytogenetic correlations in uterine
  leiomyoma. International Journal of Gynecologic Cancer (in press)
Parmiter A H, Nowell P C 1988 The cytogenetics of human malignant melanoma and
  premalignant lesions. In: Nathanson L (ed) Malignant melanoma: biology, diagnosis, and
  therapy. Kluwer Academic Publishers, Boston, pp 47–61
Pejovic T, Heim S, Mandahl N et al 1989 Consistent occurrence of a 19p + marker
  chromosome and loss of 11p material in ovarian seropapillary cystadenocarcinomas. Genes,
  Chromosomes & Cancer 1: 167–171
Pejovic T, Heim S, Mandahl N et al 1990a Trisomy 12 is a consistent chromosomal
  aberration in benign ovarian tumors. Genes, Chromosomes & Cancer 2: 48–52
Pejovic T, Heim S, Örndal C et al 1990b Simple numerical chromosome aberrations in well-
  differentiated malignant epithelial tumors. Cancer Genetics and Cytogenetics 49: 95–101
Perucca D, Szepetowski P, Simon M-P et al 1990 Molecular genetics of human bladder
  carcinomas. Cancer Genetics and Cytogenetics 49: 143–156
Prescher G, Bornfeld N, Becher R 1990 Nonrandom chromosomal abnormalities in primary
  uveal melanoma. Journal of the National Cancer Institute 82: 1765–1769
Reichmann A, Martin P, Levin B 1985 Chromosomal banding patterns in human large bowel
  adenomas. Human Genetics 70: 28–31

Rey J A, Bello M J, de Campos J M et al 1988 Chromosomal involvement secondary to −22 in human meningiomas. Cancer Genetics and Cytogenetics 33: 275–290

Rodgers C S, Hill S M, Hultén M A 1984 Cytogenetic analysis in human breast carcinoma. I. Nine cases in the diploid range investigated using direct preparations. Cancer Genetics and Cytogenetics 13: 95–119

Rodriguez E, Rao P H, Ladanyi M et al 1990 11p13-15 is a specific region of chromosomal rearrangement in gastric and esophageal adenocarcinomas. Cancer Research 50: 6410–6416

Rydholm A, Mandahl N, Heim S et al 1990 Malignant fibrous histiocytomas with a 19p+ marker chromosome have increased relapse rate. Genes, Chromosomes & Cancer 2: 296–299

Sandberg A A 1986 Chromosome changes in bladder cancer: Clinical and other correlations. Cancer Genetics and Cytogenetics 19: 163–175

Sandberg A A 1990 Chromosomes in human cancer and leukemia. Elsevier, New York

Sandberg A A, Turc-Carel C, Gemmill R M 1988 Chromosomes in solid tumors and beyond. Cancer Research 48: 1049–1059

Sandros J, Mark J, Happonen R-P et al 1988 Specificity of 6q− markers and other recurrent deviations in human malignant salivary gland tumors. Anticancer Research 8: 637–644

Sandros J, Stenman G, Mark J 1990 Cytogenetic and molecular observations in human and experimental salivary gland tumors. Cancer Genetics and Cytogenetics 44: 153–167

Scrable H J, Sapienza C, Cavenee W K 1990 Genetic and epigenetic losses of heterozygosity in cancer predisposition and progression. Advances in Cancer Research 54: 25–62

Simon D, Munoz S J, Maddrey W C et al 1990 Chromosomal rearrangements in a primary hepatocellular carcinoma. Cancer Genetics and Cytogenetics 45: 255–260

Sisley K, Rennie I G, Cottam D W et al 1990 Cytogenetic findings in six posterior uveal melanomas: involvement of chromosomes 3, 6, and 8. Genes, Chromosomes & Cancer 2: 205–209

Slater R M, de Kraker J, Voûte P A et al 1985 A cytogenetic study of Wilms' tumor. Cancer Genetics and Cytogenetics 14: 95–109

Slaughter P D, Southwick H W, Smejkal W 1953 "Field cancerization" in oral stratified squamous epithelium. Clinical implications of multicentric origin. Cancer 6: 963–968

Solis V, Pritchard J, Cowell J K 1988 Cytogenetic changes in Wilms' tumor. Cancer Genetics and Cytogenetics 34: 223–234

Sozzi G, Bertoglio M G, Pilotti S et al 1988 Cytogenetic studies in primary and metastatic neuroendocrine Merkel cell carcinoma. Cancer Genetics and Cytogenetics 30: 151–158

Speleman F, Dal Cin P, De Potter C et al 1989 Cytogenetic investigation on a case of congenital fibrosarcoma. Cancer Genetics and Cytogenetics 39: 21–24

Squire J, Gallie B L, Phillips R A 1985 A detailed analysis of chromosomal changes in heritable and non-heritable retinoblastoma. Human Genetics 70: 291–301

Sreekantaiah C, Leong S P L, Karakousis C et al 1991 Cytogenetic profile of 109 lipomas. Cancer Research 51: 422–433

Teyssier J R, Ferre D 1989 Frequent clonal chromosomal changes in human non-malignant tumors. International Journal of Cancer 44: 828–832

Tiainen M, Tammilehto L, Rautonen J et al 1989 Chromosomal abnormalities and their correlations with asbestos exposure and survival in patients with mesothelioma. British Journal of Cancer 60: 618–626

Trent J M, Thompson F H, Meyskens Jr F L 1989 Identification of a recurring site involving chromosome 6 in human malignant melanoma. Cancer Research 49: 420–423

Trent J M, Meyskens F L, Salmon S E et al 1990a Relation of cytogenetic abnormalities and clinical outcome in metastatic melanoma. New England Journal of Medicine 322: 1508–1511

Trent J M, Stanbridge E J, McBride H L et al 1990b Tumorigenicity in human melanoma cell lines controlled by introduction of human chromosome 6. Science 247: 568–571

Tsuda T, Tahara E, Kajiyama G et al 1989 High incidence of coamplification of hst-1 and int-2 genes in human esophageal carcinomas. Cancer Research 49: 5505–5508

Turc-Carel C, Limon J, Dal Cin P et al 1986 Cytogenetic studies of adipose tissue tumors. II. Recurrent translocation t(12;16) (q13;p11) in myxoid liposarcomas. Cancer Genetics and Cytogenetics 23: 291–299

Turc-Carel C, Dal Cin P, Limon J et al 1987a Involvement of chromosome X in primary cytogenetic change in human neoplasia: nonrandom translocation in synovial sarcoma. Proceedings of the National Academy of Science USA 84: 1981–1985

Turc-Carel C, Dal Cin P, Limon J et al 1987b Cytogenetic and molecular genetic studies of adipose tissue tumors. Cancer Genetics and Cytogenetics 28: 33

Turc-Carel C, Aurias A, Mugneret F et al 1988 Chromosomes in Ewing's sarcoma. I. An evaluation of 85 cases and remarkable consistency of t(11;22) (q24;q12). Cancer Genetics and Cytogenetics 32: 229–238

van den Berg E, Oosterhuis J W, de Jong B et al 1990 Cytogenetics of thyroid follicular adenomas. Cancer Genetics and Cytogenetics 44: 217–222

Viegas-Péquignot E, Flüry-Hérard A, De Cremoux H et al 1990 Recurrent chromosome aberrations in human lung squamous cell carcinomas. Cancer Genetics and Cytogenetics 49: 37–49

von Hansemann D (1890) Über asymmetrische Zelltheilung in Epithelkrebsen und deren biologische Bedeutung. Virchow's Archiv für Pathologische Anatomie 119: 299–326

Walter T A, Berger C S, Sandberg A A 1989 The cytogenetics of renal tumors. Where do we stand, where do we go? Cancer Genetics and Cytogenetics 43: 15–34

Wang-Wuu S, Soukup S, Ballard E et al 1988 Chromosomal analysis of sixteen human rhabdomyosarcomas. Cancer Research 48: 983–987

Weinberg R A 1989 Oncogenes, antioncogenes, and the molecular basis of multistep carcinogenesis. Cancer Research 49: 3713–3721

Weissman B E, Saxon P J, Pasquale S R et al 1987 Introduction of a normal human chromosome 11 into a Wilms' tumor cell line controls its tumorigenic expression. Science 236: 175–180

Weith A, Martinsson T, Cziepluch C et al 1989 Neuroblastoma consensus deletion maps to 1p36.1–2. Genes, Chromosomes & Cancer 1: 159–166

Welter C, Kovacs G, Seitz G et al 1989 Alteration of mitochondrial DNA in human oncocytomas. Genes, Chromosomes & Cancer 1: 79–82

Whang-Peng J, Lee E C 1985 Cytogenetics of human small cell lung cancer. Recent Results in Cancer Research 97: 37–46

Whang-Peng J, Knutsen T 1989 Cytogenetic studies in neoplasia (human and animal): implications, prognosis, and treatment. In: Liotta L A (ed) Influence of tumor development on the host. Kluwer Academic Publishers, Dordrecht, pp 133–175

Whang-Peng J, Bunn Jr P A, Kao-Shan C S et al 1982 A nonrandom chromosomal abnormality, del3p(14–23), in human small cell cancer (SCLC). Cancer Genetics and Cytogenetics 6: 119–134

Yaseen N Y, Watmore A E, Potter A M et al 1990 Chromosome studies in eleven colorectal tumors. Cancer Genetics and Cytogenetics 44: 83–97

Zang K 1982 Cytological and cytogenetical studies on human meningioma. Cancer Genetics and Cytogenetics 6: 249–274

Zech L, Bergh J, Nilsson K 1985 Karyotypic characterization of established cell lines and short-term cultures of human lung cancers. Cancer Genetics and Cytogenetics 15: 335–347

Zhou D J, Casey G, Cline M 1988 Amplification of human int-2 in breast cancers and squamous carcinomas. Oncogene 2: 279–282

4

The pathology of AIDS: an update

P. R. Millard   M. M. Esiri

The relentless increase in HIV infection and its inevitable progression to AIDS (Chin 1990) have stimulated worldwide interest and led to substantial advances in knowledge. International surveillance is maintained by the Global Programme on AIDS of the World Health Organization. The modes of transmitting the infection are universally the same, namely through sexual intercourse or via blood and blood products, yet distinct patterns of disease have emerged (Mann & Chin 1988). Pattern I is predominant in Western countries where homosexual and bisexual men are principally affected, along with drug addicts and haemophiliacs; heterosexual transmission, however, is increasing slowly. Pattern II is found in sub-Saharan Africa and the Caribbean: here, heterosexual and perinatal transmission are the major problems. The disease is beginning to take hold in Pattern III areas, e.g. North Africa, the Middle East and Asia, mainly through contact with infected individuals from Pattern I and II countries. In Bangkok, for example, an explosive epidemic is taking place amongst prostitutes and drug addicts. Further differences exist in the manifestations of the disease, i.e. infectious complications and tumours. In Uganda, for example, the predominant manifestation of AIDS is weight loss, hence the term 'slim disease' (Goodgame 1990). This review highlights some recent advances in our knowledge of AIDS as seen in European patients. Histopathologists continue to make important contributions not only in diagnosis but also in charting the course of the disorder and in monitoring the spectrum of changes it produces.

CENTRAL NERVOUS SYSTEM (CNS) PATHOLOGY OF HIV

Much uncertainty still surrounds the pathogenesis of HIV-inflicted damage to the CNS (Price et al 1988, Wigdahl & Kunsch 1989). Damage may occur in the form of an encephalopathy or a myelopathy or both. A practical point is that neither of these conditions can be excluded without careful microscopic examination of the relevant regions at risk. These are, chiefly, the deep white matter and the cortex of the frontal and temporal lobes of the brain for the encephalopathy, and the upper part of the spinal cord for the myelopathy (de la Monte et al 1987).

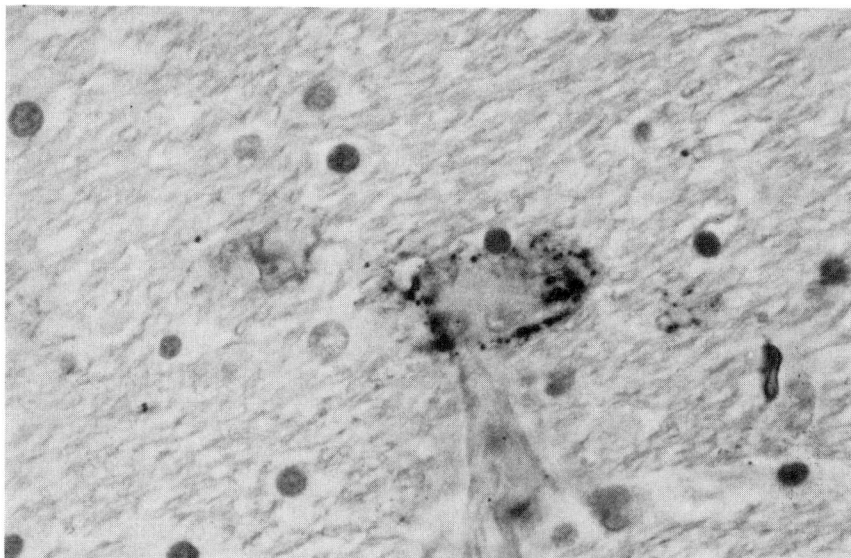

Fig. 4.1 Multinucleated giant cell in cerebral white matter from a patient with HIV encephalopathy. The section has been exposed to monoclonal antibody to p24 protein of HIV. Reaction product is seen around the margins of the multinucleated cell. (Courtesy of Dr C. C. Morris.) × 480.

HIV encephalopathy

HIV encephalopathy occurs in 20 to 30% of those with AIDS and has been firmly linked to the presence of HIV in macrophages, microglia and macrophage-derived multinucleated giant cells in the brain (Fig. 4.1). It remains unknown how this infection leads to the predominantly white matter damage (Fig. 4.2) which amounts to destruction in the most severely affected patients. Neuroglial cell infection can be produced in vitro, but it is difficult to demonstrate in vivo, and claims to have done so are not universally accepted. Infection of glial cell lines in vitro results in only a low level of infection and shows unusual features. Thus, infection is not blocked by monoclonal antibodies to the HIV-1 binding region of CD4, nor by a soluble form of CD4 receptor (Clapham et al 1989). Infection of astrocytes could not be demonstrated in primary human brain cultures in which infection of microglial cells was readily established (Watkins et al 1990). This makes the relevance of tumour cell line studies to the in vivo situation doubtful.

Most investigators consider that damage to myelin occurs through release of toxic products of the infected macrophage-derived cells. Such products might be encoded by host cell or virus genes. For example, proteases liberated by activated macrophages are known to denature myelin basic protein (Cammer et al 1978), and tumour necrosis factor can cause

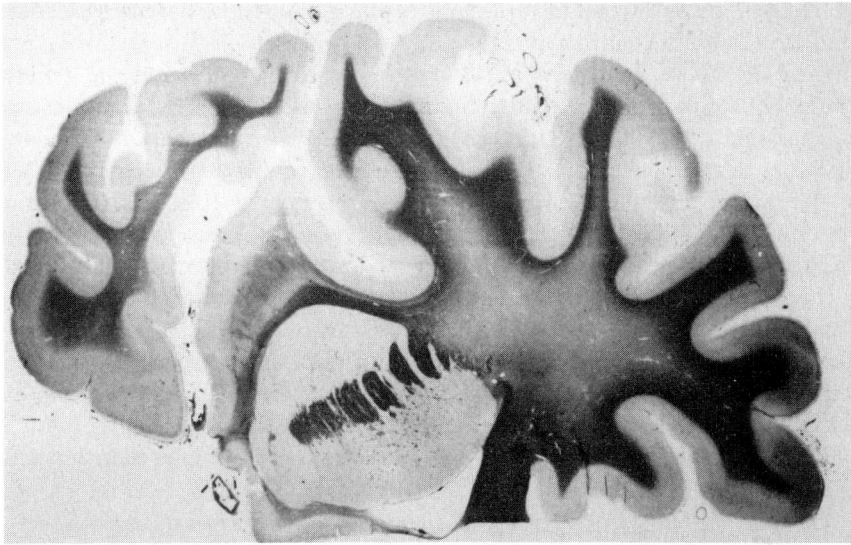

Fig. 4.2   Myelin-stained cerebral hemisphere section from a patient with HIV encephalopathy. Diffuse pallor of myelin staining is present in the frontal lobe. (Reproduced by permission from *Greenfields Neuropathology* Edward Arnold, London.)

oligodendrocyte death in vitro (Robbins et al 1987). Viral products might also have a detrimental effect on neuronal metabolism. The viral envelope glycoprotein gp 120 shows homologies with neuroleukin, a neurotrophic factor and lymphokine, and with the neuropeptide VIP (Gurney et al 1986, Brenneman et al 1988). Thus, by competing with these normal CNS molecules for specific receptors, gp 120 could compromise normal neuronal maintenance and survival. It has been recognized for several years that cortical atrophy occurs in neurologically affected AIDS sufferers, and brain weights in such patients are lower than those with no HIV encephalopathy (Navia et al 1986). Although most neuropathological studies have failed to document cortical nerve cell loss in AIDS, some have demonstrated this both in adults (Navia et al 1986, Ketzler et al 1990) and in children (Sharer et al 1986, Giangaspero et al 1989) with AIDS encephalopathy. If nerve cell loss makes a significant contribution to the manifestations of AIDS encephalopathy, the likelihood of reversing these with anti-viral therapy must be slight since, although myelin damage may be partially reparable, nerve cells cannot be replaced. Some studies have suggested that neurological symptoms in AIDS patients can be reversed by anti-viral treatment (Yarchoan et al 1987, Portegies et al 1989), but in carefully controlled studies the improvement has been slight (Schmitt et al 1988).

It is a striking fact that, whereas in blood the principal host cell of HIV is the CD4+ lymphocyte, in the brain it is the macrophage. It seems reasonable to suppose that this shift in cell tropism may be reflected in altered genetic determinants of the virus in the CNS. The polymerase chain reaction (PCR) is an appropriate technique with which to search for such alterations but so far there are no clear indications that a specific genetic sequence controls neurovirulence of the virus. However, a molecular comparison of HIV DNA extracted from CNS tissue and from blood using PCR has demonstrated an unusually high level of unintegrated viral DNA in the brain (Pang et al 1990). The significance of this observation is uncertain, but high levels of unintegrated viral DNA in vitro are usually associated with super-infection or re-infection, and with a cytopathic effect.

Increasing experience of HIV+ children has shown that they can be divided neurologically into two groups: one in which there is progressive neurological deterioration and another with little or no progressive disease (Dickson et al 1989, Wiley et al 1990). Virus can generally only be demonstrated in the brain at autopsy in those with a progressive neurological course, although in almost all patients there is brain damage with gliosis.

HIV myelopathy

HIV myelopathy usually occurs in AIDS subjects who also have an encephalopathy. It is, however, distinct from and less common than encephalopathy. The pathology consists of vacuolation and loss of myelin in the white matter particularly of the lateral and posterior columns, which is maximal at the cervical or thoracic levels (Fig. 4.3). It mimics quite closely the pathology of subacute combined degeneration of the cord due to vitamin B_{12} or folate deficiency (Petito et al 1985). This has led to an interesting suggestion that HIV myelopathy may be due to alterations in methyl group metabolism. Preliminary measurements of cerebrospinal fluid levels of 5-methyltetra-hydro-folate, s-adenosyl methionine and neopterins in a small group of children with myelopathy due to congenital HIV infection support this suggestion (Surtees et al 1990). The abnormally high levels of neopterins found by these investigators could have been released from local, activated macrophages and could have inhibited folate metabolism and led to the myelin damage. If there is any truth in this hypothesis, treatment with methyl group donors such as betaine and methionine might be expected to alleviate or prevent symptoms of HIV myelopathy.

HIV myelopathy is widely considered as the spinal cord counterpart of HIV encephalopathy and therefore it might be expected to be closely correlated with local presence of the virus in the spinal cord. HIV has been isolated from the spinal cord of a patient with vacuolar myelopathy (Ho et al 1985) and two studies have shown HIV in multinucleated and mononucleated macrophages in the vicinity of the spinal cord lesions (Eilbott et al 1989, Maier et al 1989). However, in larger series with and without myelopathy (Grafe & Wiley 1989, Rosenblum et al 1989) there was no close association between myelopathy and the detection of HIV. These obser-

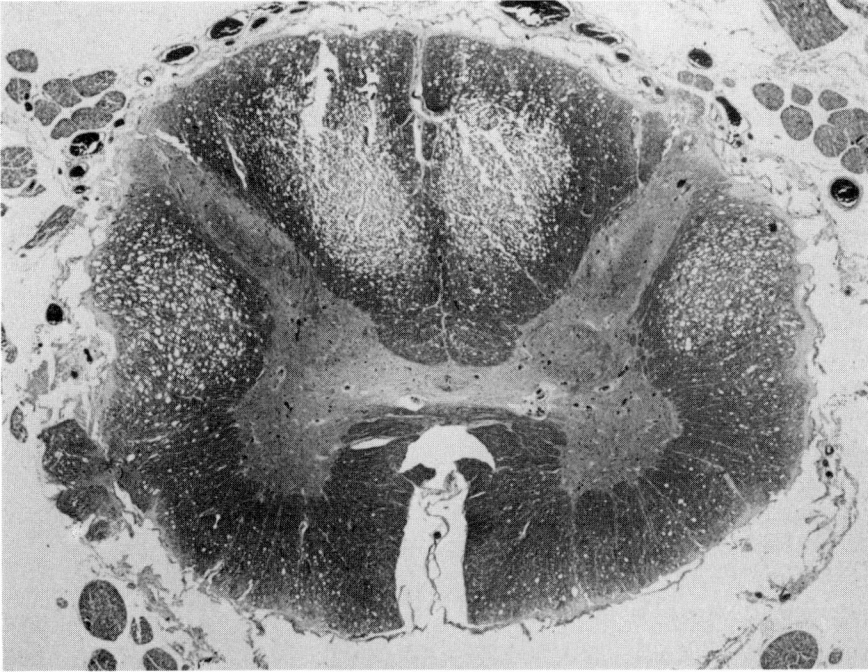

Fig. 4.3 Low power view of cervical spinal cord from a patient with HIV myelopathy. Note vacuolar change and myelin pallor in lateral and posterior columns. (Courtesy of Dr S. Levine, and Munksgaard, Copenhagen.)

vations lend further weight to the view that the myelopathy is only indirectly related to HIV infection.

Peripheral nerve pathology in HIV infection

Peripheral neuropathy is a common complication of HIV infection (Michaels et al 1988). The forms of clinical presentation and pathology are diverse and almost certainly the different types have different aetiologies. The autonomic as well as the somatic sensory and motor components of the peripheral nervous system may be involved (Griffin et al 1988). The three main types of somatic neuropathy are a painful sensory neuropathy with ganglionitis in patients with AIDS (Snider et al 1983), a mixed sensory and motor polyneuropathy or mononeuritis multiplex associated with an arteritis in pre-AIDS subjects (Lipkin et al 1985) and an acute demyelinating polyneuropathy associated with pleocytosis of the cerebrospinal fluid (Cornblath et al 1987), that is also seen before AIDS develops. Although HIV has been cultured from peripheral nerve and identified ultra-structurally in axons, it is only seldom detected in peripheral neuropathy. Cytomegalovirus has been more frequently linked to the development of this complication of HIV infection (Grafe & Wiley 1989). The demyelinating neuropathy, which is generally reversible and has been favourably influenced by plasmaphoresis, resembles the Guillain–Barré syndrome and is thought to have an autoimmune basis.

GASTROINTESTINAL TRACT AND WEIGHT LOSS

One of the most arresting features of many AIDS patients is a profound cachexia, that often exceeds that of most cancer patients. The weight loss, from analogy with prisoners of war (Nutritional Reviews 1990), is sufficient in some cases to cause death and is particularly common in Africa where AIDS is known as 'slim disease' (Serwadda et al 1985). Although infections and tumours outside the gastrointestinal tract and their treatment (Membreno et al 1987) could contribute to this, their role is not seen as substantial, and explanations centre upon the gastrointestinal tract itself (Kotler et al 1985, Smith et al 1988). Hepatic (Schaffner 1990) and pancreatic (Dowell et al 1990) disorders may adversely affect the gut but any part these have in weight loss is not considered significant.

Gastrointestinal tract

Between 50 and 90% of AIDS patients in the USA have gastrointestinal symptoms. The underlying disorders include infections, tumours and an HIV-related enteropathy, all of which may present as intractable diarrhoea (Santangelo & Krejs 1986, Smith et al 1988) and malabsorption (Kotler et al 1984, Modigliani et al 1985, Harriman et al 1989). Microorganisms have been identified from only about half of those with diarrhoea (Dryden & Shanson 1988). These include protozoa, bacteria, viruses and fungi and frequently more than one type of organism (Laughon et al 1988). The incidence of different organisms varies according to the thoroughness of the investigation and the types of samples examined. Cryptosporidiosis, for example, is best recognized from the oocyte stages in stool samples stained with a modified Ziehl–Neelsen method and is easily missed in tissue sections at light and electron microscopy because of its patchy distribution (Soave & Johnson 1988). *Mycobacterium avium intracellulare* is easily identified in Ziehl–Neelsen preparations of both stools and tissues (Damsker & Bottone 1985). Viruses may defeat routine laboratory methods and become apparent only with molecular biological techniques, blotting methods and polymerase chain reaction, which by their extreme sensitivity can result in false positive findings. The unexpected must be anticipated from any sample and the dilemma is often faced of deciding if the organism is the cause of symptoms and if so, whether it necessitates medical intervention. The range of organisms in the HIV + homosexual is similar to that in the HIV − homosexual (Baker & Peppercorn 1982, Laughon et al 1988) but venereal infection and organisms which are symptomless or produce self-limiting illnesses are less common in the former.

Histopathological features

Biopsy and autopsy reports of gastrointestinal tract changes related to AIDS provide conflicting observations. Minor degrees of inflammation can occur producing oesophagitis (Stamm & Grant 1988), gastritis (Lake-Bakaar et al 1988, Stamm & Grant 1988), jejunitis (Batman et al 1989), colitis (Rotterdam et al 1983, Jarry et al 1990) and proctitis (Bishop et al 1987) with and without microorganisms, and no unique response has been related to any one microorganism. A loss of T-helper and an inversion of the ratio of T-helper:T-suppressor cells are evident mirroring systemic changes in T-cells but they are sometimes more profound (Rodgers et al 1986, Bishop et al 1987, Jarry et al 1990). Intra-epithelial T8 lymphocytes are increased in number (Kotler et al 1986) and are activated (Weber & Dobbins 1986). Associated with these T lymphocyte changes is a depletion of NK cells, IgA plasma cells and macrophages (Kotler et al 1986). Morphometric studies show a mild partial villous atrophy and crypt hyperplasia with and without microorganisms (Kotler et al 1984, Batman et al 1989, Ullrich et al 1989). Careful examination has revealed apoptosis in the large and small bowel epithelium similar to that in graft versus host disease and viral infections (Kotler et al 1984, 1986, Batman et al 1989, Mathan et al 1990). Electron microscopy has shown evidence of autonomic nerve degeneration in the lamina propria (Griffin et al 1988).

Tumours are mainly represented by Kaposi's sarcoma and B-cell non-Hodgkin's lymphomas (Santangelo & Krejs 1986, Levine 1990). These occur in any part of the gastrointestinal tract and may be multifocal but they are rarely sufficiently diffuse to produce malabsorption and diarrhoea. Squamous cell carcinomas related to human papillomavirus (HPV) occur in the anogenital area.

Weight loss

The weight loss, in contrast to that seen in starvation, is due to loss of lean body mass rather than of fat (Kotler et al 1985, Nutritional Reviews 1990) and it is maximal during the last nine months of life (Nutritional Reviews 1990). Death has been related to malnutrition in a linear pattern (Kotler 1989). It may arise from difficulty in eating due to oral-oesophageal lesions (fungus, viral ulceration and tumour), physical blocking of the mucosal surfaces by microorganisms or tumour (Modigliani et al 1985), protozoa, and, theoretically, secretagons and bacterial overgrowth. Surprisingly, there is no evidence for the latter (Batman et al 1989) despite gastric secretory changes likely to enhance such overgrowth (Lake-Bakaar et al 1988). Immunodeficiency is a further putative factor since wasting due to protein and trace element deficiency occurs in some primary immuno-deficiency states. Together, these agencies may produce a chain of worsening anorexia and increasing hypermetabolism (Colman & Grossman 1987).

Low levels of secretory IgA may encourage protozoal and some bacterial infections (Kotler et al 1984) by permitting mucosal adherence, while the local cellular immune deficit may underlie other bacterial and viral infections (Kotler 1989). IgA loss also permits increased antigen absorption and thereby local T-cell activation which, with the increase in intra-epithelial lymphocytes and the uncontrolled action of T-suppressor cells, may produce isolated enterocyte destruction and villous atrophy (Kotler et al 1984, Weber & Dobbins 1986). Additional agencies include tumour necrosis factor and cytokines from macrophages and 'consumption' in tuberculous patients (Kotler 1989). Tumour necrosis factor experimentally impairs fat storage and increases hepatic synthesis of fatty acids and triglycerides which are raised in HIV + patients but any clinical relevance remains unclear (Nutritional Reviews 1990).

The HIV virus has been shown within lymphocytes and macrophages in the lamina propria (Harriman et al 1989, Jarry et al 1990) and in an increasing amount in the terminal stages of AIDS. Claims have also been made for its presence in colonic epithelium, notably the enterochromaffin cells (Nelson et al 1988). Support for these observations is the known anal and oral transmission of the virus; alternatively, gut infection may become established via recirculating infected mononuclear cells (Jarry et al 1990). However, more important than the local presence of HIV as a cause of gastrointestinal lesions may be the autonomic nerve degeneration attributed to HIV. This feature precedes the onset of AIDS, gastrointestinal infections and symptoms (Griffin et al 1988) and an early effect may be subclinical malabsorption, notably of B_{12} (Harriman et al 1989).

PNEUMOCYSTIS CARINII

This organism is the most important cause of morbidity amongst AIDS sufferers and certainly the main cause of death; almost 80% of patients experience one or more episodes of clinically significant infection (Masur et al 1989, Glatt & Chirgwin 1990). The source and life history of the organism and its mode of injury to the lung, however, remain unknown and debate persists over taxonomy. Efforts to prevent and treat infection have been only partially successful and they have produced new patterns of infection (Ravalli et al 1990).

Biology

Initial confusion with trypanosomes resulted in an early classification amongst the protozoa which was supported by failure to grow the organism on fungus culture media and, clinically, a partial response to antiprotozoal agents (Masur et al 1989, Glatt & Chirgwin 1990). Electron microscopic studies failed to distinguish between a fungus and a protozoon (Haque et al 1987, Yoshida 1989) and only since the introduction of molecular biological techniques has firm evidence emerged from rRNA sequences which established the organism as a fungus (Edman et al 1988, Masur et al 1989, Stringer et al 1989). Similar techniques have also revealed species differences and interspecies variations (Masur et al 1989). Demonstration of chitin in all forms of the organism provides additional evidence for inclusion with the fungi (Walker et al 1990).

The histopathologist recognizes the infection in smear or tissue preparations stained either by nonspecific methods, e.g. Grocott or Giemsa, or with specific antibodies (Linder et al 1987). Either approach identifies different forms over which no agreement in terminology exists. The terms used here are: trophozoite (2–5 μm diameter), cyst (4–6 μm diameter) and intracystic bodies (1 μm or less) (Yoshida 1989). The thin projections extending from the trophozoites that are seen only by electron microscopy are referred to as filopodia. All forms in the lungs are simple and include a poorly formed nucleus, immature mitochondria and endoplasmic reticulum but no clear Golgi apparatus (Haque et al 1987, Yoshida 1989, Millard et al 1990) (Fig. 4.4). It is assumed that trophozoites develop from intracystic

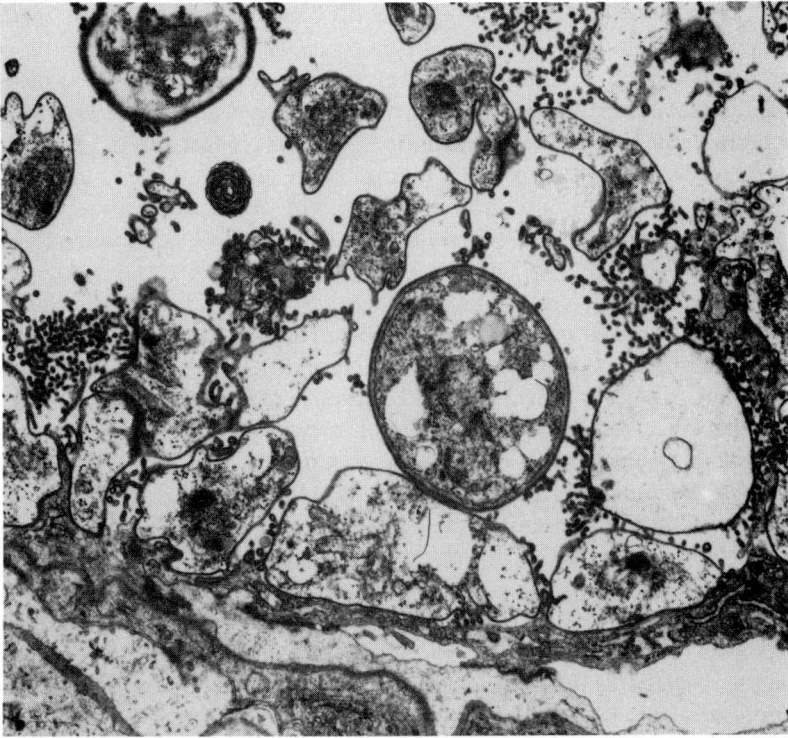

Fig. 4.4 Ultrastructural appearances of *Pneumocystis carinii* in rat lung air sac. Most forms are trophozoites which show a nucleus, poorly developed cytoplasmic organelles and filopodia extending from their surfaces and lying within the air space. A cyst form with enclosed intracystic bodies is also present. × 10 400.

bodies released by cyst rupture. The vast number of trophozoites in contrast to cysts makes this questionable and either trophozoite division is occurring or further infection is taking place. Division is not commonly witnessed (Yoshida 1989). Air-borne infection is demonstrable experimentally but no source of air contamination has been identified (Hughes 1989). The high incidence of antibodies in young children and most adults supports the view that adult infection arises from reactivated latent infection (Masur et al 1989, Glatt & Chirgwin 1990). Local epidemics may occur but never uniformly amongst all potential patients; however, this favours inhalation as a possible exogenous route in addition. Latent organisms in the lungs of either healthy or immunosuppressed adults not suffering from *P. carinii* pneumonia have not been demonstrated (Millard & Heryet 1988, Wakefield et al 1990). Specimens from infected patients include trophozoites and cysts but in experimental models trophozoites are the only forms recognized initially (Millard et al 1990) and these may be the free existing forms. Alternatively, other as yet unrecognized forms in the life cycle may exist.

Pathogenicity

The cause of death in AIDS patients with *P. carinii* pneumonia and the mechanism of respiratory embarrassment are both unclear. The organism is only pathogenic if the cellular immune response is incompetent (Masur et al 1989). The risk is greatest when T4 lymphocyte levels in HIV + patients fall below 200 cells per ml of blood. The effect of changes in numbers of macrophages, polymorphs, NK cells or other T cell subsets is unclear (Phair et al 1990).

Infected lungs reveal a spectrum of changes but common to all is a patchy distribution. The amount of lung tissue involved appears insufficient to cause either respiratory embarrassment or death (Maxfield et al 1986) and the concept of suffocation from loss of alveolar air space is thus untenable. At autopsy the lung is a graveyard of therapeutic intervention including drugs and oxygen therapy, as well as infection by other microorganisms and it is hence difficult to evaluate the damage caused directly by *P. carinii*. In experimental studies, pneumocyte damage is minimal and late and it affects both Type I and Type II pneumocytes (Yoshida 1989, Millard et al 1990). It is not unequivocally the result of contact between the organism and the pneumocytes since this is not always close and does not involve intracellular penetration. In vitro studies do, however, show that any attachment depends upon the pneumocyte having an intact cytoskeleton and that, once achieved, division of the cell is inhibited (Limper & Martin 1990). Damage is not mediated directly via the filopodia. These have contact neither with pneumocytes nor with other trophozoites; their function seems to be nutritional associated with an increase in surface area. It is evident from culture studies that pneumocyte damage is not produced either by growth inhibiting substances or from an excessive uptake of nutrients by the microorganism (Limper & Martin 1990).

Comparison with the adult respiratory distress syndrome and other conditions provoking intrapulmonary arteriovenous shunting with progressive hypoxaemia offer alternative explanations of lung damage (Maxfield et al 1986). These include a role for surfactant (Sheehan et al 1986), an unidentified component of the frothy intra-alveolar exudate (Millard et al 1990), and the associated inflammatory reaction. The surface carbohydrates of *P. carinii* may trigger these latter responses by the chemical activation of complement (Lu et al 1990). Respiratory impairment has been related to the neutrophil polymorph component in bronchial alveolar lavage specimens rather than to the numbers of *P. carinii* (Limper et al 1989).

Microscopic appearances

These have been described at light (Weber et al 1977) and electron microscopy (Yoshida 1989) and have varied little amongst different groups of immunocompromised patients. It has been suggested that the organism is only related to Type I pneumocytes but this is probably due to the timing of the examination and the greater surface area of the air spaces normally occupied by these cells by comparison with Type II cells (Millard et al 1990). Organisms overlie both types of pneumocytes at all stages of the disorder but predominantly Type II cells and their regenerative forms in the end stages. Contact between organisms and pneumocytes may involve direct anchorage (Haque et al 1987) but such occurrences are uncommon, possibly artefactual, and are not supported by preliminary freeze fracture scanning electron microscopy studies. The lung response, too, varies in the course of the disease but includes no unique features other than presence of the organism (Weber et al 1977).

Variants that are emerging in AIDS patients are probably the effect of treatment, including prophylactic, and particularly the use of aerosols of pentamidine (Northfelt 1989). Fluctuations in immunocompetence may also be instrumental. Miliary dissemination, nodules, cavitation (Barrio et al 1986), pneumothorax (Martinez et al 1988) and extrapulmonary spread (Northfelt 1989, Ravalli et al 1990) all occur more frequently and, concurrently, granulomas (Cuppes et al 1989) (Fig. 4.5). These face the histopathologist with a taxing diagnostic choice in which monoclonal antibodies against *P. carinii* (Linder et al 1987) are helpful in differentiating these granulomas from those due to acid fast bacilli or histoplasma. Extrapulmonary spread of *P. carinii* prior to AIDS was rare and mainly confined to mediastinal lymph nodes. Diffuse organ involvement has been seen in AIDS but the mechanism and the role of aerosol therapy are both unclear. Vascular dissemination rather than interstitial spread is probable since organisms have been recognized in vessels (Glatt & Chirgwin 1990, Ravalli et al 1990) and are only rarely found in the septal tissues of the lung.

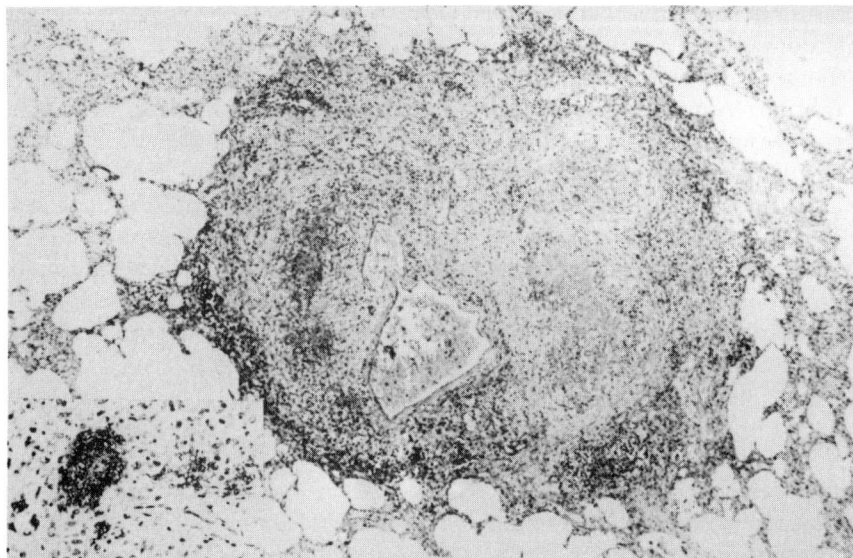

Fig. 4.5   A granuloma in the lung associated with *Pneumocystis carinii*. H & E × 160. The organisms could only be demonstrated by a specific antibody (insert × 500).

The organisms may penetrate the vasculature directly (although neither motility nor digestive enzymes are universally accepted) or enter as a result of the associated inflammatory destruction. Alternatively, macrophage carriage could be responsible since in most electron microscopic studies (Haque et al 1987, Yoshida 1989) occasional organisms have been found in these cells.

KAPOSI'S SARCOMA

Prior to the recognition of HIV, Kaposi's sarcoma provided a marker of AIDS in homosexuals, as it both preceded and antedated the immuno-deficiency state. Diagnostic difficulties emerged with further experience, and debate on the origin, pathogenesis and cause of the tumour has grown.

Diagnosis

Dermatologists describe patches, plaques and nodules but realise that a spectrum of histological features occurs in all lesions (Santucci et al 1988). Once fully developed, the slit-like spaces lined by flattened cells and supported by groups of spindle cells which are admixed with red cells and haemosiderin, are characteristic. A diagnostic though rare feature (Francis et al 1986) is the presence of eosinophilic globules in the cytoplasm of spindle cells (Fig. 4.6). A mononuclear cell response including plasma cells appears and in this T-helper cells are diminished, their proportion

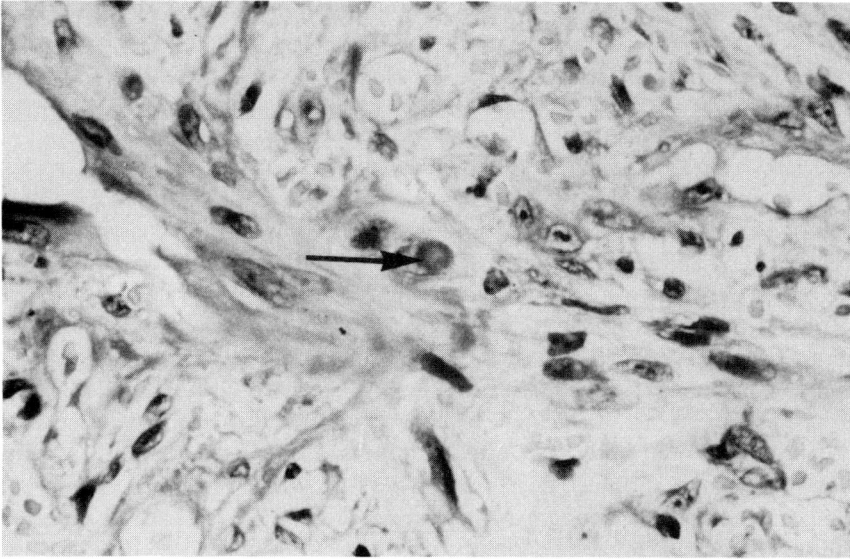

Fig. 4.6 Kaposi's sarcoma in the skin with an intracytoplasmic inclusion (arrow) within one cell. H & E × 340.

corresponding with those in the circulation in AIDS cases (Francis et al 1986, Santucci et al 1988).

The appearance of Kaposi's sarcoma in an HIV + patient means that AIDS has developed and the prognosis is poor. Consequently, biopsy is necessary in potential early lesions. The histological diagnosis can be difficult and is easily missed without multiple levels (Francis et al 1986). Changes may be restricted to irregular or jagged, slightly dilated channels lined by plump cells which dissect the dermal collagen. The appearances are identical to those seen in tumours unassociated with HIV at a similar stage and may also be seen in clinically uninvolved skin in HIV + patients (De Dobbeleer et al 1987, Ruszczak et al 1987). At this stage, spindle cells, red cells and haemosiderin are not conspicuous and the characteristic haemorrhagic macroscopic appearance is absent. Pyogenic granuloma, stasis dermatitis, bacillary (epithelioid) angiomatosis (Berger et al 1989) and pseudo Kaposi's sarcoma (Landthaler et al 1989) have all provided differential diagnostic difficulties.

Vascular or lymphatic endothelium?

Clinically, the tumour is vascular and a cause of haemorrhage particularly in the gastrointestinal tract and the lungs (Garay et al 1987, Barrison et al 1988). Some HIV − and HIV + patients manifest substantial local oedema and arguments persist as to whether the tumour is vascular or lymphatic in origin (Dorfman 1988). Electron microscopy supports an endothelial origin but its interpretation is not unequivocal and studies using histochemical and immunochemical methods have failed to resolve the matter (Facchetti et al 1988, Green et al 1988, Roth et al 1988, Massarelli et al 1989). Difficulties arise from the use of frozen or paraffin sections or of monoclonal or polyclonal antibodies and the age of the lesions studied. The most widely used antibody has been that to Factor VIII related antigen (Facchetti et al 1988), a component of vascular endothelium. However, this antigen is not expressed by all normal vascular endothelium either at different anatomical sites or at different periods of development, or even in all vascular tumours (Rutgers et al 1986). No reliable antibody for lymphatic endothelium has emerged and its recognition may rest upon negative staining. The development of lymphatics and their relationship with the circulation is unclear although direct communication exists between the thoracic duct and the vena cava and lymphatico-venous anastomoses are postulated in the dermis and submucosal regions (Dictor & Andersson 1988, Facchetti et al 1988). The early lesions of Kaposi's sarcoma appear particularly at these sites and the early irregular channels clearly mimic small lymphatics. Later lesions may be more complex with an associated vascular response to the tumour. This may be the source of the red cells although these may also come from reflux from the venous channels and subsequent leakage through the walls of lymphatics. Such a hypothesis unifies a role for lymphatic and vascular endothelium and is not incompatible with the differing results of immuno-cytochemical and histochemical studies. A variant of this view perceives the tumour as arising from dermal dendrocytes, cells closely allied to endothelial cells, following activation by HIV (Nickoloff & Griffiths 1989).

Tumour or reactive response?

The term sarcoma implies a malignant and highly metastatic tumour; a course clearly not followed in many examples of Kaposi's sarcoma (Costa & Rabson 1983, Brooks 1986, Penn 1986). Spontaneous regression may also occur. Chromosome studies have failed to identify a constant or unique abnormality (Bovi et al 1986, Saikevych et al 1987). Tumours at sites of injury, the distribution in dependent regions and predominance in the skin where trauma may have occurred raise the possibility of an initial reactive response which later progresses to a true tumour. The striking reduction in the proportion of Kaposi's sarcoma amongst HIV+ homosexuals (Des Jarlais et al 1987, Bernstein et al 1989, Rutherford et al 1989, Lifson et al 1990), a phenomenon attributed to reduced promiscuity and potential exposure to infection, could also support this viewpoint. Parallels for such a course exist in AIDS, e.g. the progression of reactive lymphoid responses, initially polyclonal and later monoclonal, to B cell lymphomas (Levine 1990).

A concept advanced is that an angiogenic stimulus induces the reactive response (Levy & Ziegler 1983, Bovi et al 1986, Brooks 1986, Azzarelli et al 1988). This may also involve spermatozoa (Stein-Werblowsky & Ablin 1990), infections or excessive liberation of cytokines. The latter may originate from T-cells (Davies et al 1990) or the tumour cells themselves (Nakamura et al 1988, Salahuddin et al 1988, Ensoli et al 1989). Cytokines similar to fibroblast growth factors have been identified from the tumour cells as well as their controlling oncogene (Bovi & Basilico 1987, Bovi et al 1987, Salahuddin et al 1988, Werner et al 1989). These factors are believed to exert a paracrine and an autocrine effect upon the tumour cells (Ensoli et al 1989) thereby strengthening the belief that Kaposi's sarcoma is a reactive response, certainly in its early phases.

Stimulus and promoting factors

No cause for Kaposi's sarcoma has been identified and, in common with many tumours, a multi-factorial basis is probable. The remarkable male predominance and restriction to certain racial types in Europe clearly raise the possibility of a genetic basis (Ross et al 1985, Gross & Safai 1989) but HLA studies have not revealed a consistent pattern (Melbye et al 1987). The geographical clustering of many AIDS and non-AIDS patients implies an infective basis (Dictor & Attewell 1988, Beral et al 1990).

Cytomegalovirus (CMV) has been implicated in Kaposi's sarcoma (Giraldo & Beth 1986). Antibodies to CMV have been found in a high percentage of HIV− and HIV+ patients, but they are equally present amongst those without Kaposi's sarcoma and in non-homosexual HIV+ patients, e.g. haemophiliacs, in whom Kaposi's sarcoma is rare. Early in situ DNA studies overlooked homologies between human and herpes virus DNA and so claimed an association for Kaposi's sarcoma. Others have demonstrated that CMV is not confined to the tumour but is present in unaffected tissues (Hashimoto et al 1987, Grody et al 1988). Improved methodology has confirmed that CMV is not present in Kaposi's sarcoma in substantial copy numbers but the possibility remains that very low or undetectable numbers might exist, possibly in only a few cells (Ambinder et al 1987, Hashimoto et al 1987, Grody et al 1988, Van den Berg et al 1989). A 'hit and run' mechanism may also operate (Boldogh et al 1990). No association has been found between the tumour and HIV, hepatitis B virus or Epstein–Barr virus, which are all commonly found in Kaposi's sarcoma patients (Civantos et al 1982, Bovi et al 1986, Craighead et al 1988, Jahan et al 1989), although the HIV tat gene is present in some tumour cell cultures (Vogel et al 1988).

An unidentified virus has been proposed (Mortimer 1987, Craighead et al 1988) and strong circumstantial evidence advanced that this is a retrovirus (Mittelman et al 1985, Dictor & Jarplid 1988). This evidence comes from avian haemangiomatosis, a disorder similar to Kaposi's sarcoma but related to a retrovirus of the lymphoid leukosis group. The hypothesis is that such a virus is spread in a similar fashion to HIV but requires a large dose to establish infection. If the virus is encountered by an immunocompetent individual, resistance develops and any subsequent loss of immune competence is not followed by tumour formation. Such an explanation would account for the almost total absence of Kaposi's sarcoma amongst HIV + haemophiliacs (Maurin et al 1988), its low incidence in HIV + intravenous drug abusers and the high level amongst HIV + homosexuals where near coincident infection with HIV is assumed. Whether such a virus acts as the initiator of the tumour process or as a cofactor similar to the Epstein–Barr virus and B cell lymphomas, is difficult to unravel.

Other potential cofactors are the multiple infections experienced by most HIV + homosexuals (Marmor et al 1982) although neither individually nor collectively can any be incriminated (Lifson et al 1990). Recreational drugs, especially nitrates, and promiscuous sexual activity are other perceived cofactors amongst homosexuals (Marmor et al 1982, Krown 1988, Gross & Safai 1989) but this remains unproven.

CYTOMEGALOVIRUS INFECTIONS

CMV is endemic in all populations (Mach et al 1989) and particularly amongst homosexuals with rates of up to 90% (Drew 1988). Primary infection is invariably asymptomatic but, if transmitted in utero, encephalitis, microcephaly and stillbirth can develop. The virus is harmful to adults only if their immune competence, particularly the cellular arm, is impaired (Rook 1988), but even then infection cannot always be equated with symptoms or organ damage (Griffiths & Grundy 1988). In the adult, infection develops either from reactivation of the latent virus or from secondary infection. T-cells and macrophages may serve as reservoirs and sites of latency (Turtinen et al 1987) rather than endothelial cells (Smiley et al 1988, Roberts et al 1989, Sedmak et al 1990). Infection is transmitted particularly by blood where the risk increases in proportion to the amount received (Apperley & Goldman 1988) and also by grafts, and body fluids including semen.

The many different strains of the virus (Collier et al 1989, Mach et al 1989) may explain why re-infection is more likely to produce tissue damage than reactivation but the pathway for this, including a receptor for the virus, has not been unequivocally identified. Present evidence suggests that $\beta2$ microglobulin may be the cell receptor and expression of Class I HLA antigens an important component in pathogenesis (Apperley & Goldman 1988).

The virus is of particular interest because it may potentiate the effects of HIV (Griffiths & Grundy 1988).

CMV and HIV

CMV, like HIV, produces T4 lymphocyte lysis and inhibits antigen presentation (Rook 1988, Booss et al 1989, Ho et al 1990). Additionally, CMV may potentiate the lysis of HIV infected T4 cells and promote HIV dispersion (Casarealie et al 1989). Synergism may also exist through the release of lymphokines that either attract cells harbouring the second virus or support the local growth of this virus (Ho et al 1990, McKeating et al 1990). The similarity with the findings in monkeys infected with simian immunodeficiency virus concurrently infected with CMV favours these concepts (Baskin 1987). The greater propensity for CMV + haemophiliacs to progress from HIV positivity to AIDS (Webster et al 1989) further supports the hypothesis, as do the high rates of CMV positivity amongst homosexuals prior to the development of HIV positivity. Nevertheless, increased rates of CMV positivity have not been found consistently in haemophiliacs (Barnass et al 1989), drug abusers or heterosexuals with AIDS. It is not disputed that either virus increases the potential for infection by other microorganisms.

Organ damage

Pulmonary CMV infection in graft recipients has a high mortality (Apperley & Goldman 1988, Heurlin et al 1989), but not in AIDS patients (Jacobson & Mills 1988, Klatt & Shibata 1988). Death from CMV in AIDS patients has been attributed to pneumonitis, encephalitis, Addison's disease and pseudomembranous colitis (Klatt & Shibata 1988) but in all centres the commonest site of infection is the retina with blindness as a result (Drew 1988, Schmitt-Gräff et al 1990). CMV infection complicating AIDS has occurred at virtually all anatomical sites (Jacobson & Mills 1988, Klatt & Shibata 1988, Roberts et al 1989, Vinters et al 1989), some otherwise uncommon ones being the skin (Abrams & Farhood 1989, Bournerias et al 1989), gall bladder (Hinnant et al 1989), endometrium (Brodman & Deligdisch 1986), cervix (Brown et al 1988), epididymis (Randazzo et al 1986) and urinary bladder (Lucas et al 1989), but clinical symptoms and histopathological responses are not always apparent. Similar observations in other CMV + adult populations have led to the concept that the virus may not always cause disease or may do so via different mechanisms (Griffiths & Grundy 1988, Bladen 1989, Hinnant et al 1989).

Direct lysis of infected cells by the replicating virus, as in retinitis and hepatitis, is the commonest pathogenetic mechanism. This is responsive to agents blocking DNA synthesis, e.g. ganciclovir (Jacobson et al 1988). Immunopathogenic responses are considered to be the basis for many of the other effects (Griffiths & Grundy 1988). These may develop either as a result of infected cells expressing early antigens and thereby becoming liable to lysis by cytotoxic T-cells or through the virus activating clones of T- or B-cells from which autoantibodies arise. Either response may then be augmented by inflammatory responses. CMV pneumonitis in organ recipients is an end result and in these circumstances maintaining or even

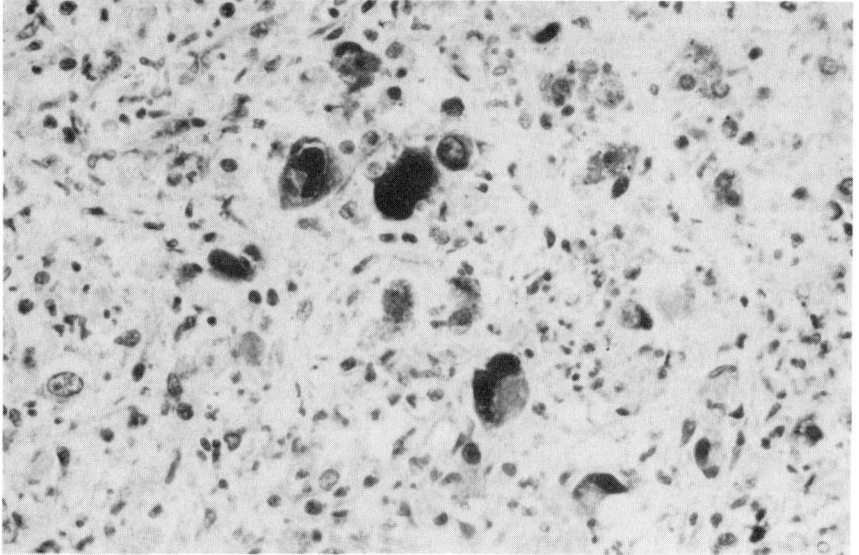

Fig. 4.7   Adrenal medulla exposed to a labelled antibody to CMV. × 260.

increasing immunosuppression may be the therapy of choice (Griffiths & Grundy 1988). Pneumonitis in AIDS patients, in contrast, is most likely the result of cytolytic damage.

Diagnosis

The 'owls eye' intranuclear inclusion body seen in haematoxylin and eosin sections is the basis for the histological diagnosis (Jesionek & Kiolemenoglou 1904). Tissue responses are neither unique (Abrams & Farhood 1989, Francis et al 1989) nor always present and the virus may be widespread or confined to a single site. A monoclonal antibody (DAKO) will label the virus in paraffin-fixed tissue (Fig. 4.7) but not at all stages of the infection (Francis et al 1989, Jiwa et al 1989) and in situ hybridization methods and the polymerase chain reaction have been used for diagnosis (Clayton et al 1989, Jiwa et al 1989, Shibata & Klatt 1989). Such techniques reveal more widespread infection but their greater sensitivity rarely adds to that of the antibody method which is easier and quicker to perform.

REFERENCES

Abrams J, Farhood A I 1989 Infection-associated vascular lesions in acquired immunodeficiency syndrome patients. Human Pathology 20: 1025–1026
Ambinder R F, Newman C, Hayward G S et al 1987 Lack of association of cytomegalovirus with endemic African Kaposi's sarcoma. Journal of Infectious Diseases 156: 193–197
Apperley J F, Goldman J M 1988 Cytomegalovirus: biology, clinical features and methods of diagnosis. Bone Marrow Transplant 3: 253–264

Azzarelli A, Mazzaferro V, Quaglivolo V et al 1988 Kaposi's sarcoma: malignant tumour or proliferative disorder? European Journal of Cancer and Clinical Oncology 24: 973–978

Baker R W, Peppercorn M A 1982 Gastrointestinal ailments of homosexual men. Medicine 61: 390–405

Barnass S, O'Toole C, Colvin B 1989 Cytomegalovirus infection and progression to AIDS. Lancet ii: 336

Barrio J L, Suarez M, Rodriquez J L et al 1986 Pneumocystis carinii pneumonia presenting as cavitating and noncavitating solitary pulmonary nodules in patients with the acquired immunodeficiency syndrome. American Review of Respiratory Diseases 134: 1094–1096

Barrison I G, Foster S, Harris J W et al 1988 Upper gastrointestinal Kaposi's sarcoma in patients positive for HIV antibody without cutaneous disease. British Medical Journal 296: 92–93

Baskin G B 1987 Disseminated cytomegalovirus infection in immunodeficient rhesus monkeys. American Journal of Pathology 129: 345–352

Batman P A, Miller A R O, Forster S M et al 1989 Jejunal enteropathy associated with human immunodeficiency virus infection: quantitative histology. Journal of Clinical Pathology 42: 275–281

Beral V, Peterman T A, Berkelman R L et al 1990 Kaposi's sarcoma among persons with AIDS: a sexually transmitted infection? Lancet 335: 123–128

Berger T G, Tappero J W, Kaymen A et al 1989 Bacillary (epithelioid) angiomatosis and concurrent Kaposi's sarcoma in acquired immunodeficiency syndrome. Archives of Dermatology 125: 1543–1547

Bernstein L, Levin D, Menck H et al 1989 AIDS-related secular trends in cancer in Los Angeles county men: a comparison by marital status. Cancer Research 49: 466–470

Bishop P E, McMillan A, Gilmour H M 1987 A histological and immunocytochemical study of lymphoid tissue in rectal biopsies from homosexual men. Histopathology 11: 1133–1147

Bladen R V 1989 Possible factors contributing to persistence of cytomegalovirus infection. Advances in Experimental Medicine and Biology 257: 27–36

Boldogh I, Abubakar S, Albrecht T 1990 Activation of proto-oncogenes: an immediate early event in human cytomegalovirus infection. Science 247: 561–564

Booss J, Dann P R, Griffith B P et al 1989 Host defense response to cytomegalovirus in the central nervous system. American Journal of Pathology 134: 71–78

Bournerias I, Boisnic S, Patey O et al 1989 Unusual cutaneous cytomegalovirus involvement in patients with acquired immunodeficiency syndrome. Archives of Dermatology 125: 1243–1246

Bovi P D, Basilico C 1987 Isolation of a rearranged human transforming gene following transfection of Kaposi sarcoma DNA. Proceedings of the National Academy of Sciences USA 84: 5660–5664

Bovi P D, Donti E, Knowles D M et al 1986 Presence of chromosomal abnormalities and lack of AIDS-retrovirus DNA sequence in AIDS-associated Kaposi's sarcoma. Cancer Research 46: 6333–6338

Bovi P D, Curatola A M, Kern F G et al 1987 An oncogene isolated by transfection of Kaposi's sarcoma DNA encodes a growth factor that is a member of the FGF family. Cell 50: 729–737

Brenneman D E, Westbook G L, Fitzgerald S P et al 1988 Neuronal cell killing by the envelope protein of HIV and its prevention by vasoactive intestinal polypeptide. Nature 335: 639–642

Brodman M, Deligdisch L 1986 Cytomegalovirus endometritis in a patient with AIDS. Mt Sinai Journal of Medicine 53: 673–675

Brooks J J 1986 Kaposi's sarcoma: a reversible hyperplasia. Lancet ii: 1309–1311

Brown S, Senekjian E K, Montag A G 1988 Cytomegalovirus infection of the uterine cervix in a patient with acquired immunodeficiency syndrome. Obstetrics and Gynecology 71: 489–491

Cammer W, Bloom B R, Norton W T et al 1978 Degradation of basic protein in myelin by neutral proteases secreted by stimulated macrophages. Proceedings of the National Academy of Sciences (USA) 75: 1554–1558

Casarealie D, Fiala M, Chang C M et al 1989 Cytomegalovirus enhances lysis of HIV-infected T-lymphocytes. International Journal of Cancer 44: 124–130

Chin J 1990 Current and future dimensions of the HIV/AIDS pandemic in women and children. Lancet ii: 221–224

Civantos F, Penneys N S, Haines H 1982 Kaposi's sarcoma: absence of cytomegalovirus antigens. Journal of Investigative Dermatology 79: 79–80

Clapham P, Weber J, Whitby D et al 1989 Soluble CD4 blocks the infectivity of diverse strains of HIV and SIV for T cells and monocytes but not for brain and muscle cells. Nature (London) 337: 368–370

Clayton F, Klein E B, Kotler D P 1989 Correlation of in situ hybridisation with histology and viral cultures in patients with acquired immunodeficiency syndrome with cytomegalovirus colitis. Archives of Pathology and Laboratory Medicine 113: 1124–1126

Collier A C, Chandler S H, Handsfield H H et al 1989 Identification of multiple strains of cytomegalovirus in homosexual men. Journal of Infectious Disease 159: 123–126

Colman N, Grossman F 1987 Nutritional factors in epidemic Kaposi's sarcoma. Seminars in Oncology 14(S3): 54–62

Cornblath D R, McArthur J C, Kennedy P G E et al 1987 Inflammatory demyelinating peripheral neuropathies associated with human T-cell lymphotropic virus type III infection. Annals of Neurology 21: 32–40

Costa J, Rabson A S 1983 Generalised Kaposi's sarcoma is not a neoplasm. Lancet i: 58

Craighead J, Moore A, Grossman H et al 1988 Pathogenetic role of HIV infection in Kaposi's sarcoma of equatorial East Africa. Archives of Pathology and Laboratory Medicine 112: 259–265

Cuppes J B, Blackie S P, Road J D 1989 Granulomatous *Pneumocystis carinii* pneumonia mimicking tuberculosis. Archives of Pathology and Laboratory Medicine 113: 1281–1284

Damsker B, Bottone E J 1985 *Mycobacterium avium–Mycobacterium intracellulare* from the intestinal tracts of patients with the acquired immunodeficiency syndrome: concepts regarding acquisition and pathogenesis. Journal of Infectious Diseases 151: 179–181

Davies A J S, Wallis V J, Morrison W I 1990 The trouble with T-cells. Lancet i: 1574–1576

De Dobbeleer G, Godfrine S, André J et al 1987 Clinically uninvolved skin in AIDS: evidence of atypical dermal vessels similar to early lesions observed in Kaposi's sarcoma: ultrastructural study in four patients. Journal of Cutaneous Pathology 14: 154–157

de la Monte S M, Ho D D, Schooley R T et al 1987 Subacute encephalomyelitis of AIDS and its relation to HTLV-III infection. Neurology 37: 562–569

Des Jarlais D C, Stoneburner R, Thomas P et al 1987 Declines in proportion of Kaposi's sarcoma among cases of AIDS in multiple risk groups in New York City. Lancet ii: 1024–1025

Dickson D W, Belman A L, Park Y D et al 1989 Central nervous system pathology in pediatric AIDS. APMIS (suppl) 8: 40–57

Dictor M, Andersson C 1988 Lymphaticovenous differentiation in Kaposi's sarcoma: cellular phenotypes by stage. American Journal of Pathology 130: 411–417

Dictor M, Attewell R 1988 Epidemiology of Kaposi's sarcoma in Sweden prior to the acquired immunodeficiency syndrome. International Journal of Cancer 42: 346–351

Dictor M, Järplid B 1988 The cause of Kaposi's sarcoma: an avian retroviral analog. Journal of the American Academy of Dermatology 18: 398–402

Dorfman R F 1988 Kaposi's sarcoma: evidence supporting its origin from the lymphatic system. Lymphology 21: 45–52

Dowell S F, Moore G W, Hutchins G M 1990 The spectrum of pancreatic pathology in patients with AIDS. Modern Pathology 3: 49–53

Drew W L 1988 Cytomegalovirus in patients with AIDS. Journal of Infectious Diseases 158: 449–456

Dryden M S, Shanson D C 1988 The microbial causes of diarrhoea in patients infected with the human immunodeficiency virus. Journal of Infection 17: 107–114

Edman J C, Kovacs J A, Masur H et al 1988 Ribosomal RNA sequence shows *Pneumocystis carinii* to be a member of the fungi. Nature 334: 519–522

Eilbott D J, Peress N, Burger H et al 1989 Human immunodeficiency virus type I in spinal cords of acquired immunodeficiency syndrome patients with myelopathy: expression and replication in macrophages. Proceedings of the National Academy of Sciences (USA) 86: 3337–3341

Ensoli B, Nakamura S, Salahuddin S Z et al 1989 AIDS—Kaposi's sarcoma-derived cells express cytokines with autocrine and paracrine growth factors. Science 243: 223–226

Facchetti F, Lucini L, Gavazzoni R et al 1988 Immunomorphological analysis of the role of blood vessel endothelium in the morphogenesis of cutaneous Kaposi's sarcoma: a study of 57 cases. Histopathology 12: 581–593

Francis N D, Parkin J M, Weber J et al 1986 Kaposi's sarcoma in acquired immune deficiency syndrome (AIDS). Journal of Clinical Pathology 39: 469–474

Francis N D, Boylston A W, Roberts A H G et al 1989 Cytomegalovirus infection in gastrointestinal tracts of patients infected with HIV-1 or AIDS. Journal of Clinical Pathology 42: 1055–1064

Garay S M, Belenko M, Fazzini E et al 1987 Pulmonary manifestations of Kaposi's sarcoma. Chest 91: 39–43

Giangaspero F, Scanabissi E, Baldacci M C et al 1989 Massive neuronal destruction in human immunodeficiency virus (HIV) encephalitis: a clinicopathological study of a pediatric case. Acta Neuropathologica 78: 662–665

Giraldo G, Beth E 1986 The involvement of cytomegalovirus in acquired immune deficiency syndrome and Kaposi's sarcoma. Progress in Allergy 37: 319–331

Glatt A E, Chirgwin K 1990 *Pneumocystis carinii* pneumonia in human immunodeficiency virus infected patients. Archives of Internal Medicine 150: 271–279

Goodgame R W 1990 AIDS in Uganda—clinical and social features. New England Journal of Medicine 323: 383–389

Grafe M, Wiley C A 1989 Spinal cord and peripheral nerve pathology in AIDS: the roles of cytomegalovirus and human immunodeficiency virus. Annals of Neurology 25: 561–566

Green T L, Meyer J R, Daniels T E et al 1988 Kaposi sarcoma in AIDS: basement membrane and endothelial cell markers. Journal of Oral Pathology 17: 266–272

Griffin G E, Miller A, Batman P et al 1988 Damage to jejunal intrinsic autonomic nerves in HIV infection. AIDS 2: 379–382

Griffiths P D, Grundy J E 1988 The status of CMV as a human pathogen. Epidemiologic Information 100: 1–15

Grody W W, Lewin K J, Naeim F 1988 Detection of cytomegalovirus DNA in classic and epidemic Kaposi's sarcoma by in situ hybridisation. Human Pathology 19: 524–528

Gross D J, Safai B 1989 Kaposi's sarcoma/AIDS cofactors. International Journal of Dermatology 28: 571–573

Gurney M E, Apatoff B R, Spear G T et al 1986 Neuroleukin: a lymphokine product of lectin-stimulated T cells. Science 234: 574–581.

Haque A, Plattner S B, Cook R T et al 1987 *Pneumocystis carinii*: taxonomy as viewed by electron microscopy. American Journal of Clinical Pathology 87: 504–510

Harriman G R, Smith D R, Horne M K et al 1989 Vitamin B12 malabsorption in patients with acquired immunodeficiency syndrome. Archives of Internal Medicine 149: 2039–2041

Hashimoto H, Müller H, Müller F 1987 In situ hybridisation analysis of cytomegalovirus lytic infection in Kaposi's sarcoma associated with AIDS: a study of 14 autopsy cases. Virchow's Archiv A (Pathological Anatomy) 411: 441–448

Heurlin N, Brattstrom C A, Tyden G et al 1989 Cytomegalovirus the predominant cause of pneumonia in renal transplant patients. Scandinavian Journal of Infectious Diseases 21: 245–253

Hinnant K, Schwartz A, Rotterdam H et al 1989 Cytomegaloviral and cryptosporidial cholecystitis in two patients with AIDS. American Journal of Surgical Pathology 13: 57–60

Ho D D, Rota T R, Schooley R T et al 1985 Isolation of HTLV III from cerebrospinal fluid and neural tissues of patients with neurological syndromes related to the acquired immunodeficiency syndrome. New England Journal of Medicine 313: 1493–1497

Ho W, Harouse J M, Rando R E et al 1990 Reciprocal enhancement of gene expression and viral replication between human cytomegalovirus and human immunodeficiency virus type 1. Journal of General Virology 71: 97–103

Hughes W T 1989 Animal models for *Pneumocystis carinii* pneumonia. Journal of Protozoology 36(1): 41–45

Jacobson M A, Mills J 1988 Serious cytomegalovirus disease in the acquired immunodeficiency syndrome (AIDS): clinical findings, diagnosis, and treatment. Annals of Internal Medicine 108: 585–594

Jacobson M A, O'Donnell J J, Porteous D et al 1988 Retinal and gastrointestinal disease due to cytomegalovirus in patients with the acquired immune deficiency syndrome: prevalence, natural history, and response to ganciclovir therapy. Quarterly Journal of Medicine 67: 473–486

Jahan N, Razzaque A, Greenspan J et al 1989 Analysis of human KS biopsies and cloned cell lines for cytomegalovirus, HIV 1, and other selected DNA virus sequences. AIDS Research Human Retroviruses 5: 225–231

Jarry A, Cortez A, René E et al 1990 Infected cells and immune cells in the gastrointestinal tract of AIDS patients: an immunohistochemical study of 127 cases. Histopathology 16: 133–140

Jesionek A, Kiolemenoglou B 1904 Ueber einen Befund von protozoënartigen gebilden in den organeneines hereditärluetischen fötus. Munchener Medizinische Wochenschrift 15: 1905–1907

Jiwa N M, Raap A K, Van de Rijke F M et al 1989 Detection of cytomegalovirus antigens and DNA in tissues fixed in formaldehyde. Journal of Clinical Pathology 42: 749–754

Ketzler S, Weis S, Haug H et al 1990 Loss of neurons in the frontal cortex in AIDS brains. Acta Neuropathologica 80: 90–94

Klatt E C, Shibata D 1988 Cytomegalovirus infection in the acquired immunodeficiency syndrome. Archives of Pathology and Laboratory Medicine 112: 540–544

Kotler D P 1989 Intestinal and hepatic manifestations of AIDS. Advances in Internal Medicine 34: 43–72

Kotler D P, Gaetz H P, Lange M et al 1984 Enteropathy associated with the acquired immunodeficiency syndrome. Annals of Internal Medicine 101: 421–428

Kotler D P, Wang J, Pierson N 1985 Body composition studies in patients with the acquired immunodeficiency syndrome. American Journal of Clinical Nutrition 42: 1255–1265

Kotler D P, Weaver S C, Terzakis J A 1986 Ultrastructural features of epithelial cell degeneration in rectal crypts of patients with AIDS. American Journal of Surgical Pathology 10: 531–538

Krown S E 1988 AIDS-associated Kaposi's sarcoma: pathogenesis, clinical course and treatment. AIDS 2: 71–80

Lake-Bakaar G, Quadros E, Beidas S et al 1988 Gastric secretory failure in patients with the acquired immunodeficiency syndrome (AIDS). Annals of Internal Medicine 109: 502–504

Landthaler M, Stolz W, Eckert F et al 1989 Pseudo-Kaposi's sarcoma occurring after placement of arteriovenous shunt. Journal of the American Academy of Dermatology 21: 499–505

Laughon B E, Druckman D A, Vernon A et al 1988 Prevalence of enteric pathogens in homosexual men with and without acquired immunodeficiency syndrome. Gastroenterology 94: 984–993

Levine A M 1990 Lymphoma in acquired immunodeficiency syndrome. Seminars in Oncology 17: 104–112

Levy J A, Ziegler J L 1983 Acquired immunodeficiency syndrome is an opportunistic infection and Kaposi's sarcoma results from secondary immune stimulation. Lancet ii: 78–80

Lifson A R, Darrow W W, Hessol N A et al 1990 Kaposi's sarcoma in a cohort of homosexual and bisexual men: epidemiology and analysis for co-factors. American Journal of Epidemiology 131: 221–231

Limper A H, Martin W J 1990 Pneumocystis carinii: inhibition of lung growth mediated by parasite attachment. Journal of Clinical Investigation 85: 391–396

Limper A H, Offord K P, Smith T F et al 1989 Pneumocystis carinii pneumonia: differences in lung parasite number and inflammation in patients with and without AIDS. American Review of Respiratory Diseases 140: 1204–1209

Linder E, Lundin L, Vorma H 1987 Detection of Pneumocystis carinii in lung-derived samples using monoclonal antibodies to an 82 KDa parasite component. Journal of Immunological Methods 98: 57–62

Lipkin W I, Parry G, Kiprov D et al 1985 Inflammatory neuropathy in homosexual men with lymphadenopathy. Neurology 35: 1479–1483

Lu J, Thiel S, Wiedemann H et al 1990 Binding of the pentames/hexames forms of mannan-binding protein to zymosan activates the proenzyme $C1r_2$ $C1s_2$ complex of the classical pathway of complement, without involvement of C1q. Journal of Immunology 144: 2287–2294

Lucas S B, Par D C, Wright E et al 1989 AIDS presenting as cytomegalovirus cystitis. British Journal of Urology 64: 429–430

Mach M, Stamminger T, Jahn G 1989 Human cytomegalovirus: recent aspects from molecular biology. Journal of General Virology 70: 3117–3146

McKeating J A, Griffiths P D, Weiss R A 1990 HIV susceptibility conferred to human fibroblasts by cytomegalovirus-induced Fc-receptor. Nature 343: 659–661

Maier H, Budka H, Lassmann H et al 1989 Vacuolar myelopathy with multinucleated giant cells in the acquired immune deficiency syndrome (AIDS). Light and electron microscopic distribution of human immunodeficiency virus (HIV) antigens. Acta Neuropathologica 78: 497–503

Mann J M, Chin J 1988 AIDS: global perspective. New England Journal of Medicine 319: 302–303

Marmor M, Laubenstein L, William D C et al 1982 Risk factors for Kaposi's sarcoma in homosexual men. Lancet i: 1083–1087

Martinez C M, Romanelli A, Mullen M P et al 1988 Spontaneous pneumothoraces in AIDS patients receiving aerosolised pentamidine. Chest 94: 1317–1318

Massarelli G, Scott C A, Ibba M et al 1989 Immunocytochemical profile of Kaposi's sarcoma cells: their reactivity to a panel of antibodies directed against different tissue cell markers. Applied Pathology 7: 34–41

Masur H, Lane H C, Kovacs J A et al 1989 Pneumocystis pneumonia: from bench to clinic. Annals of Internal Medicine 111: 813–826

Mathan M, Griffin G E, Miller A et al 1990 Ultrastructure of the jejunal mucosa in human immunodeficiency virus infection. Journal of Pathology 161: 119–127

Maurin N, Kierdorf H, Hofstaedter F 1988 Fatal cases of AIDS in a haemophiliac (with Kaposi's sarcoma) and his female partner. Thrombosis and Haemostasis 59: 343

Maxfield R A, Sorkin I B, Fazzini E P et al 1986 Respiratory failure in patients with acquired immunodeficiency syndrome *Pneumocystis carinii* pneumonia. Critical Care Medicine 14: 443–449

Melbye M, Kestens L, Biggar R J et al 1987 HLA-studies of endemic Kaposi's sarcoma patients and matched controls: no association with HLA-DR5. International Journal of Cancer 39: 182–184

Membreno L, Irony I, Dere W et al 1987 Adenocortical function in acquired immunodeficiency syndrome. Journal of Clinical Endocrinology and Metabolism 65: 482–487

Michaels J, Sharer L R, Epstein L G 1988 Human immunodeficiency virus type I (HIV-1) infection of the nervous system: a review. Immunodeficiency Review 1: 71–104

Millard P R, Wakefield A E, Hopkin J M 1990 A sequential ultrastructural study of rat lungs infected with *Pneumocystis carinii* to investigate the appearances of the organism, its relationships and its effects on pneumocytes. Journal of Experimental Pathology 71: 895–904

Millard P R, Heryet A R 1988 Observations favouring *Pneumocystis carinii* pneumonia as a primary infection: a monoclonal antibody study on paraffin sections. Journal of Pathology 154: 365–370

Mittelman A, Wong G, Safai B et al 1985 Analysis of T cell subsets in different clinical subgroups of patients with the acquired immune deficiency syndrome. Comparison with the "classic" form of Kaposi's sarcoma. American Journal of Medicine 78: 951–956

Modigliani R, Bories C, Le Charpentier Y et al 1985 Diarrhoea and malabsorption in acquired immune deficiency syndrome: a study of four cases with special emphasis on opportunistic protozoan infestations. Gut 26: 179–187

Mortimer P P 1987 Viral cause of Kaposi's sarcoma? Lancet i: 280–281

Nakamura S, Salahuddin S Z, Biberfeld P et al 1988 Kaposi's sarcoma cells: long-term culture with growth factor from retrovirus-infected CD4+ T cells. Science 242: 426–430

Navia B A, Cho E-S, Petito C K et al 1986 The AIDS dementia-complex II. Neuropathology. Annals of Neurology 19: 525–535

Nelson J A, Reynolds-Kohler C, Margaretten W et al 1988 Human immunodeficiency virus detected in bowel epithelium from patients with gastro-intestinal symptoms. Lancet i: 259–262

Nickoloff B J, Griffiths C E M 1989 The spindle-shaped cells in cutaneous Kaposi's sarcoma. American Journal of Pathology 135: 793–800

Northfelt D W 1989 Extrapulmonary pneumocystosis in patients taking aerosolised pentamidine. Lancet ii: 1454

Nutritional Reviews 1990 What do we know about the mechanism of weight loss in AIDS? Nutrition Reviews 48: 153–155

Pang S, Koyanagi Y, Miles S et al 1990 High levels of unintegrated HIV-1 DNA in brain tissue of AIDS dementia patients. Nature (London) 343: 85–89

Penn I 1986 The occurrence of malignant tumours in immunosuppressed states 1968–1984. Progress in Allergy 37: 259–300

Petito C K, Navia B A, Cho E-S et al 1985 Vacuolar myelopathy pathologically resembling subacute combined degeneration in patients with AIDS. New England Journal of Medicine 312: 874–879

Phair J, Muñoz A, Detels R et al 1990 The risk of *Pneumocystis carinii* pneumonia among men infected with human immunodeficiency virus Type I. New England Journal of Medicine 322: 161–165

Portegies P, de Gans J, Lange J M A et al 1989 Declining incidence of AIDS dementia complex after introduction of Zidovudine treatment. British Medical Journal 299: 819–821

Price R W, Brew B, Sidtis J et al 1988 The brain in AIDS: central nervous system HIV-1 infection and AIDS dementia complex. Science 239: 586–592

Randazzo R F, Hulette C M, Gottlieb M S et al 1986 Cytomegaloviral epididymitis in a patient with the acquired immune deficiency syndrome. Journal of Urology 136: 1095–1097

Ravalli S, Garcia R L, Vincent R A et al 1990 Disseminated *Pneumocystis carinii* infection in the acquired immunodeficiency syndrome. New York State Journal of Medicine 90: 155–157

Robbins D S, Yasaman S, Drysdale B et al 1987 Production of cytotoxic factor for oligodendrocytes by stimulated astrocytes. Journal of Immunology 139: 2593–2597

Roberts W H, Sneddon J M, Waldman J et al 1989 Cytomegalovirus infection of gastrointestinal endothelium demonstrated by simultaneous nucleic acid hybridisation and immunohistochemistry. Archives of Pathology and Laboratory Medicine 113: 461–464

Rodgers V D, Fassett R, Kagnoff M F 1986 Abnormalities in intestinal mucosal T-cells in homosexual populations including those with the lymphadenopathy syndrome and acquired immunodeficiency syndrome. Gastroenterology 90: 552–558

Rook A H 1988 Interactions of cytomegalovirus with the human immune system. Review of Infectious Diseases 10(S3): 460–467

Rosenblum M, Scheck A C, Cronin B A et al 1989 Dissociation of AIDS-related vacuolar myelopathy and productive HIV-1 infection of the spinal cord. Neurology 39: 892–896

Ross R K, Casagrande J T, Dworsky R L et al 1985 Kaposi's sarcoma in Los Angeles, California. Journal of the National Cancer Institute 75: 1011–1015

Roth W K, Werner S, Risau W et al 1988 Cultured, AIDS-related Kaposi's sarcoma cells express endothelial cell markers and are weakly malignant in vitro. International Journal of Cancer 42: 767–773

Rotterdam H, Lerner C W, Tapper M L 1983 Biopsies of digestive tract in patients with acquired immunodeficiency syndrome. Laboratory Invest 48: 72A

Ruszczak Z, da Silva A M, Orfanos C E 1987 Angioproliferative changes in clinically noninvolved, perilesional skin in AIDS-associated Kaposi's sarcoma. Dermatologica 175: 270–279

Rutgers J L, Wieczorek R, Bonetti F et al 1986 The expression of endothelial cell surface antigens by AIDS-associated Kaposi's sarcoma: evidence for a vascular endothelial cell origin. American Journal of Pathology 122: 493–499

Rutherford G W, Schwarcz S K, Lemp G F et al 1989 The epidemiology of AIDS-related Kaposi's sarcoma in San Francisco. Journal of Infectious Diseases 159: 569–572

Saikevych I A, Mayer M, White R L et al 1987 Cytogenetic study of Kaposi's sarcoma associated with acquired immunodeficiency syndrome. Archives of Pathology and Laboratory Medicine 112: 825–828

Salahuddin S Z, Nakamura S, Biberfeld P et al 1988 Angiogenic properties of Kaposi's sarcoma-derived cells after long-term culture in vitro. Science 242: 430–433

Santangelo W C, Krejs G J 1986 Gastrointestinal manifestations of the acquired immunodeficiency syndrome. American Journal of Medical Science 292: 328–334

Santucci M, Pimpinelli N, Moretti S et al 1988 Classic and immunodeficiency-associated Kaposi's sarcoma. Archives of Pathology and Laboratory Medicine 112: 1214–1220

Schaffner F 1990 The liver in HIV infection. Progress in Liver Diseases 9: 603–623

Schmitt F A, Bigley J W, McKinnis R et al 1988 Neuropsychological outcome of Zidovudine (AZT) treatment of patients with AIDS and AIDS-related complex. New England Journal of Medicine 319: 1573–1578

Schmitt-Gräff A, Neuen-Jacob E, Rettig B et al 1990 Evidence for cytomegalovirus and human immunodeficiency virus infection of the retina in AIDS. Virchows Archiv A (Pathological Anatomy) 416: 249–253

Sedmak D D, Roberts W H, Stephens R E et al 1990 Inability of cytomegalovirus infection of cultured endothelial cells to induce HLA class II antigen expression. Transplantation 49: 458–462

Serwadda D, Sewankambo N K, Carswell J W 1985 Slim disease: a new disease in Uganda and its association with HTLV-III infection. Lancet ii: 849–852

Sharer L R, Enstein L G, Cho E-S et al 1986 Pathologic features of AIDS encephalopathy in children: evidence for LAV/HTLV-III infection of brain. Human Pathology 17: 271–284

Sheehan P M, Stokes D L, Yeh Y et al 1986 Surfactant phospholipids and lavage phospholipase A2 in experimental *Pneumocystis carinii* pneumonia. American Review of Respiratory Diseases 134: 526–531

Shibata D, Klatt E C 1989 Analysis of human immunodeficiency virus and cytomegalovirus infection by polymerase chain reaction in the acquired immunodeficiency syndrome. Archives of Pathology and Laboratory Medicine 113: 1239–1244

Smiley M L, Mar E, Huang E 1988 Cytomegalovirus infection and viral-induced transformation of human endothelial cells. Journal of Medical Virology 25: 213–226

Smith P D, Lane H C, Gill V J et al 1988 Intestinal infections in patients with the acquired immunodeficiency syndrome (AIDS): etiology and response to therapy. Annals of Internal Medicine 108: 328–333

Snider W D, Simpson D M, Nielson G et al 1983 Neurological complications of acquired immunodeficiency syndrome: analysis of 50 patients. Annals of Neurology 14: 403–418

Soave R, Johnson W D 1988 *Cryptosporidium* and *Isospora belli* infections. Journal of Infectious Diseases 157: 225–229

Stamm B, Grant J W 1988 Biopsy pathology of the gastrointestinal tract in human immunodeficiency virus-associated disease: a 5 year experience in Zürich. Histopathology 13: 531–540

Stein-Werblowsky R, Ablin R J 1990 Aetiology of Kaposi's sarcoma. Lancet ii: 627

Stringer S L, Stringer J R, Blase M A et al 1989 *Pneumocystis carinii*: sequence from ribosomal RNA implies a close relationship with fungi. Experimental Parasitology 68: 450–461

Surtees R R, Hyland K, Smith I 1990 Central nervous system methyl-group metabolism in children with neurological complications of HIV infection. Lancet i: 619–621

Turtinen L W, Saltzman R, Jordan M C et al 1987 Interactions of human cytomegalovirus with leukocytes in vivo: analysis by in situ hybridisation. Microbial Pathogenesis 3: 287–297

Ullrich R, Zeitz M, Heise W et al 1989 Small intestinal structure and function in patients infected with human immunodeficiency virus (HIV): evidence for HIV-induced enteropathy. Annals of Internal Medicine 111: 15–21

Van den Berg F, Schipper M, Jiwa M et al 1989 Implausibility of an aetiological association between cytomegalovirus and Kaposi's sarcoma shown by four techniques. Journal of Clinical Pathology 42: 128–131

Vinters H V, Kwok M K, Ho H W et al 1989 Cytomegalovirus in the nervous system of patients with the acquired immune deficiency syndrome. Brain 112: 245–268

Vogel J, Hinrichs S H, Reynolds R K et al 1988 The HIV tat gene induces dermal lesions resembling Kaposi's sarcoma in transgenic mice. Nature 335: 606–611

Wakefield A E, Pixley F J, Banerji S et al 1990 Detection of *Pneumocystis carinii* with DNA amplification. Lancet ii: 451–453

Walker A N, Garner R E, Horst M N 1990 Immunocytochemical detection of chitin in *Pneumocystis carinii*. Infection and Immunity 58: 412–415

Watkins B A, Dora H H, Kelly W B et al 1990 Specific tropism of HIV-1 for microglial cells in primary human brain cultures. Science 2: 549–553

Weber J R, Dobbins W O 1986 The intestinal and rectal epithelial lymphocyte in AIDS: an electron-microscopy study. American Journal of Surgical Pathology 10: 627–638

Weber W R, Askin F B, Dehner L P 1977 Lung biopsy in *Pneumocystis carinii* pneumonia. A histopathologic study of typical and atypical features. American Journal of Clinical Pathology 67: 11–19

Webster A, Cook D G, Emery V C et al 1989 Cytomegalovirus infection and progression towards AIDS in haemophiliacs with human immunodeficiency virus infection. Lancet ii: 63–65

Werner S, Hofschneider P H, Stürzl M et al 1989 Cytochemical and molecular properties of Simian virus 40 transformed Kaposi's sarcoma-derived cells: evidence for the secretion of a member of the fibroblast growth factor family. Journal of Cell Physiology 141: 490–502

Wigdahl B, Kunsch C 1989 Role of HIV in human nervous system dysfunction: AIDS. Research in Human Retroviruses 5: 369–374

Wiley C A, Belman A L, Dickson D W et al 1990 Human immune deficiency virus within the brains of children with AIDS. Clinical Neuropathology 9: 1–6

Wilkes M S, Felix J C, Fortin A H et al 1988 Value of necropsy in acquired immunodeficiency syndrome. Lancet ii: 85–88

Yarchoan R, Berg G, Brouwers P et al 1987 Response of human immunodeficiency-virus-associated neurological disease to 3-azido-3'deoxythymidine. Lancet ii: 132–135

Yoshida Y 1989 Ultrastructural studies of Pneumocystis carinii. Journal of Protozoology 36: 53–60

5

T-cell malignant lymphomas

I. Lauder

In Western Europe and North America T-cell lymphomas are not common and probably constitute between 10 and 20% of lymphomas excluding those that arise primarily in the skin (Lauder et al 1985, Smith et al 1988a, Hollema & Poppema 1989). This review will concentrate almost entirely on T-cell lymphomas not primarily affecting the skin although of course secondary involvement is common in most forms of T-cell lymphoma (Stansfeld 1985). Considerable geographical differences in frequency do exist and this has resulted in some interesting epidemiological studies which have provided important clues as to the aetiology of some forms of T-cell malignancy.

AETIOLOGY

Viruses

Retroviruses have long been known to cause leukaemia and lymphoma in animals and following the detection of such a virus from a patient with cutaneous T-cell lymphoma (Poiesz et al 1981) it was found subsequently in patients with adult T-cell leukaemia in Japan and lymphoma in the Caribbean (adult T-cell leukaemia/lymphoma, ATL). The virus is a type C retrovirus, containing a reverse transcriptase of 90 kDa and was designated human T-cell leukaemia/lymphoma virus (HTLV-I). The virus is unusual in that it is capable of infecting and transforming T-cells. Once infected, the T-cells assume prolonged in vitro growth even in the absence of T-cell growth factor (Sarin & Gallo 1985). It has subsequently been found to be endemic in several parts of the world (Gallo et al 1983) and can be associated with a variety of T-cell malignancies as indicated in the updated Kiel classification. Nuclear irregularities are no longer regarded as being characteristic of T-cell lymphomas but in the so-called Caribbean lymphoma (O'Brien et al 1983) the nuclear pattern is often so unusual that it may provide the first clue as to an HTLV-I aetiology in an individual case (Fig. 5.1).

A recent study in Taiwan has shown that T-cell malignancy constitutes 39% of non-Hodgkin's lymphoma (NHL) (Su et al 1988). About one fifth of

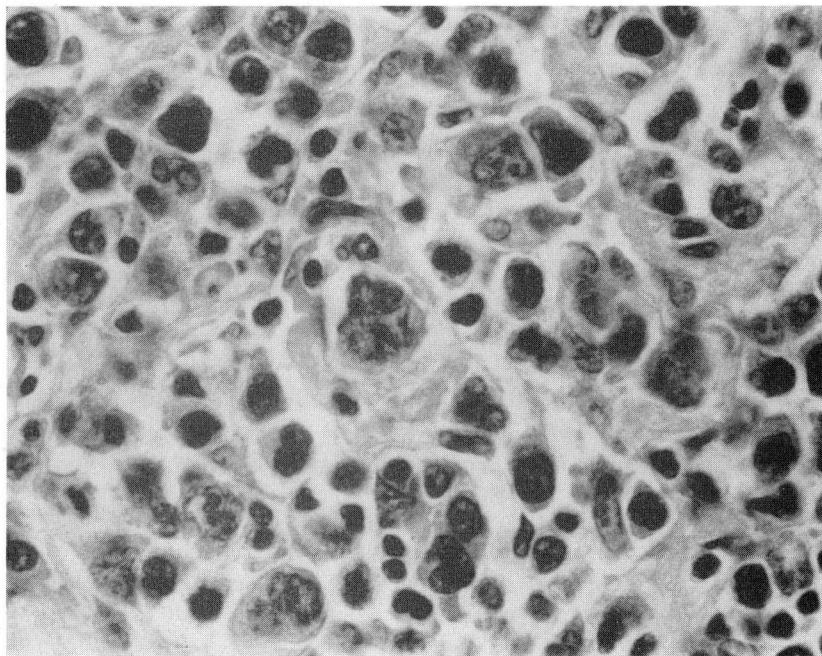

Fig. 5.1   A high power view of a mediastinal lymph node from a 58-year-old West Indian woman. Serology was positive for HTLV-I and a TCR β gene rearrangement was demonstrated. Note the marked irregularities of nuclear outline best seen in the large centrally situated cell. H & E × 900.

the cases reported were HTLV-I positive and displayed some of the typical clinical features—skin involvement, hypercalcaemia and a rapidly progressive clinical course. The HTLV-I negative cases were similar to peripheral T-cell lymphoma as seen in Europe. Although both primary cutaneous T-cell lymphoma and secondary cutaneous involvement in ATL are common in Japan, the clinical and pathological features suggest that these two are two distinct entities (Nagatini et al 1990). In general, histology proved to be unreliable in distinguishing HTLV-I positive from HTLV-I negative cases. A related virus (HTLV-II) causes a T-cell variant of hairy cell leukaemia (Kalyanaraman et al 1982). There is a possibility that other retroviruses will be discovered so that most, if not all, forms of T-cell malignancy may prove to be of viral aetiology.

The Epstein–Barr virus (EBV) is perhaps best known as a putative aetiological agent in B-cell neoplasia such as Burkitt's lymphoma but evidence is now accumulating for a role in T-cell malignancy. Two cases of 'Burkitt-like' T-lymphoblastic lymphoma have also been reported (Oliver et al 1988) one of which showed the classic jaw presentation of Burkitt's lymphoma. Somewhat surprisingly, the prognosis appeared to be better than that of the equivalent B-cell disease. Lethal midline granuloma is one

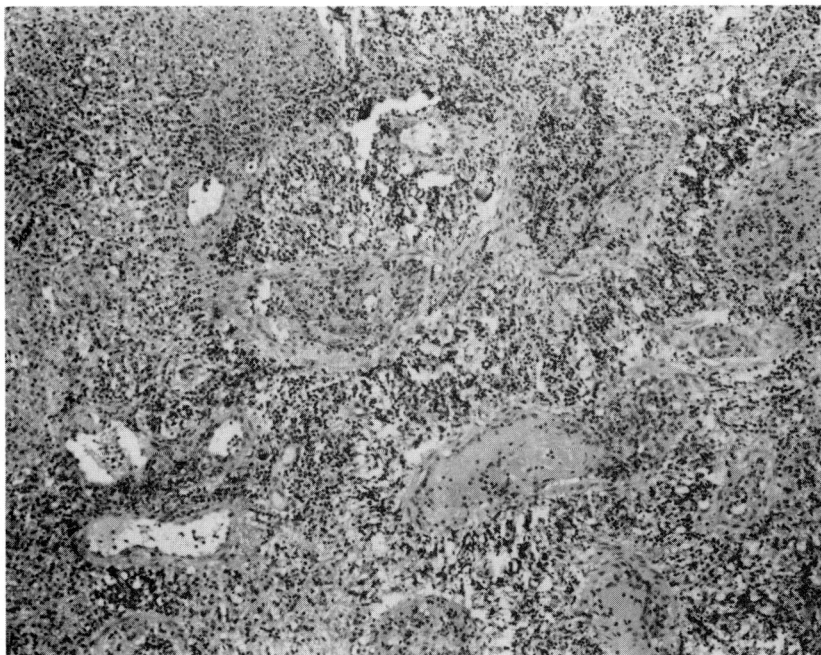

Fig. 5.2 A nasal biopsy from an 8-year-old boy. Note the presence of tumour cells in and around several medium sized blood vessels. A TCR β gene rearrangement confirmed an angiocentric T-cell lymphoma. H & E × 90.

form of angiocentric lymphoma now shown to be of T-cell lineage (Fig. 5.2). In a high proportion of these cases it is possible to demonstrate EBV in the lesions (Harabuchi et al 1990) and although this does not establish an aetiological role for EBV it certainly indicates the need for further study in this tumour. Other supportive evidence comes from study of a patient with chronic EBV infection who after a 6-year period developed an EBV positive T-cell lymphoma (Bonagura et al 1990). The tumour contained EBNA and also linear replicating EBV DNA.

T-cell neoplasia has been observed in a number of patients with immunosuppression (Garvin et al 1988, Kemnitz et al 1990, Brown et al 1991) including AIDS (Shorrock et al 1990). In view of the well established role of EBV in the development of B-cell neoplasia in such patients it would be interesting to know if this virus was also present in T-cell neoplasia. The study by Kemnitz et al (1990) included a detailed virological assessment in which neither EBV nor any other viral genome could be discovered. Southern blot analysis for EBV can now be undertaken in DNA extracted from fixed tissues (Libetta et al 1990) and such methodology could be used retrospectively to examine the potential role of EBV in T-cell neoplasia. Such studies should include cutaneous T-cell lymphomas where serological evidence also indicates a higher incidence of EBV positivity than in controls

(Lee et al 1990) and also the Burkitt-like T-lymphoblastic lymphomas described above.

Other aetiological agents

Many epidemiological studies have demonstrated the importance of radiation in the development of lymphoma (Bernard 1988) although few studies have looked specifically at T-cell neoplasia. In experimental models, irradiation of the thymus can be used to induce T-cell lymphomas and this could be utilized as a model for the study of the biology of such lymphomas and the role of growth factors (Gjerset et al 1990).

In experimental models, lymphomas also develop as part of a graft versus host disease (GVH) in which either the transferred T-cells become neoplastic or alternatively they act on recipient immune cells. The role of the immune system in lymphomagenesis has been reviewed by Habeshaw (1988).

DIAGNOSIS

Histological appearances

The histological diagnosis and classification of T-cell malignancy presents considerable difficulty. It is perhaps hardly surprising that morphological features alone are unsatisfactory when one considers that in the peripheral blood it is virtually impossible by morphological means to distinguish T-cells from B-cells let alone detect either of the two main cell subsets. A number of histological and cytological features have been said to be suggestive of T-cell lymphoma. These include prominent post-capillary venules, sparing of B-cell areas, irregularities in nuclear outline, clear cytoplasm and the presence of other cells such as eosinophils, histiocytes (including epithelioid cells), plasma cells and interdigitating reticulum cells (Stansfeld 1985). Whilst these features may be helpful, none of them is truly diagnostic. Nuclear irregularities (Burke et al 1985, Weiss et al 1985) and clear cytoplasm (Stansfeld 1985) may be seen in B-cell lymphomas and the other cell types in many benign, as well as malignant T-cell proliferations presumably as a result of cytokine production. Clear cells in both T- and B-cell neoplasms are related in some cases to the presence of giant multivesicular bodies (Eyden et al 1990). In other instances a signet ring appearance in B-cell lymphomas is associated with immunoglobulin production (Kim et al 1978).

The pattern of infiltration is often helpful in that peripheral T-cell lymphomas tend to occupy microanatomical sites normally associated with T-cells at least in the early stages. In lymph nodes this will be the paracortex and interfollicular zones and in the spleen the periarterial lymphoid sheath. Topographical localization, whilst interesting for what it tells us about the normal homing properties of lymphocytes, must be viewed with some caution. In the spleen, for instance, a number of B-cell neoplasms including BCLL and ML-CB/CC may commonly involve the T-cell areas (Van Krieken et al 1989) but it is unusual for them to destroy totally the architecture of T-cell areas.

An increase in vascularity is often seen in T-cell lymphomas and the arborizing pattern shown by reticulin preparations is still a helpful feature of angioimmunoblastic lymphadenopathy (AIL). Vascular changes, however, are nonspecific and prominent post-capillary venules may be seen in B-cell neoplasia, Hodgkin's disease and a number of reactive conditions of which infectious mononucleosis is perhaps the most likely to be mistaken for T-cell neoplasia.

In lymphoepithelioid T-cell lymphoma (Lennert's lymphoma) clusters of pale staining epithelioid cells are scattered across a diffusely effaced node architecture. Their presence is possibly related to the production of cytokines by the T-cell component. Considerable caution should be taken in making this diagnosis as not only are similar changes seen in Hodgkin's disease but in a series of 11 cases diagnosed on histology, three were eventually found to be of B-cell origin (Spier et al 1988). The distinction is important since cases shown to be of T-cell origin have a much worse prognosis. Hodgkin's disease is occasionally misdiagnosed as T-cell lymphoma in cases where diagnostic Reed-Sternberg cells are few and the converse is also true since Hodgkin's-like cells are often observed in T-cell lymphomas. The determination of full immunophenotype and genotype is essential in difficult cases.

The ready availability of antibodies with defined specificities against a wide range of T-cell antigens has considerably alleviated such diagnostic problems. Such antibodies are extremely useful in providing an indication of the lineage of a particular lymphoid proliferation but they do not give unequivocal evidence of a clonally restricted population of T-cells which, in most instances, would indicate malignancy. Whereas with B-cell lymphomas, even in paraffin sections, it is now usually possible to infer the presence of malignancy by the demonstration of light chain restriction, no similar feature or property is currently available for T-cell proliferations.

The use of paraffin section markers has considerably aided the diagnosis of T-cell neoplasia. Following initial observations with small numbers of antibodies (West et al 1986) several groups have now extended this approach by using many more (Hall et al 1988, Myskow et al 1988). In the latter series all 33 T-cell lymphomas reacted with either CD43 (MT1) or CD45 RO (UCHL1) or with both. The former authors suggested that a small panel including CD45 (LCA), CD20 (L26), MB2, CD43, CD45 RO provide good discrimination between T- and B-cell lymphomas and can usefully be combined with non-lineage specific antibodies such as CD15, CD30 and antibodies directed against epithelial and macrophage antigens. To this list, one would now wish to add CD3 as the antibodies against this antigen are probably the best, and most useful, of those currently available (Mason et al 1989).

Those who employ only a limited panel of antibodies and who are unfamiliar with the immunostaining pattern in other lymphomas can readily fall into a number of diagnostic pitfalls. In lymphoblastic lymphomas problems may arise in that failure to express leucocyte common antigen (CD45) may lead to an initial impression of a non-lymphoid tumour. Expression of CD43 (MTI) may be interpreted as indicating a T-cell lineage whereas it is frequently expressed on the surface of B-lymphoblastic lymphoma cells. When CD15 is used positive staining may be thought to indicate Hodgkin's disease although it is now well recognized that T-cells may also express this antigen (Wieczorek et al 1985). Myeloid cells show strong expression of this antigen and granulocytic sarcoma is liable to be mistaken for a T-cell lymphoma unless this is borne in mind. The expression of CD15 antigen can be seen in up to 50% of all forms of T-cell neoplasia. As occasional multinucleated cells may also be seen in T-cell neoplasia the possibility of confusion with Hodgkin's disease is readily apparent. The CD15 antigen is present in several other tissues and it certainly cannot be considered to be a reliable marker of Hodgkin's disease (Angel et al 1989) although it is on occasions a useful screening test.

Even in those cases in which there is unequivocally a great excess of T-cells, this does not necessarily indicate T-cell malignancy. Hodgkin's disease may include a large, and often predominant, number of T-cells (Angel et al 1987) and it is now acknowledged that some B-cell lymphomas may include many T-cells, a phenomenon which has been designated 'T-cell-rich B-cell disease' (Ramsay et al 1988, Ng et al 1989). It is the author's view that although paraffin section markers are helpful in suggesting T-cell lymphoma it is always preferable that this is accompanied by full immunophenotyping on frozen sections and with immunogenetic analysis which is invaluable in distinguishing T-cell lymphoma from Hodgkin's disease (Gledhill et al 1990).

Yet another problematical area is the distinction between T-cell and histiocytic lymphomas—the term being used here in its true sense and not as in the outdated terminology of the Rappaport classification. Not only may these cells show some common cytological features, particularly in the more immature and pleomorphic variants, but they also often share markers such as CD4 and enzymes e.g. α1-antitrypsin (Wright 1988). Enteropathy associated lymphoma (Fig. 5.3) was originally erroneously designated as 'malignant histiocytosis of the intestine' (Isaacson et al 1982) whereas most recent investigations all point towards a T-cell origin (Isaacson et al 1985). Use of a monoclonal antibody (HML-1) directed against human intestinal T-cells, confirmed that lymphomas arising in association with ulcerative jejunitis and coeliac disease are derived from intestinal mucosal T-cells (Stein et al 1988). Even phagocytosis, a phenomenon long associated with histiocytes, may be seen in some T-cell lymphomas (Kadin et al 1981). In

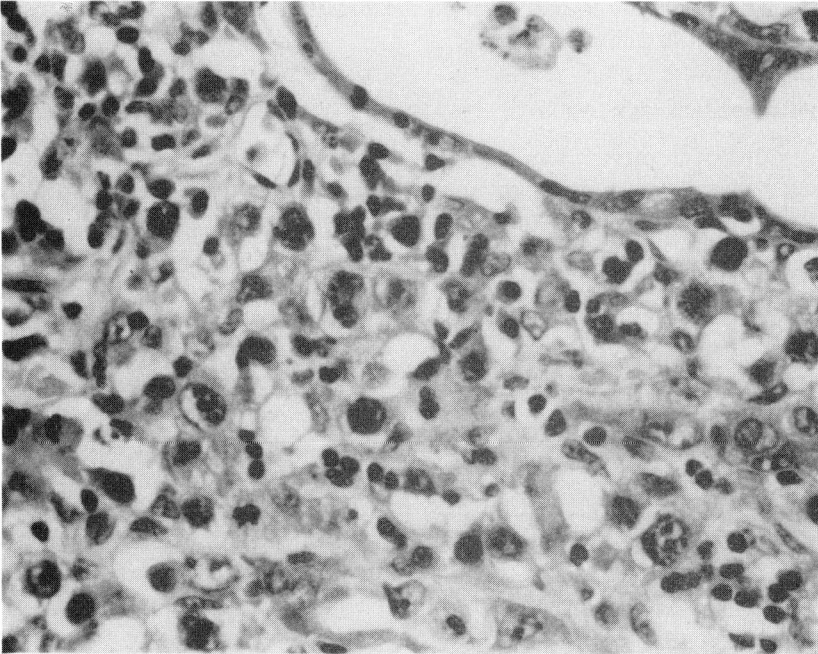

Fig. 5.3 An ulcerative lesion in the jejunum of a 43-year-old coeliac disease patient. Note the highly pleomorphic and polymorphic infiltrate. Many of the large atypical cells illustrate the difficulty in distinguishing between T-cells and histiocytes. A TCR β rearrangement was demonstrated. H & E × 360.

other instances, undoubted T-cell neoplasia is associated with activation of histiocytes so that even 'classical' phagocytic disorders such as histiocytic medullary reticulosis (HMR) may be examples of T-cell lymphoma (Falini et al 1990). The widespread distribution of the malignant cells in the liver, spleen and bone marrow, often with cutaneous involvement, is also reminiscent of so-called malignant histiocytosis and HMR (Sun et al 1990). True histiocytic lymphoma is, in fact, extremely rare and in one recent series of 925 non-Hodgkin's lymphomas only four cases were finally accepted as of histiocytic origin (Ralfkiaer et al 1990).

Given all the difficulties inherent in making a diagnosis of T-cell lymphoma it is surprising that a number of studies have advocated fine needle aspiration cytology (FNA) for diagnosis. However, where this technique has been applied, it has usually been accompanied by a whole battery of other investigations including flow cytometry (Katz et al 1989) and detailed immunophenotyping (Oertel et al 1988). FNA may occasionally be helpful for confirming involvement of a particular anatomical site and can provide valuable material for genotyping. Histopathologists should ensure that all suspected lymphoid malignancies are sent unfixed and fresh to their departments so that both immunophenotyping and genotyping can be carried out in difficult cases.

Immunophenotyping

The value of immunophenotyping is best considered by examining how a variety of antibody and enzyme markers can be used to study normal T-cell differentiation (Knowles 1989) and by showing that such studies in T-cell neoplasia give a good indication of the degree of differentiation in a particular neoplastic proliferation.

The first marker to be used for T-cells was the formation of rosettes when incubated with sheep erythrocytes. Table 5.1 illustrates how the current range of antibodies against defined CD antigens can be combined with demonstration of the enzyme terminal deoxynucleotidyl transferase (TDT) to provide a clear picture of normal T-cell differentiation. Before commenting on how the pattern of maturation can be used in analysing differentiation in T-cell malignancy, it should be noted that CD2, 5 and 7 can be regarded as pan T-antigens expressed throughout most stages of T-cell differentiation. TDT production is normally only seen at the pre-thymic and thymic phases of differentiation but is not normally seen in peripheral T-cells. CD4 and CD8 are expressed in the helper/inducer and cytotoxic/suppressor subsets respectively and dual expression outside of the thymus is abnormal. Table 5.1 also shows the neoplastic equivalents of the normal phases of differentiation with a basic distinction between thymic and peripheral T-cell neoplasia. It is important to note that none of the neoplastic 'boxes' shown should be regarded as rigid. Thus, whilst in

Table 5.1 Immunophenotyping of T-cells during normal maturation and differentiation with their neoplastic equivalents

Marker	Pro-thymocyte	Immature thymocyte	Common thymocyte	Mature thymocyte	Helper inducer	Cytotoxic suppressor
TDT	+	+	+	+	−	−
CD2	+	+	+	+	+	+
CD7	+	+	+	+	(+)	(+)
CD5	−	−	+	+	+	+
CD1	−	−	+	−	−	−
CD3	−	−	+ cytoplasmic	+ cytoplasmic + SM	+ SM	+ SM
CD4	−	−	(+)	+ OR	+	−
CD8	−	−	(+)	+	−	+
Neoplastic equivalent	Pre thymic	Thymic			Peripheral	
	ALL	Lymphoblastic lymphoma			Peripheral T-cell lymphoma	

general it is true that T-ALL does in most cases express a prothymocyte phenotype, one third may express common thymocyte antigens. Likewise the phenotype of T-lymphoblastic lymphoma, which constitutes 80% of all lymphoblastic lymphomas, is most commonly that of the common thymocyte but may, as the table illustrates, occasionally express either immature thymocyte or mature thymocyte phenotype (Knowles 1989).

The peripheral T-cell lymphomas (PTCL) are a heterogeneous group of lymphomas and their immunophenotype is diverse. They are distinguished from the more immature neoplasms by their failure to express CD1 and by the lack of TDT positivity. The most helpful feature is the loss of one or more of the major T-cell antigens (CD2, CD3, CD5 or CD7). Only about a quarter of PTCL exhibit their full range of normal antigens (Picker et al 1987) and in a fifth of cases, three of the major antigens are lost. There is always a danger in using negative staining patterns in making a primary diagnosis of malignancy but the loss of one or more of the major T-cell antigens is perhaps the most helpful immunological criterion for T-cell malignancy. Abnormal patterns of expression may be of use but predominance of T-cells and apparent subset restriction (e.g. CD4) are extremely unreliable and many non-neoplastic skin diseases show both T-cell predominance and CD4 restriction.

An alternative to the use of antibodies against CD antigens is to use reagents directed against the T-cell receptor. A variety of these are now available including $\beta F1$ which recognizes the β subunit of TCR, $\delta TCS1$ the δ subunit and WT31 the $\alpha\beta$ subunits. In a series of 28 cases (20 thymic, 8 peripheral) none showed positivity with $\delta TCS1$, 16 were positive with $\beta F1$ and four of the eight PTCL cases showed WT31 positivity (Mori et al 1990). It was concluded that WT31 was only of limited value in PTCL in contrast to at least one previous study by Campana et al (1989). It is also theoretically possible to detect clonality in a T-cell population by the use of clonotypic antibodies. However, a large number of antibodies would be required because of the number of possible variable region gene products. Using a range of antibodies described as 'almost clonotypic', Charley et al (1990) found that all of the cells in one of three cases of Sezary syndrome were stained positively by one particular antibody. Further such reagents may become available but they are likely to be superseded by more specific and sensitive methods such as the polymerase chain reaction (PCR).

Genotyping

The T-cell component of the immune system has evolved to provide a wide diversity of cell mediated responses to a vast number of potential antigens, most of which are derived from intracellular microorganisms. Whereas B cells can recognize soluble antigens, T-cells recognize antigen only when presented together with gene products of the major histocompatibility complex (MHC). This phenomenon of MHC class restriction (Zinkernagel

& Doherty 1975) requires in the case of helper (CD4) cells co-recognition of class II MHC products whereas with cytotoxic (CD8) cells class I MHC products must be co-recognized. In vitro, some TCR $\gamma\delta$ cells appear to exhibit normal cytotoxicity but the situation in vivo remains to be resolved (Haas et al 1990).

Knowledge of the structure of the T-cell receptor patterns is crucial to an understanding of T-cell malignancy and will therefore be explained first.

THE T-CELL RECEPTOR (TCR)

By producing monoclonal antibodies directed against individual T-cell clones (anticlonotypic antibodies) it was possible to immunoprecipitate a protein of 90 kDa which on reduction was found to be a heterodimer of 50 kDa and 40 kDa respectively (Acuto & Reinherz 1985). These are designated to α and β chains of the TCR and they are normally disulphide linked. Subsequent progress has been considerably enhanced by the cloning of the relevant genes with the β chain genes (Yanagi et al 1984), and the α chain genes respectively (Kronenberg et al 1986, Toyonaga & Mak 1987). Detailed analysis showed sequence homology with a number of other genes (immunoglobulins, MHC Class I and II, CD2, CD3, CD4, CD8, CD28, Thy-1, N-CAM, CEA) now collectively known as the immunoglobulin gene superfamily (Hunkapiller & Hood 1989). It should be noted that this evolutionary homology does not necessarily imply common functionality or genetic control.

About 95% of peripheral T-cells express the $\alpha\beta$ disulphide linked heterodimer TCR. An alternative heterodimer — TCR $\gamma\delta$ —, is present only on 1–5% of peripheral T-cells but it is of importance in normal T-cell maturation and differentiation (Fowlkes & Pardoll 1989). Studies of the development of T-cells in mice have shown that TCR $\gamma\delta$ appears at about 14 days of gestation and is followed 2–4 days later by TCR $\alpha\beta$.

The T-cell receptor appears to determine specificity for both MHC and antigen and is expressed close to the CD3 antigen complex which consists of four or five polypeptides. After recognition of antigen by the receptor it seems that the CD3 complex is involved in signal transduction which gives rise to activation of protein kinase C and transcription of genes such as interferon γ and interleukin 2 (Weiss et al 1986). Cells which express TCR $\gamma\delta$ usually either fail to express CD4 or CD8 or express only CD8 (Borst et al 1988). Expression of CD8 appears to increase on activation and the cells are thought to be predominantly cytotoxic in type. The most recent evidence suggests that the TCR $\gamma\delta$ lymphocytes are an important component of the lymphoid population associated with epithelia and their role in a variety of gastrointestinal diseases is currently under investigation (Lancet 1991).

The genes encoding for each of the four possible chains have been mapped (Table 5.2) and only two chromosomes, 7 and 14, are involved. The mechanism by which diversity is generated is best exemplified by the study

Table 5.2 The T-cell receptor proteins

	Size (kDa)	Segments			Chromosome
		V	D	J	
TCR α	50	75	0	50	14q11
TCR β	40	25	2	12	7q35
TCR γ	35	7	0	2	7p15
TCRδ	45–50	10	2	2	14q11

of the organization of genes involved. For the sake of simplicity only the β chain genes will be examined here: the others are broadly similar and similar combinatorial events take place.

The genes encoding for TCR β are illustrated in Fig. 5.4. As with the immunoglobulin genes, they are composed of discontinuous segments of DNA and the assembly of the functioning gene requires the process of gene rearrangement and recombination as originally suggested for the immunoglobulin genes by Tonegawa (1983). There are perhaps 100 Vβ genes, a much smaller number of diversity (D) segment and joining (J) segment genes and two constant region genes. Recombination of the genes results first in D-J joining which normally precedes V to D rearrangement. Within the thymus, δ and γ chain arrangements normally occur before β chain (Born et al 1986).

Diversity is generated by several mechanisms, the most obvious of which is the number of combinatorial possibilities of Vβ, Dβ, Jβ, and Cβ genes. Further diversity is facilitated by considerable flexibility in the precise site at which nucleotides join (junctional diversity) and also by a process in which random nucleotides are added during joining. These so called 'N-regions' can vary between 1 and more than 10 nucleotides ('N-region diversity'). With immunoglobulin genes further diversity is generated by mutation of variable segment genes but this mechanism does not appear to operate for TCR chains. Taking into account all the possible combinations and the various diversification mechanisms it has been calculated that the mouse has the capacity to produce some 2.9×10^{22} receptors (Hunkapiller & Hood 1989).

In reactive conditions the T-cell response is polyclonal. Under these circumstances the Cβ1 region is very frequently rearranged. Because any genetic rearrangement will result in alterations of restriction enzyme sites, appropriate treatment of extracted DNA followed by electrophoresis, Southern blotting and application of a suitable radioactive probe, will demonstrate the pattern of rearrangement (Fig. 5.5). With restriction enzyme EcoRI, polyclonal proliferations usually show a reduction in the 12.0 kb band, because of the preference for rearrangement by the Cβ1 gene.

In suspected T-cell neoplasia by far the most useful immunogenetic

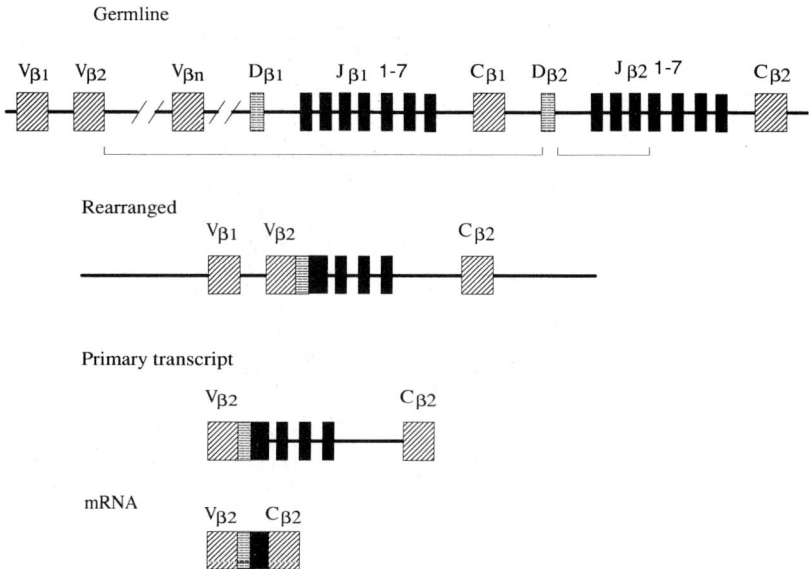

Fig. 5.4   Germ-line and representative rearranged conformation of the TCR β chain gene. Brackets below the germ-line gene cluster indicate sequences deleted to produce the rearranged conformation illustrated. Once a productive rearrangement has taken place by recombination of the variable (V), diversity (D) and joining (J) gene clusters, transcription of the recombined segment takes place. Primary transcripts are modified by differential splicing to include the appropriate constant region gene Cβ2 in the sequence illustrated.

method is analysis of TCR β rearrangements. In the large series reported by Reis et al (1988) more than 95% of the T-cell malignancies showed this form of gene rearrangement. Negative results are most frequent in the most immature neoplasms or in cases in which the proportion of malignant cells falls below the detection sensitivity level of about 1–5%. In the former situation, analysis of TCRγ and TCRδ may be helpful since it will be recalled that TCRγ and TCRδ rearrangements normally occur before TCRβ. It is claimed that TCRδ rearrangements are useful for the determination of clonality even in the most immature T-cell neoplasms which may not show other TCR gene rearrangements (Kimura et al 1989). Whilst this method may well be of use in determining clonality in difficult cases, it is unfortunately not lineage specific and a high proportion of immature B-cell neoplasms also show TCRδ rearrangements. Another problem is a number of presumed benign conditions which may commonly show TCRβ rearrangements. These include lymphomatoid papulosis, pityriasis lichenoides et varioliformis acuta, granulomatous slack skin and pagetoid reticulosis (Knowles 1989). Some of these diseases may eventually turn out to be indolent forms of T-cell lymphoma rather analogous to the relationship between some forms of so-called 'pseudolymphoma' and the

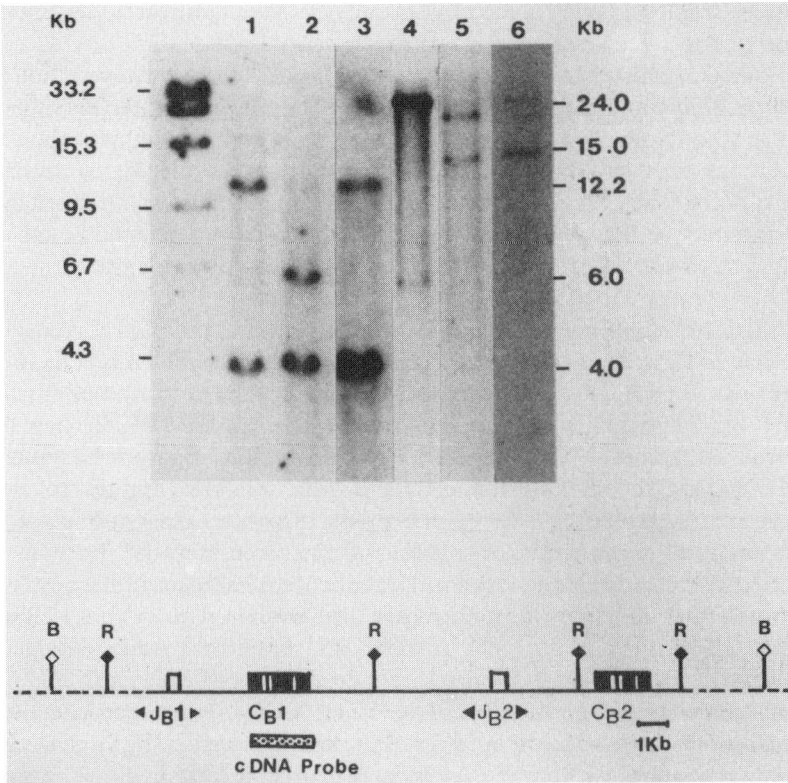

Fig. 5.5   Southern blot analysis of the T-cell receptor β chain gene using the Jurkat constant region cDNA probe. The partial map of the B chain gene in germ line configuration shows the joining (J) and constant (C) regions, the sites of cleavage by the restriction endonucleases BamHI (B) and EcoRI (R) and the Cβ1 and Cβ2 regions that hybridize with the probe. Above, the left hand track shows bacteriophage lambda DNA size standards followed by six tracks of human DNA digested with the restriction endonucleases EcoRI, tracks 1–3, and BamHI tracks 4–6. Each set of tracks shows the results of digestion of germ line DNA from placenta (1,4), DNA from a peripheral blood sample from a patient with T-ALL (2,5) and lymph node DNA from a patient with T-cell lymphoma (3,6). The EcoRI digest shows germ line bands at 12.2 kb and 4.0 kb in the placenta DNA track 1. The blood sample DNA in track 2 shows deletion of the 12.2 kb Cβ1 fragment leaving only a weak germ line and a rearranged band at 6.0 kb. The lymph node DNA track 3 also shows a weaker than expected 12.2 kb band due to T-cell receptor gene rearrangements into the Cβ2 fragment. The BamHI digest shows a 24.0 kb germ line band in the placenta DNA track 4. The blood DNA in track 5 shows two rearranged bands at 21 kb and 14 kb (5). There is a single 15 kb rearranged band which is predominant in the lymphoma DNA sample (6). The T-ALL case demonstrates rearrangement of both alleles of T-cell receptor β chain gene, one into the Cβ1 region and the other into the Cβ2 region. The lymphoma case has a single rearrangement into the Cβ2 region. (Courtesy of Dr J. H. Pringle, Department of Pathology, Leicester University.)

long term development of B-cell lymphomas of the mucosa associated lymphoid tissue.

The problem of detecting clonality when the population of malignant cells is very low, e.g. <1% as in minimal residual disease in some bone marrow samples, may be solved by the polymerase chain reaction technique. Using primers recognizing conserved sequences of the variable, diversity and joining segment genes McCarthy et al (1991) have shown that it is possible to demonstrate clonal restriction in about three quarters of cases. This methodology may also be applicable to heavy and light chain genes (McCarthy et al 1990) and should theoretically be applicable to relatively poor quality DNA extracted from fixed tissues. An additional advantage of this method is the rapidity with which it can be performed, i.e. 48 h compared to the 7–14 days which are usually required for the equivalent Southern blotting method.

Whilst the detection of a clonal TCR gene rearrangement is currently the best way of diagnosing T-cell malignancy, there are problems. The first is that of so-called lineage infidelity and the second, the detection of apparent clonal rearrangements in presumed benign disorders which has been referred to. About 10% of T-cell neoplasms exhibit apparent heavy chain gene rearrangements and the converse situation also applies to B-cell neoplasms (Reis et al 1988). Of the many possible explanations for this phenomenon the most plausible is one of 'mistaken identity': both T- and B-cell gene rearrangements use similar if not identical recombinase enzymes and the signal or trigger sequences are also similar. Under these circumstances it is not surprising that mistakes are sometimes made. Analysis of RNA transcripts shows that only rarely do full length inappropriate T- or B-transcripts appear so that complete (VDJ) TCRβ rearrangements do not normally occur in B-cell neoplasms. For similar reasons, light chain gene rearrangements are rarely if ever seen in T-cell neoplasia since complete heavy chain gene rearrangement must preceed that of the light chain genes.

The process of gene rearrangement, and the intense recombinase enzyme activity which accompanies it, probably accounts for another property of T-cell neoplasms namely their high incidence of chromosomal abnormalities especially chromosomes 7 and 14 which harbour the four TCR chain genes (Table 5.2). By way of example, inT-CLL 80% of cases show a 14q32 translocation either t(14;14)(q1;q32) or inv (14)(q11;q32) (Ueshima et al 1984). Most of the translocations appear to involve an oncogene and for a fuller account of this interesting topic two recent articles provide useful information (Reis et al 1988, Russo et al 1988).

CLASSIFICATION

No article on T-cell neoplasia would be complete without some mention of the difficulties in classifying such neoplasms. From what has already been said it will be apparent that morphology is not a satisfactory way and the author's own preference would be for a scheme based on a combination of immuno- and geno-typing. Even when full phenotyping and genotyping are available, the considerable morphological heterogeneity of peripheral T-cell lymphomas is also reflected in the heterogeneous results of sophisti-

Table 5.3   Updated Kiel classification of non-Hodgkin's lymphomas

B	T
Low grade	*Low grade*
Lymphocytic—chronic lymphocytic and prolymphocytic leukaemia; hairy-cell leukaemia	Lymphocytic—chronic lymphocytic and prolymphocytic leukaemia
	Small, cerebriform cell—mycosis fungoides, Sézary's syndrome
Lymphoplasmacytic/cytoid (LP immunocytoma)	Lymphoepithelioid (Lennert's lymphoma)
Plasmacytic	Angioimmunoblastic (AILD, LgX)
Centroblastic/centrocytic	T zone
—follicular	
—diffuse	
Centrocytic	Pleomorphic, small cell (HTLV-1)
High grade	*High grade*
Centroblastic	Pleomorphic, medium and large cell (HTLV-1)
Immunoblastic	Immunoblastic (HTLV-1)
Large cell anaplastic (Ki-1 +)	Large cell anaplastic (Ki-1 +)
Burkitt lymphoma	
Lymphoblastic	Lymphoblastic
Rare types	*Rare types*

cated immunological and molecular biological investigations (Smith et al 1988b).

Our clinical colleagues however require us to apply labels which will give them information regarding prognosis and treatment. In Europe, the updated Kiel classification (Table 5.3) was published in 1988 in the format of a letter to the *Lancet* (Stansfeld et al 1988). It was derived from a previous study by Japanese, Chinese and European pathologists (Suchi et al 1987). In line with the previously published Kiel classification for B-cell lymphomas this updated classification shows high grade and low grade categories.

The Kiel classification may not prove easy to apply. With the help of marker studies and in the absence of the proliferation centres seen in BCLL a diagnosis of TCLL is not usually difficult, particularly when accompanied by the relevant haematological information. Most of the other types present serious difficulties in assignment to the most appropriate category. Cell types are often mixed, some degree of pleomorphism is common and vascularity is usually increased. It is difficult to decide whether or not the case should be assigned to high or low grade categories and decisions as to the final category are often rather arbitrary. The reasons for this are not difficult to discern. When using the Kiel classification for B-cell lymphomas we have very well defined cytological and morphological criteria which most pathologists can readily assimilate and use. Thus, most pathologists now have a clear mental picture of a centrocyte or centroblast but would struggle to bring to mind similar pictures of pleomorphic small, medium, and large T-cells.

Apart from personal prejudices, it is also worth remembering that few formal assessments have been made of the T-cell part of the updated Kiel classification. Even advocates of the Kiel system have been forced to be critical and one recent comparison with other classifications comments that, although the updated Kiel classification is the best in current use, 'the proposed classification of T-cell lymphomas, can only be regarded as provisional' (Falzon & Isaacson 1990). An assessment of inter- and intra-observer reproducibility of the updated Kiel classification has recently been published (Hastrup et al 1991). This study at Aarhus looked at 100 peripheral T-cell lymphomas and four observers examined the material on two occasions. Using kappa statistics the level of inter-observer repro-ducibility was low and the authors concluded that reproducibility of the updated Kiel classification is inadequate in its present form. They also emphasized the need for more objective criteria for the various morpho-logical categories. Attempts have also been made to apply the Working Formulation (WF) to comparative studies of B- and T-cell lymphomas (Cheng et al 1989). The WF does not even include any formal distinction between T- and B-cell neoplasms and this exercise appears to be neither scientifically valid nor intellectually satisfying.

At least two further entities need to be added to the updated Kiel classification of T-cell lymphomas. One is the enteropathy associated T-cell lymphoma mentioned above and the other is angiocentric T-cell lymphoma. These aggressive tumours may occur in the skin, nose and nasopharyngeal region and may well also include lymphomatoid granulomatosis (Chan et al 1988). The infiltrate tends to be pleomorphic and polymorphic and is often accompanied by widespread coagulative necrosis. It may penetrate in and around nerves and extend into the subcutaneous tissue. In Japan 75% of lymphomas arising in the nasal mucosa were of T-cell type, more than half were HTLV-1 positive and these latter cases carried a particularly poor prognosis (Uchinozo et al 1990).

PROGNOSIS

The lack of a single agreed classification system and the frequent difficulties in diagnosis and categorization do not make a comparison easy between different series. One study in Austria has looked at 75 cases using the updated Kiel classification (Chott et al 1990). Although 37% of patients experienced a complete remission, survival was poor with a median rate of 23 months. Peripheral T-cell lymphomas of pleomorphic medium and large cell type were the most aggressive with a median survival rate of 8 months. At diagnosis, three quarters of cases were stage III or IV and bad prognostic indicators were Ki-67 positivity and the presence of 'B' symptoms.

In Japan, the poor overall response rate and survival of all cases of malignant lymphoma is largely attributed to the considerable excess of HTLV-1 induced cases (Shimize et al 1989). In one North American study the picture was less clear cut. The most striking difference was in Stage IV cases with a 3-year survival of 44% for B-cell but 0% for T-cell lymphomas. The prognosis is so bad in this latter group that other and more drastic forms of therapy should perhaps be contemplated and the value of bone-marrow transplantation and targeted monoclonal antibodies ('magic bullets') are currently under consideration.

REFERENCES

Acuto O, Reinherz E L 1985 The human T-cell receptor, structure and function. New England Journal of Medicine 312: 1100–1111
Angel C A, Warford A, Campbell A C et al 1987 The immunohistology of Hodgkin's disease—Reed-Sternberg cells and their variants. Journal of Pathology 153: 21–30
Angel C A, Warford A, Day S J et al 1989 Comparative quality assessment in immuno-cytochemistry: pilot study of CD15 staining in paraffin wax embedded tissue in Hodgkin's disease. Journal of Clinical Pathology 42: 1096–1100
Bernard S M 1988 Epidemiology of malignant lymphomas. In: Habeshaw J A, Lauder I (eds) Malignant lymphomas. Churchill Livingstone, Edinburgh, pp 6–31
Bonagura V R, Katz B Z, Edwards B L et al 1990 Severe chronic EBV infection associated with specific EBV immunodeficiency and an EBNA + T-cell lymphoma containing linear, EBV DNA. Clinical Immunology and Immunopathology 57: 32–44
Born W, Rathbun G, Tucker P et al 1986 Synchronised rearrangement of T-cell gamma and beta chain genes in fetal thymocyte development. Science 234: 479–482
Borst J, van Dongen J, Bolhuis R L H et al 1988 Distinct molecular forms of human T-cell receptor gamma/delta detected on viable T-cells by a monoclonal antibody. Journal of Experimental Medicine 167: 1625–1644
Brown L A, Wiselka M, Campbell A et al 1991 High grade T-cell lymphoma following treatment with cyclosporin A. Histopathology (in press)
Burke J S, Warnke R A, Connors J M et al 1985 Diffuse malignant lymphoma with cerebriform nuclei: a B-cell lymphoma studied with monoclonal antibodies. American Journal of Clinical Pathology 83: 753–759
Campana D, Janossy G, Coustan-Smith et al 1989 The expression of T-cell receptor associated proteins during T-cell ontogeny in man. Journal of Immunology 142: 57–66
Chan J K, Ng C S, Ngan K C et al 1988 Angiocentric T-cell lymphoma of the skin. An aggressive lymphoma distinct from mycosis fungoides. American Journal of Surgical Pathology 12: 861–876
Charley M, McCoy J P, Deng J S et al 1990 Anti-V region antibodies as 'almost clonotypic' reagents for the study of cutaneous T-cell lymphomas and leukemias. Journal of Investigative Dermatology 95: 614–617
Cheng A-L, Chen Y-C, Wang C-H et al 1989 Direct comparisons of peripheral T-cell lymphoma with diffuse B-cell lymphoma of comparable histological grades—should peripheral T-cell lymphoma be considered separately? Journal of Clinical Oncology 7: 725–731
Chott A, Augustin I, Wrba F et al 1990 Peripheral T-cell lymphomas: a clinicopathologic study of 75 cases. Human Pathology 21: 1117–1125
Eyden B P, Cross P A, Harris M 1990 The ultrastructure of signet-ring cell non-Hodgkin's lymphoma. Virchows Archiv A (Pathological Anatomy) 417: 395–404
Falini B, Pileri S, De-Solas I et al 1990 Peripheral T-cell lymphoma associated with haemophagocytic syndrome. Blood 75: 434–444
Falzon M, Isaacson P G 1990 Histological classification of the non-Hodgkin's lymphoma. Blood Reviews 4: 111–115
Fowlkes B J, Pardol D M 1989 Molecular and cellular events of T-cell development. Advances in Immunology 44: 207–264

Gallo R C, Sliski A, Wong-Staal F 1983 Origin of human T-cell leukaemia/lymphoma virus. Lancet ii: 2962–2963

Garvin A J, Self S, Sahome E A et al 1988 The occurrence of a peripheral T-cell lymphoma in a chronically immunosuppressed renal transplant patient. American Journal of Surgical Pathology 12: 64–70

Gjerset R A, Yeargin J, Volkman S K et al 1990 Insulin-like growth factor-I supports proliferation of autocrine thymic lymphoma cells with a pre-T-cell phenotype. Journal of Immunology 145: 3497–3501

Gledhill S, Krajewski A S, Dewar A E et al 1990 Analysis of T-cell receptor and immunoglobulin gene rearrangements in the diagnosis of Hodgkin's and non-Hodgkin's lymphoma. Journal of Pathology 161: 245–254

Haas W, Kaufman S, Martinez A C 1990 The development and function of γδ T-cells. Immunology Today II: 340–343

Habeshaw J A 1988 The immune system and lymphoma. In: Habeshaw J A, Lauder I (eds) Malignant lymphomas. Churchill Livingstone, Edinburgh, pp 48–88

Hall P A, d'Ardenne J, Stansfeld A G 1988 Paraffin section immunohistochemistry. 1. Non-Hodgkin's lymphoma. Histopathology 13: 149–160

Harabuchi Y, Yamanaka N, Kataura A et al 1990 Epstein–Barr virus in nasal T-cell lymphomas in patients with lethal midline granuloma. Lancet 335: 128–130

Hastrup N, Hamilton-Dutoit S, Ralfkiaer E et al 1991 Peripheral T-cell lymphomas: an evaluation of reproducibility of the updated Kiel classification. Histopathology 18: 99–105

Hollema H, Poppema S 1989 T-lymphoblastic and peripheral T-cell lymphomas in the northern part of the Netherlands. Cancer 64: 1620–1628

Hunkapiller T, Hood L 1989 Diversity of the immunoglobulin gene super family. Advances in Immunology 44: 1–63

Isaacson P G, Jones D B, Sworn M J et al 1982 Malignant histiocytosis of the intestine: report of three cases with immunological and cytochemical analysis. Journal of Clinical Pathology 35: 510–516

Isaacson P G, O'Connor N T J, Spencer J et al 1985 Malignant histiocytosis of the intestine: a T-cell lymphoma. Lancet ii: 688–691

Kadin M E, Kamoun M, Lamberg J 1981 Erythrophagocytic Tγ lymphoma—a clinicopathological entity resembling malignant histiocytosis. New England Journal of Medicine 304: 648–653

Kalyanaraman V S, Sarngadharan M G, Robert-Guroff M et al 1982 A new subtype of human T-cell leukaemia virus (HTLV-II) associated with a T-cell variant of hairy cell leukemia. Science 218: 571–573

Katz R L, Gritsman A, Cabanillas F et al 1989 Fine-needle aspiration cytology of peripheral T-cell lymphoma. A cytologic, immunologic, and cytometric study. American Journal of Clinical Pathology 91: 120–131

Kemnitz J, Cremer J, Gebel M et al 1990 T-cell lymphoma after heart transplantation. American Journal of Clinical Pathology 94: 95–101

Kim H, Dorfman R F, Rappaport H 1978 Signet ring cell lymphoma—a rare morphologic and functional expression of nodular (follicular) lymphoma. American Journal of Surgical Pathology 2: 119–132

Kimura N, Takihara Y, Akiyoshi T et al 1989 Rearrangement of T-cell receptor δ chain gene as a marker of lineage and clonality in T-cell lymphoproliferative disorders. Cancer Research 49: 4488–4492

Knowles D M 1989 Immunophenotypic and antigen gene rearrangement analysis in T-cell neoplasia. American Journal of Pathology 143: 761–785

Kronenberg M, Siu G, Hood L et al 1986 The molecular genetics of the T-cell antigen receptor and T-cell antigen recognition. Annual Review of Immunology 4: 529–591

Lancet 1991 Editorial: Gamma/delta T-cell receptor. Lancet 337: 207–208

Lauder I, Bird C C, Child J A et al 1985 Surface membrane phenotypic expression and treatment response of malignant lymphomas. Journal of Pathology 145: 259–268

Lee P Y, Charley M, Tharp M et al 1990 Possible role of Epstein–Barr virus infection in cutaneous T-cell lymphoma. Journal of Investigative Dermatology 95: 309–312

Libetta C M, Pringle J H, Angel C A et al 1990 Demonstration of Epstein–Barr viral DNA in formalin fixed paraffin-embedded samples of Hodgkin's disease. Journal of Pathology 161: 255–260

Mason D Y, Cordell J L, Brown M et al 1989 Detection of T-cells in paraffin wax embedded tissue using antibodies against a peptide sequence from the CD3 antigen. Journal of Clinical Pathology 42: 1194–1200

McCarthy K P, Sloane J P, Wiedemann L M 1990 Rapid method for distinguishing clonal from polyclonal B-cell populations in surgical biopsy specimens. Journal of Clinical Pathology. 43: 429–432

McCarthy K P, Sloane J P, Kabarowski J H S et al 1991 The rapid detection of clonal T-cell proliferations in patients with lymphoid disorders. American Journal of Pathology (in press)

Mori N, Oka K, Yoda Y et al 1990 T-cell receptor expression in the T-cell malignancies. American Journal of Clinical Pathology 93: 495–501

Myskow M W, Krajewski A S, Salter D M et al 1988 Paraffin section immunophenotyping of non-Hodgkin's lymphoma, using a panel of monoclonal antibodies. American Journal of Clinical Pathology 90: 564–574

Nagatini T, Matsuzaki T, Iemoto G et al 1990 Comparative study of cutaneous T-cell lymphoma and adult T-cell leukemia/lymphoma. Clinical, histopathologic, and immunohistochemical analysis. Cancer 66: 2380–2386

Ng C S, Chan J K C, Hui P K et al 1989 Large B-cell lymphomas with a high content of reactive T-cells. Human Pathology 20: 1145–1154

O'Brien C, Lampert I A, Catovsky D 1983 The histopathology of adult T-cell lymphoma/leukaemia in blacks from the Caribbean. Histopathology 7: 349–364

Oertel J, Oertel B, Kastner M et al 1988 The value of immunocytochemical staining of lymph node aspirates in diagnostic cytology. British Journal of Haematology 70: 307–316

Oliver J D, Grogan T M, Payne C M et al 1988 Burkitt's-like lymphoma of T-cell type. Modern Pathology 1: 15–22

Picker L J, Weiss L M, Medeiros L J et al 1987 Immunophenotypic criteria for the diagnosis of non-Hodgkin's lymphoma. American Journal of Pathology 128: 181–201

Poiesz B J, Ruscetti F W, Reitz M S et al 1981 Isolation of a new type-C retrovirus (HTLV) in primary uncultured cells of a patient with Sézary T-cell leukaemia. Nature 294: 268–271

Ralfkiaer E, Delsol G, O'Connor N T J et al 1990 Malignant lymphoma of true histiocytic origin. A clinical, histological, immunophenotypic and genotypic study. Journal of Pathology 160: 9–17

Ramsay A S, Smith W J, Isaacson P G 1988 T-cell rich B-cell lymphoma. American Journal of Surgical Pathology 12: 433–443

Reis M D, Griesser H, Mak T W 1988 Gene rearrangements in leukemias and lymphomas. Recent Advances in Haematology 5: 99–120

Russo G, Haluska F G, Isobe M et al 1988 Molecular basis of B- and T-cell neoplasia. Recent Advances in Haematology 5: 121–130

Sarin P S, Gallo R C 1985 T-cell malignancies and human T-cell leukemia (lymphotropic) retroviruses (HTLV). Haematopoietic Stem Cell Physiology 184: 445–456

Shimizu K, Hamajima N, Ohnishi K et al 1989 T-cell phenotype is associated with decreased survival in non-Hodgkin's lymphoma. Japanese Journal of Cancer 80: 720–726

Shorrock K, Ellis I O, Finch R G 1990 T-cell lymphoma associated with human immuno-deficiency (HIV) infection. Histopathology 16: 189–191

Smith J L, Jones D B, Bell A J et al 1988a Correlation between histology and immuno-phenotype in a series of 322 cases of non-Hodgkin's lymphoma. Haematology and Oncology 7: 37–48

Smith J L, Haegert D G, Hodges E et al 1988b Phenotypic and genotypic heterogeneity of peripheral T-cell lymphoma. British Journal of Cancer 58: 723–729

Spier C M, Lippman S M, Miller T P et al 1988 Lennert's lymphoma. A clinicopathological study with emphasis on phenotype and its relationship to survival. Cancer 61: 517–524

Stansfeld A G 1985 Lymph node biopsy interpretation. Churchill Livingstone, Edinburgh

Stansfeld A G, Diebold J, Noel H et al 1988 Updated Kiel classification for lymphomas. Lancet i: 292–293

Stein H, Dienemann D, Sperling M et al 1988 Identification of a T-cell lymphoma category derived from intestinal-mucosa-associated T-cells. Lancet ii: 1053–1054

Su I-J, Wang C-H, Cheng A-L et al 1988 Characterization of the spectrum of postthymic T-cell malignancies in Taiwan. A clinicopathologic study of HTLV-I-positive and HTLV-I-negative cases. Cancer 61: 2060–2070

Suchi T, Lennert K, Tu L-Y et al 1987 Histopathology and histochemistry of peripheral
   T-cell lymphomas: a proposal for their classification. Journal of Clinical Pathology 40:
   995–1015
Sun T, Brody J, Susin M et al 1990 Extranodal T-cell lymphoma mimicking malignant
   histiocytosis. American Journal of Haematology 35: 269–274
Tonegawa S 1983 Somatic generation of antibody diversity. Nature 302: 575–581
Toyonaga B, Mak T W 1987 Genes of the T-cell antigen receptor in normal and malignant
   T-cells. Annual Review of Immunology 5: 585–620
Uchinozo A, Fukuda K, Itoh K et al 1990 A clinical and immunological study on non-
   Hodgkin's malignant lymphoma in the nasosinus region. Nippon Jibiinkoka Gakkai Kaiho
   93: 554–565
Ueshima Y, Rowley J D, Variakojis D et al 1984 Cytogenetic studies on patients with chronic
   T-cell leukemia/lymphoma. Blood 63: 1028–1031
Van Krieken J H J M, Feller A C, Velde J et al 1989 The distribution of non-Hodgkin's
   lymphoma in the lymphoid compartments of the human spleen. American Journal of
   Surgical Pathology 13: 757–765
Weiss A, Imboden J, Hardy K et al 1986 The role of the T3/antigen receptor complex in
   T-cell activation. Annual Review of Immunology 4: 593–619
Weiss R L, Kjeldsberg C R, Colby T V et al 1985 Multilobated B-cell lymphomas.
   Haematology and Oncology 3: 79–86
West K P, Warford A, Fray L et al 1986 The demonstration of B-cell, T-cell and myeloid
   antigens in paraffin sections. Journal of Pathology 150: 89–101
Wieczorek R, Burke J S, Knowles D M 1985 Leu-M1 antigen expression in T-cell neoplasia.
   American Journal of Pathology 12: 374–380
Wright D H 1988 Histiocytic malignancies. In: Habeshaw J A, Lauder I (eds) Malignant
   lymphomas. Churchill Livingstone, Edinburgh, pp 217–238
Yanagi Y, Yoshikai, Leggett K et al 1984 A human T-cell-specific cDNA clone encodes a
   protein having extensive homology to immunoglobulin chains. Nature 308: 145–149
Zinkernagel R M, Doherty P C 1975 H-2 compatibility requirement for T-cell-mediated lysis
   of target cells infected with lymphocytic choriomeningitis virus. Different cytotoxic T-cell
   specificities are associated with structures coded for in H-2K or H-2D. Journal of
   Experimental Medicine 141: 1427–1437

6

Soft tissue tumours: an update

C. D. M. Fletcher

Soft tissue tumours remain a source of diagnostic anxiety and confusion among many histopathologists, largely because distinctive new entities continue to be described with monotonous regularity. This has necessitated repeated and radical changes to the classification and nomenclature of connective tissue neoplasms over the last 25 years. Increasing sub-categorization has, however, allowed a greater insight into the biology and natural history of different tumour types, and hence it has provided a more rational basis upon which to predict prognosis and to plan treatment. It has also helped to dispel the widespread misconception that soft tissue sarcomas form a particularly aggressive and almost invariably fatal group of tumours. It must always be remembered that the average 5 year survival figure of 65% for all sarcomas is substantially better than that of the most common carcinomas. Accurate classification has also established the cornerstone upon which molecular or genetic studies are based, since findings such as oncogene amplification, gene expression or a reciprocal translocation are far more valuable when correlated with the clinical and histological features. This chapter aims to address recent advances in our knowledge of soft tissue neoplasia under the general headings of new entities, conceptual changes and the impact of new technology.

NEW ENTITIES

Under this heading, some of the more important soft tissue tumours which have been first recognized or accurately delineated over the last 5 years or so are described.

Spindle cell haemangioendothelioma

Spindle cell haemangioendothelioma was first described as a 'low grade variant of angiosarcoma' by Weiss & Enzinger (1986). It most often presents superficially in the distal extremities (especially hands and feet) of adolescents or young adults of either sex (Weiss & Enzinger 1986, Scott & Rosai 1988, Fletcher et al 1991) but, overall, has a wide age range. Approximately 50% of patients either present with, or later develop, multiple lesions and

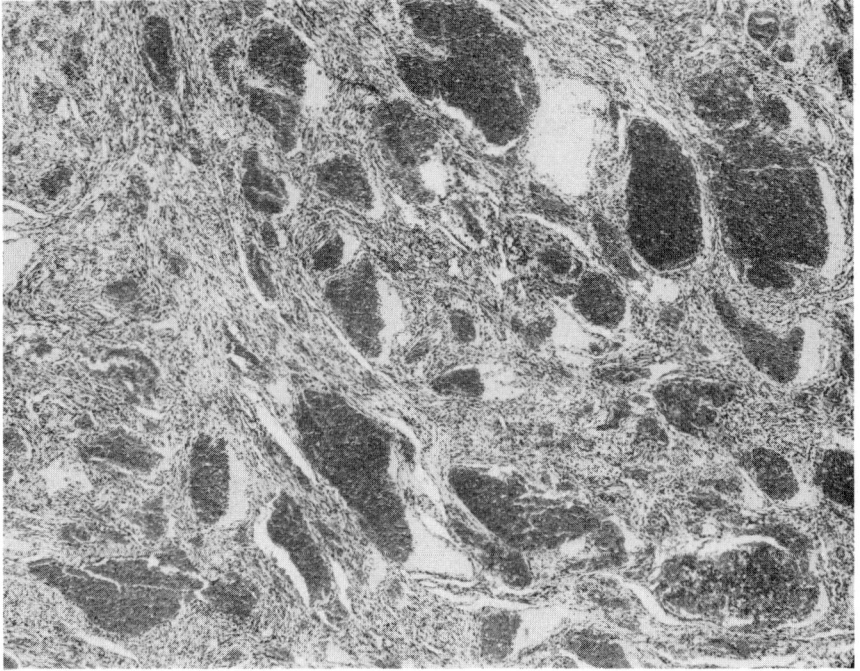

Fig. 6.1 Spindle cell haemangioendothelioma. Note in this case the almost even admixture of blood-filled cavernous spaces and intervening spindle cell areas. H & E × 40. (Reproduced with permission from Fletcher et al 1991.)

generally in the same anatomical region. A small proportion of patients have clinical evidence of an associated developmental (usually vascular) anomaly, such as congenital lymphoedema, Klippel–Trenaunay syndrome or Maffucci's syndrome. New lesions (or so-called recurrences) tend to develop in previously unaffected skin or soft tissue and to spread proximally in a clinically alarming fashion but long-standing lesions may also regress spontaneously (Fletcher et al 1991). To date, only a single case has been reported to metastasize (Weiss & Enzinger 1986), and there is good reason to believe that this example had, in fact, transformed to a biologically separate post-irradiation sarcoma.

Macroscopically, each individual lesion usually appears as a reddish-blue, dermal or subcutaneous nodule which seldom exceeds 2 cm in diameter. On sectioning, gaping vascular spaces, sometimes containing thrombi, may be seen.

Histologically, the lesion has a characteristic and consistent appearance. The cardinal features are thin-walled, dilated vascular spaces and inter-vening solid, spindle cell areas, admixed in variable proportions (Fig. 6.1). The vascular spaces are generally lined by a single layer of bland-looking endothelium and the main point of concern is the solid element. This

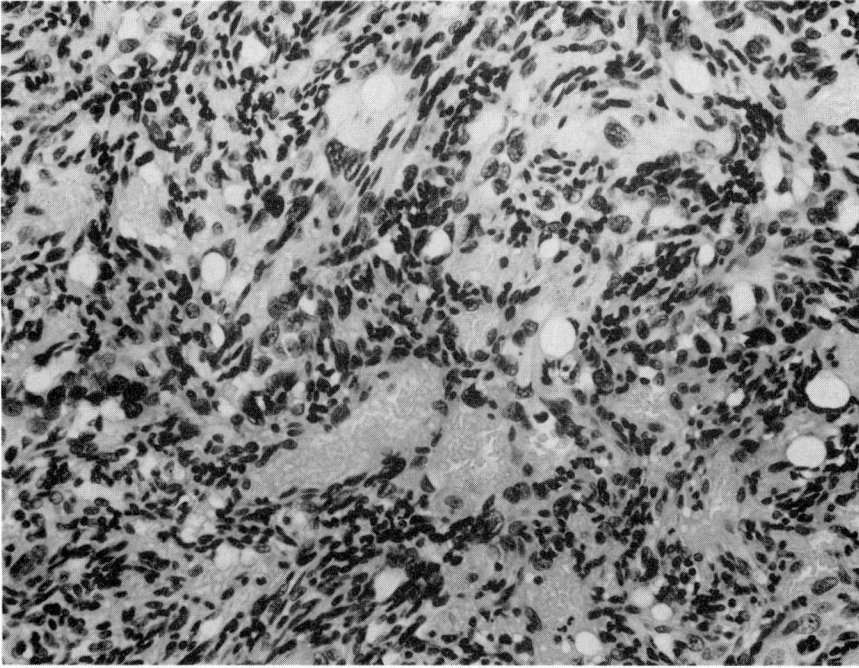

Fig. 6.2 Spindle cell haemangioendothelioma. The solid areas are composed of bland spindle cells, admixed with cells containing plump vesicular nuclei and cells showing cytoplasmic vacuolation, a useful distinguishing feature from Kaposi's sarcoma. H & E × 250.

consists mainly of cells with ill-defined eosinophilic cytoplasm which have either tapering, spindle-shaped nuclei or plump, vesicular ('epithelioid') nuclei (often with a single nucleolus), along with a small number of rounded cells, the cytoplasm of which is entirely occupied by a single large vacuole or 'lumen' (Fig. 6.2). There is little or no nuclear pleomorphism and mitoses are few. Within these solid areas slit-like spaces are frequently present, some of which are lined by eosinophilic cells as above and they contain red blood cells.

Other distinctive features are: (1) the common presence of elongated papillary structures, covered by plump endothelial cells, which typically project into the cavernous spaces; (2) smooth muscle bundles (often best demonstrated immunohistochemically) either at the periphery of cavernous spaces or dispersed irregularly in the solid areas; and (3) the almost invariable finding of malformed thick or thin-walled vessels (often very suggestive of arteriovenous shunting) which are generally distributed at the periphery of the nodule(s). Combining the dubious nature of the single case associated with metastasis with the clinical or histological evidence that these lesions are often associated with either a malformed vasculature or a local anomaly of blood flow, it has been suggested that spindle cell haemangioendotheliomas should not be regarded as malignant and may not even be truly neoplastic (Fletcher et al 1991). This would also be borne out by the fact that these lesions seem not to genuinely recur (i.e. not at the previous site of excision) and also that they have been flow cytometrically diploid in all cases examined personally to date.

Bacillary angiomatosis

First described under the rubric 'epithelioid angiomatosis' (Cockerell et al 1987), this is a distinctive, often multifocal, reactive vascular proliferation which is almost invariably associated with the acquired immunodeficiency syndrome (AIDS). Bacillary angiomatosis appears to affect predominantly patients in the homosexual or intravenous drug abuse groups (Koehler et al 1988, LeBoit et al 1989). Clinically, it most often presents with multiple cutaneous, superficial subcutaneous or mucosal vascular nodules or papules, which closely mimic Kaposi's sarcoma. Rare cases of a deep soft tissue mass (Schinella & Greco 1990) and visceral, osseous or lymph node involvement have been described. Recognition of this entity is of particular value since it responds impressively to antibiotics, particularly erythromycin (Skaniawski et al 1990), but, if left untreated, it is potentially fatal (Cockerell et al 1987).

Histologically, bacillary angiomatosis bears a superficial resemblance to pyogenic granuloma (lobular capillary haemangioma) or epithelioid hae-mangioma, depending on the depth of the lesion (LeBoit et al 1989, Walford et al 1990). It is generally composed of small, capillary-sized vessels, often arranged in a lobular pattern, set in a variably oedematous or fibrotic stroma. The endothelial lining is typically plump with pale eosinophilic cytoplasm and vesicular nuclei (hence 'epithelioid') and it sometimes shows cytoplasmic vacuolation. Endothelial cells may be large enough to obliterate the vascular lumina, giving the lesion a solid appearance and, in these cases, reticulin staining is useful to demonstrate the vascular architecture. Pleomorphism may be striking and normal mitoses are often evident. A characteristic and diagnostically helpful feature is the presence of neutro-phil polymorphs and/or polymorph nuclear debris, often arranged in clusters, within the stroma which typically contains plump fibroblasts (Fig. 6.3). Another distinctive feature is the finding of amphophilic granular debris, often resembling fibrin, either adjacent to or occasionally within vascular lumina. Staining by the Warthin–Starry technique demonstrates numerous, small rod-shaped bacilli, which may either correspond to the granular debris as above or lie loosely in the stroma.

Stoler et al (1983) were the first to identify these bacilli and they have subsequently been confirmed as the causative agent (Cockerell & Friedman-Kien 1988, Koehler et al 1988, LeBoit et al 1988). They are currently believed to be closely related to, if not identical with, the cat-scratch bacillus. It is of interest to note the striking histological similarities between bacillary angiomatosis and another vasoformative lesion induced by bacilli,

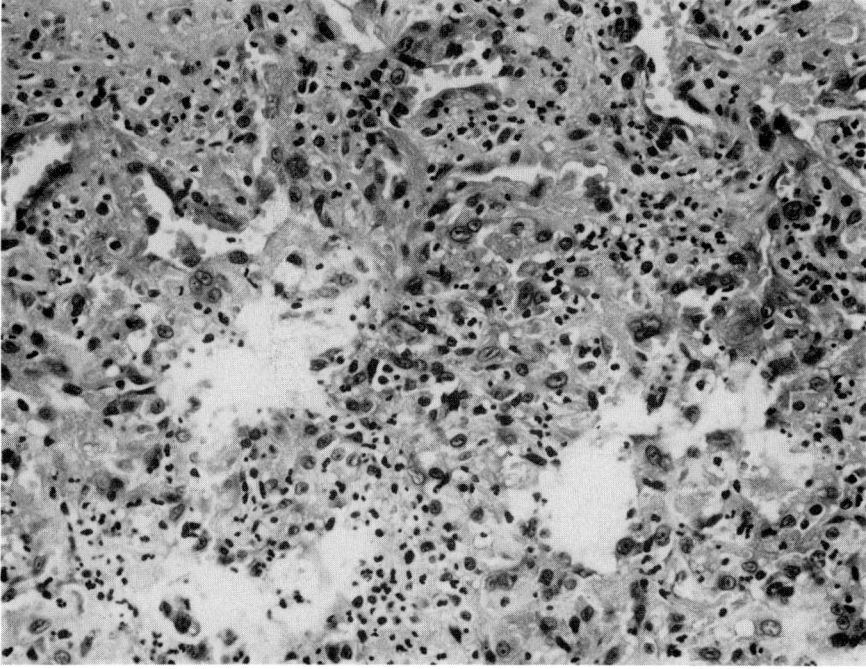

Fig. 6.3 Bacillary angiomatosis. Note the markedly epithelioid appearance of the endothelial cells and the prominent infiltrate of neutrophil polymorphs. H & E × 250.

namely verruga peruana. This represents a characteristic phase of Oroya fever (due to *Bartonella bacilliformis*), a condition which is largely confined to the South American subcontinent (Arias-Stella et al 1986, 1987).

Glomeruloid haemangioma

This recently described vascular lesion (Chan et al 1990) merits brief mention because of its implications for systemic disease. Patients present with multiple cutaneous vascular nodules or papules, again clinically reminiscent of Kaposi's sarcoma. Histologically, it is characterized by a lobular proliferation of thin-walled capillaries within the lumina of numerous ectatic dermal vessels. A diagnostic feature is the presence, within the intercapillary stroma, of plump, epithelioid endothelial cells, many of which contain intracytoplasmic eosinophilic globules, probably corresponding to immunoglobulin. The clinical significance of glomeruloid haemangioma is its close association with multicentric Castleman's disease (angiofollicular lymphoid hyperplasia) complicated by POEMS (poly-neuropathy, organomegaly, endocrinopathy, monoclonal gammopathy, skin lesions) syndrome. The haemangiomas may precede any clinical evidence of Castleman's disease or its other systemic manifestations and

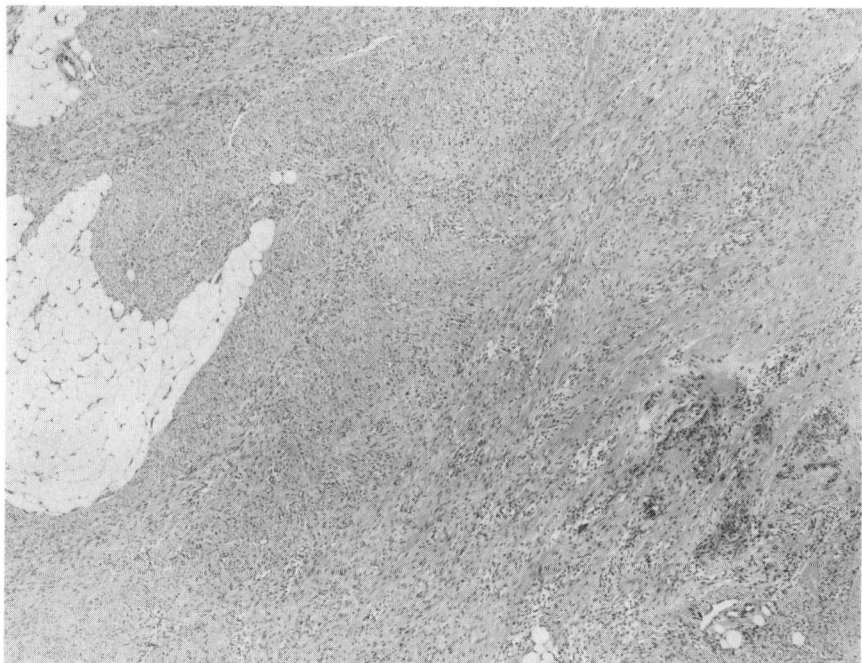

Fig. 6.4   Plexiform fibrohistiocytic tumour. The fibroblastic component, centred on the dermal/subcutaneous junction, closely resembles a fibromatosis. H & E × 40.

therefore thorough investigation and careful follow-up are indicated in any case of glomeruloid haemangioma.

Plexiform fibrohistiocytic tumour

This further addition to the family of so-called 'fibrohistiocytic' neoplasms was first described in a series of 65 cases by Enzinger & Zhang (1988). Plexiform fibrohistiocytic tumour, in the majority of cases, develops before the age of 30 and is commonest in young children. Females are affected more often than males. The single most frequent site is the upper limb, particularly the forearm/elbow region, but the anatomical distribution is wide. The lesion, which is almost invariably solitary, presents as a slowly growing, ill-defined, firm dermal or subcutaneous nodule. Because of the poorly circumscribed, infiltrative nature of most cases, many lesions tend, at least initially, to be inadequately excised and this almost certainly accounts for the high local recurrence rate. Two patients developed local lymph node metastases but, to date, there has been no report of systemic spread or death.

Macroscopically, these tumours tend to have an ill-defined appearance, usually consisting of ramifying, pale, fibrous trabeculae and/or nodular foci, the whole of which rarely exceeds 3–4 cm in maximum diameter.

Plexiform fibrohistiocytic tumour has a distinctive histological appearance

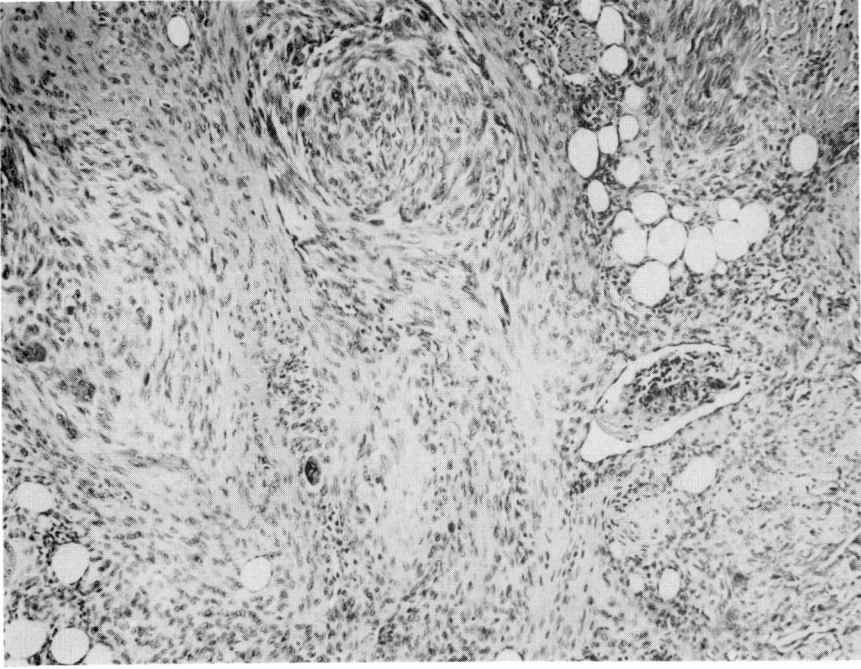

Fig. 6.5   Plexiform fibrohistiocytic tumour. This more 'histiocytic' looking example shows ill-defined aggregates of plump cells with vesicular nuclei and a few osteoclast-like giant cells. Note also the focus of vascular invasion, as may occasionally be seen. H & E × 100.

but there is a wide spectrum depending on the relative proportions of the two principal components. These consist, respectively, of infiltrating fibroblastic fascicles and of nodules or aggregates of plump, eosinophilic histiocyte-like cells. The 'fibroblastic' component, when predominant, closely resembles fibromatosis, being usually only moderately cellular with bland, monomorphic nuclei (Fig. 6.4). It differs from fibromatosis in two significant ways: first, it is superficially located, generally being centred on the dermal/subcutaneous junction, and, second, it has an unusual growth pattern typified by numerous ramifying trabeculae which seem to 'anas- tomose' in a random fashion, leaving islands of normal tissue trapped within the lesion. The 'histiocytic' component, which is effectively the diagnostic feature, may take the form of either ill-defined aggregates or discrete nodules. These are composed of plump, usually eosinophilic, epithelioid cells with vesicular nuclei associated with variable numbers of osteoclast- like multinucleate cells and chronic inflammatory cells (Fig. 6.5). Within or adjacent to these nodules, there is often striking extravasation of red blood cells and, occasionally, extensive haemosiderin deposition. Some of these nodules, particularly in older patients, may undergo marked peripheral or, less often, total hyalinization. There is no significant nuclear pleomorphism and mitoses are few but, in a minority of cases, vascular invasion may be evident.

This distinctive neoplasm was classified as 'fibrohistiocytic' because of the histiocyte-like appearance of the epithelioid nodular element and its immunohistochemical positivity for alpha-1-antitrypsin and alpha-1-antichymotrypsin in some cases. These enzymes have, however, been entirely discredited as histiocytic markers (Soini & Miettinen 1988, 1989). Personal experience of about 15 cases has shown that the epithelioid nodular element co-expresses smooth muscle actin and CD68 (a reputedly reliable marker of monocyte/macrophage differentiation). The significance of these results is as yet uncertain but clearly they set this entity apart from the other so-called fibrohistiocytic tumours. It is interesting to note that cytogenetic analysis of a single case has revealed a complex karyotype including an ill-defined translocation and two deletions (Smith et al 1990).

Deep benign fibrous histiocytoma

Although briefly mentioned in the standard text on soft tissue tumours (Enzinger & Weiss 1988), it is not widely appreciated that benign fibrous histiocytoma may arise in deep soft tissues and the clinicopathological features of such lesions have only been delineated recently (Fletcher 1990).

Deep benign fibrous histiocytoma is predominantly a tumour of adulthood and is commoner in males. Occasional cases do, however, present in childhood or even infancy. The anatomical distribution is wide but the most frequently affected sites are the lower limb or head and neck region. The tumour develops as a slowly growing, painless mass, more often situated in the deep subcutis than within skeletal muscle and occasional cases are intra-abdominal. Despite their worrying histological features, these tumours seem only to recur after inadequate excision.

Macroscopically, in contrast to their cutaneous counterparts, deep fibrous histiocytomas are well circumscribed or pseudoencapsulated and commonly measure 5 cm or more in diameter. The cut surface is firm, pale to tan coloured and may occasionally show cystic change or haemorrhage, but necrosis is not a feature.

Histologically, these lesions more closely resemble dermatofibrosarcoma than cutaneous fibrous histiocytoma, but they lack the ill-defined, infiltrative margins of the former. Tumour cells are monomorphic, spindle-shaped and palely eosinophilic with either tapering or plump, vesicular nuclei. They show limited mitotic activity and are characteristically arranged in a storiform pattern (Fig. 6.6). The stroma may show varying degrees of myxoid change or hyalinization and the hyaline collagen often has a brightly eosinophilic, wiry appearance or a stellate 'amianthoid' configuration. Inflammatory cells are usually sparse. Foamy (xanthoma) cells or osteoclast-like multinucleate giant cells are seen in a third or so of cases. The vasculature is inconspicuous in most examples but a marked, branching, haemangiopericytoma-like pattern may be seen in some (Fig. 6.7). Rarely,

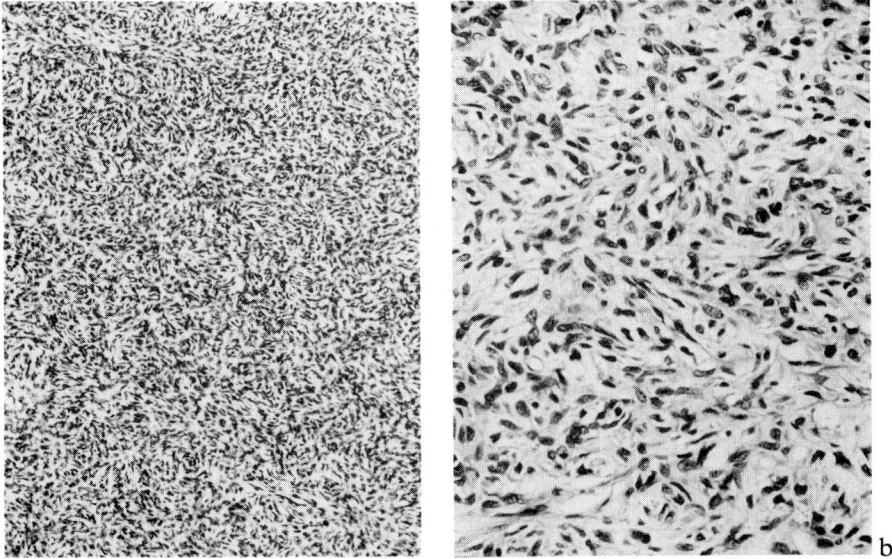

Fig. 6.6 Deep benign fibrous histiocytoma. **(a)** Note the storiform dermatofibrosarcoma-like pattern. These lesions, however, do not have irregular infiltrative margins. H & E × 90. **(b)** Closer examination reveals the mixed tapering and vesicular nuclei of the spindle cell population. Inflammatory cells are sparse. H & E × 225. (Both **(a)** and **(b)** reproduced with permission from Fletcher 1990.)

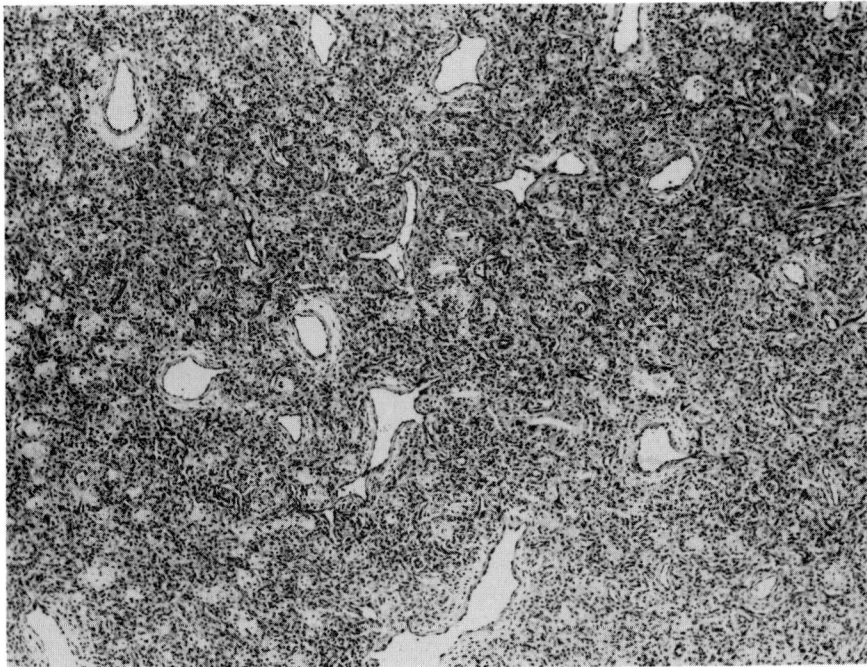

Fig. 6.7 Deep benign fibrous histiocytoma: a striking vascular pattern that may be confused with haemangiopericytoma. H & E × 63. (Reproduced with permission from Fletcher 1990.)

small foci of suppurative necrosis or vascular invasion may be evident but there is no evidence to date that these 'worrisome' features correlate with malignant behaviour; nevertheless, it is perhaps wise to be guarded about prognosis in such cases.

As with other so-called fibrohistiocytic tumours, there is no evidence that these lesions show true monocyte/macrophage differentiation (Fletcher 1990) and their histogenesis is entirely unknown. However, the term deep benign fibrous histiocytoma is useful if only because it reflects a morphological pattern with which all histopathologists are familiar.

Intranodal myofibroblastoma

Although strictly speaking this is a tumour of lymph nodes, intranodal myofibroblastoma warrants description here because of its overt connective tissue morphology which may stimulate a mistaken diagnosis of metastatic sarcoma.

Intranodal myofibroblastoma was first described simultaneously under two different names (Suster & Rosai 1989, Weiss et al 1989). It most often presents as a solitary mass of variable duration in the groin of adults.

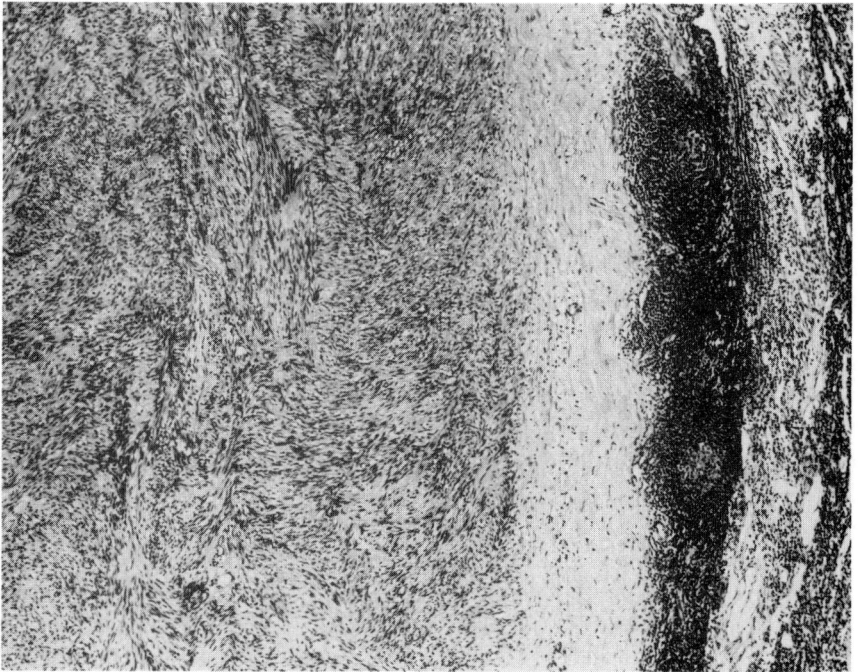

Fig. 6.8   Intranodal myofibroblastoma. A hyaline fibrous capsule separates this spindle cell tumour from the overlying attenuated lymph node cortex. H & E × 63. (Reproduced with permission from Fletcher & Stirling 1990.)

Although this anatomical location was originally considered to be a characteristic feature, cases have subsequently been described in the submandibular region (Fletcher & Stirling 1990) and, as time passes, this tumour may prove to have a wide topographical distribution. The clinical behaviour is entirely benign and there seems to be no tendency for even local recurrence, irrespective of the adequacy of excision.

Histologically, the tumour typically replaces almost all of the affected lymph node and is separated from a thin layer of residual cortical tissue by a dense hyaline capsule (Fig. 6.8). A nodal region may not be evident in some cases. The tumour is composed of short, interlacing bundles of pale eosinophilic spindle cells with vesicular, generally tapering nuclei, many of which contain a small nucleolus. Pleomorphism is absent and mitoses are few. Nuclear palisading may be marked focally and most cases bear a resemblance to either a schwannoma or a smooth muscle tumour. Other distinctive features are the presence of widespread interstitial haemorrhage, nodules of hyaline collagen with a rather stellate outline (so-called amianthoid fibres) (Fig. 6.9) and globular, fuchsinophilic intracytoplasmic inclusions which are probably composed of actin. Myxoid change and metaplastic bone may occasionally be seen.

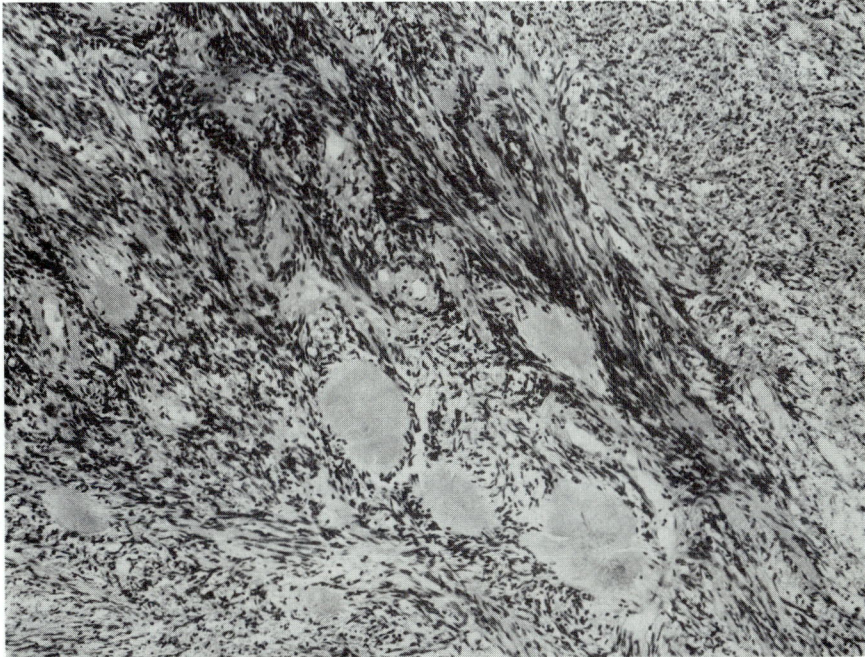

Fig. 6.9 Intranodal myofibroblastoma. The majority of cases show this striking 'amianthoid' pattern of hyalinization, which often appears to commence in blood vessel walls. H & E × 100.

Immunohistochemically, tumour cells express pan-muscle actin (HHF-35) and smooth muscle actin (IA4) but are desmin and S-100 negative. Together with the ultrastructural findings (Suster & Rosai 1989, Fletcher & Stirling 1990), these results support myofibroblastic differentiation. Previously, most of these lesions had been classified as lymph node schwannomas (Enzinger & Weiss 1988, Weiss et al 1989), an entity which may no longer exist.

Extra-renal rhabdoid tumour

This is the only truly new type of frankly malignant soft tissue tumour to be described in recent years and whether or not it is a genuinely discrete entity remains a matter of controversy. The term 'rhabdoid tumour' was originally coined for a group of paediatric renal tumours which were distinct from the subtype of Wilms tumour showing rhabdomyosarcomatous differentiation (Haas et al 1981). Histologically comparable lesions arising in soft tissue were recognized later (Gonzalez-Crussi et al 1982, Lynch et al 1983) and increasing numbers were reported (Tsuneyoshi et al 1985, Sotelo-Avila et al 1986, Kent et al 1987). Similar tumours have now been described at a wide variety of sites, including many visceral organs (Fletcher & McKee 1990).

Extra-renal rhabdoid tumours are commonest in young children but may present over a wide age range. They are typically large, rapidly growing masses which are usually insensitive to modern adjunctive therapies and the majority of patients die with disseminated disease in a short time.

Histologically, these tumours are usually arranged in a diffuse sheet-like pattern and tend to show widespread necrosis. The tumour cells are relatively small and round with copious eosinophilic cytoplasm (hence the resemblance to rhabdomyoblasts) and ovoid vesicular nuclei, which characteristically contain a prominent eosinophilic nucleolus. The diagnostic *sine qua non* is the presence, within the cytoplasm of many of these cells, of spherical, eosinophilic hyaline inclusions (Fig. 6.10), which may be weakly PAS-positive and diastase resistant. These inclusions correspond ultrastructurally to dense paranuclear aggregates of intermediate filaments. Areas of some tumours may show a more nonspecific spindle cell or anaplastic morphology. The characteristic inclusions are almost always vimentin and keratin positive but antigen expression by these tumours has proved to be amazingly heterogeneous, so that almost every conceivable group of markers has been reported as positive (Fletcher & McKee 1990, Carter et al 1989).

Current opinion favours the view that this phenotypic diversity simply reflects the shared morphology of a wide range of different neoplasms and that extrarenal rhabdoid tumour is not a discrete entity. This hypothesis is also borne out by the demonstration of typical rhabdoid cells in a variety of specific types of sarcoma (Tsuneyoshi et al 1987) and the author has recently seen a pigmented metastatic melanoma which showed the classical

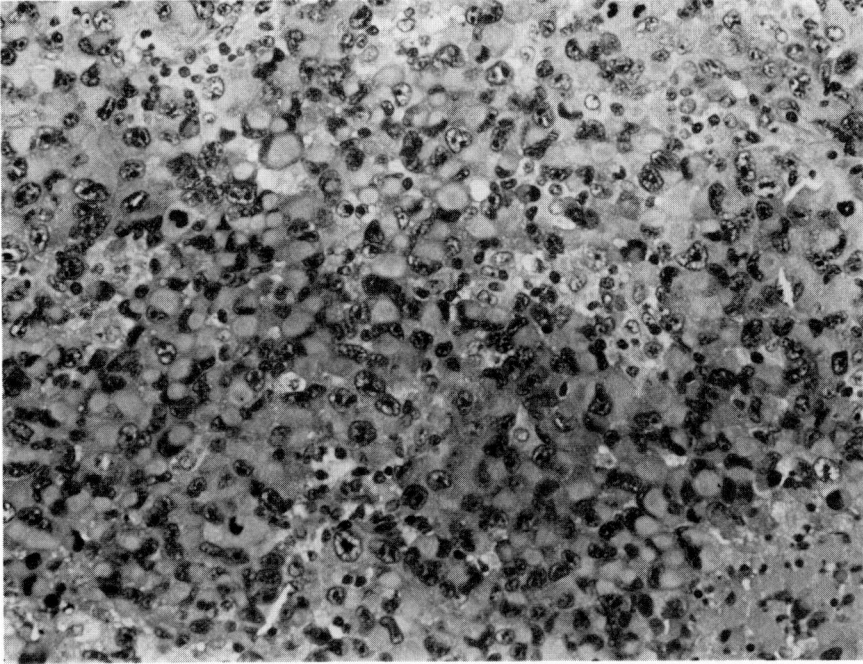

Fig. 6.10   Extra-renal rhabdoid tumour. These lesions, whether a discrete entity or not, share a common morphology characterized by striking hyaline intracytoplasmic inclusions and large vesicular nuclei with prominent nucleoli. H & E × 250.

rhabdoid morphology and immunophenotype in a lymph node metastasis (Bittesini et al 1991). Interestingly and in some ways surprisingly, renal rhabdoid tumours remain a uniform entity (Weeks et al 1989a,b).

Ossifying fibromyxoid tumour

This unusual and uncommon tumour was first delineated in a recent series of 59 cases from the Armed Forces Institute of Pathology (Enzinger et al 1989). Ossifying fibromyxoid tumour most often presents as a slowly growing mass in the deep subcutis or muscle of the proximal extremities of middle-aged adults, predominantly males. Radiological examination may reveal soft tissue calcification and, occasionally, erosion of underlying bone. Local recurrence is common after simple excision and may be multiple. In the original series, one recurrent lesion was said to have transformed to a well differentiated extraskeletal osteosarcoma and one other patient developed a probable metastasis in the contralateral thigh. No death has yet been reported.

Macroscopically, the mass is usually lobulated, well circumscribed and firm with a thick fibrous pseudocapsule. Most examples measure less than

5 cm in diameter but are occasionally much larger. The cut surface is generally pale and gritty to cut.

Histologically, a dense fibrous capsule is almost invariably present, which may include small islands of tumour and, in or adjacent to the deep aspect of this capsule, most cases have an incomplete peripheral shell of lamellar bone. Deeper in the tumour, trabeculae of bone or dense hyaline collagen are seen and impart a multilobular appearance to it. Tumour cells are generally small and round with indistinct, pale eosinophilic cytoplasm and small, vesicular nuclei. They are set in a rather loose fibromyxoid stroma, may show a trabecular growth pattern and exhibit only limited mitotic activity. Recurrences tend to be more cellular and have a more infiltrative growth pattern.

The histogenesis of ossifying fibromyxoid tumour remains a matter of speculation, but, based on S-100 positivity in 70% of cases, the presence of sulphated acid mucopolysaccharides and limited ultrastructural evidence, either a chondroid or neural origin seem most likely.

CONCEPTUAL CHANGES

Under this heading, an attempt is made to outline and explain some of the major changes that have occurred over recent years in our understanding or attitude to specific groups of tumours.

Well differentiated liposarcoma and atypical lipoma

It has gradually become apparent that well differentiated liposarcoma, in a histologically pure form, does not metastasize (Evans et al 1979, Kindblom et al 1982, Azumi et al 1987). This begs the question as to whether the term sarcoma is justified. Evans et al (1979) were the first to suggest the alternative term atypical lipoma but, in doing so, they limited its use specifically to lesions arising at accessible sites and amenable to wide excision, i.e. in the deep soft tissue of a limb. Histologically comparable tumours arise in the retroperitoneum which are usually inoperable and often kill by local recurrence alone. The term well differentiated liposarcoma (whether adipocytic, sclerosing or inflammatory) may justifiably be retained for lesions at this site.

The principal inference from this change is that if these lesions are completely and widely excised with an adequate margin of normal tissue, then the patient, for all practical purposes, is cured. This, however, raises several important points. First, before this confident outlook is conveyed to the patient, it is absolutely vital that the excised tumour is thoroughly sampled to exclude the presence of a higher grade or dedifferentiated component which would confer a quite different prognosis. Second, the surgeon must not be allowed to underestimate the significance of a diagnosis of atypical lipoma. Irrespective of terminology, if excision is marginal or inadequate, these tumours run at least a 30% risk of local recurrence. This might not appear too serious in view of the low grade nature of the tumour, but there is a significant risk that recurrence may be complicated by progression to a high grade or dedifferentiated liposarcoma (Fig. 6.11). In other words, undertreatment of a potentially curable neoplasm may leave one dealing with an aggressive sarcoma which metastasizes in around 50% of cases. Third, in order to avoid meaningless confusion, the term atypical lipoma should not be used to encompass the clinicopathologically distinct spindle cell and pleomorphic lipomas, which are exclusively subcutaneous in origin, very rarely recur and show no tendency to dedifferentiate.

The term atypical lipoma has also been employed (Kindblom et al 1982) to describe a group of fatty tumours arising in deep soft tissue which, although lacking in lipoblasts, show variation in adipocyte size, hyperchromasia of nuclei and often contain bizarre, frequently multinucleate cells in the stroma which may be extensively fibrotic (Fig. 6.12). Purists might argue that such lesions should not be grouped with well differentiated liposarcoma. Experience has shown, however, that this type of atypical lipoma also has an appreciable local recurrence rate and may also progress to a high grade or dedifferentiated liposarcoma.

Malignant fibrous histiocytoma

It is perhaps predictable and, to some, a source of unwanted confusion that malignant fibrous histiocytoma (MFH) should be discussed in a review of this type. Following the inadvertently ill-conceived introduction of this diagnostic term almost 30 years ago (for review, see Fletcher 1987), the concept of MFH has blossomed so that it is currently said to have five subtypes—pleomorphic/storiform, myxoid, giant cell, inflammatory and angiomatoid. Of these, the pleomorphic/storiform variant reputedly accounts for around 70% of the total number of cases and is widely regarded and accepted as the commonest single soft tissue sarcoma of late adult life (Enzinger 1986). Although this diagnosis was not widely employed until the 1970s (Kempson & Kyriakos 1972, Weiss & Enzinger 1978) and the initial reaction among histopathologists was antipathetic, MFH has become an extremely popular term to use not least, one suspects, because it provides an element of diagnostic convenience.

Pleomorphic MFH was originally regarded as a tumour of fibroblasts, histiocytes, mixed 'fibrohistiocytic' cells and undifferentiated mesenchymal cells, although confusion always prevailed as to which was the true 'progenitor cell'. The concept of such a 'cell' in soft tissue tumours is no longer thought to be viable by many, and patterns of differentiation or gene expression are beginning to form a more reliable basis for tumour classification. Irrespective of these niceties, markers such as lysozyme, alpha-1-antitrypsin and alpha-1-antichymotrypsin were long thought to be indicative of histiocytic differentiation and therefore a clue to the diagnosis

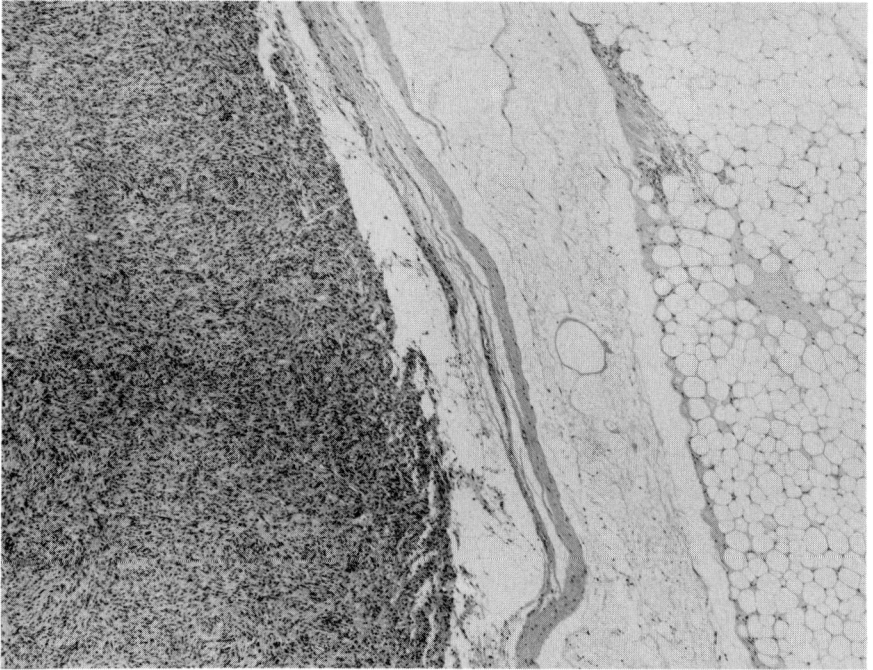

Fig. 6.11   Dedifferentiated liposarcoma in a local recurrence of a well differentiated liposarcoma in the thigh. Note the typically abrupt transition form low grade tumour on the right to high grade sarcoma on the left. H & E × 40.

of MFH. However, the specificity of these antigens has now been thoroughly discredited (Soini & Miettinen 1988, 1989) and further studies have gone on to show that MFH does not express any of the true immunophenotypic or enzyme histochemical characteristics of monocyte/macrophage differentiation (Wood et al 1986, Fletcher 1987). In fact MFH has proved to be extremely heterogeneous not only immunohistochemically (Lawson et al 1987, Hirose et al 1989, Miettinen & Soini 1989), but also ultrastructurally (Jabi et al 1987, Goodlad & Fletcher 1991) and by cytogenetic analysis (Molenaar et al 1989).

These findings, taken in conjunction with the clear and astute demonstration by Brooks (1986a) that a range of other specified sarcomas may, if they 'dedifferentiate', adopt a morphological pattern indistinguishable from pleomorphic MFH, raise the possibility that it represents the non-specific final common pathway in the progression of many different sarcomas. One must then consider, whether or not MFH should be retained as an entity at all. In the author's view it should not, the principal reason being that if optimally fixed and prepared tissue is available, combined with thorough sampling, then by careful histological, immuno-histochemical and ultrastructural analysis a specific, definable line of differentiation can be

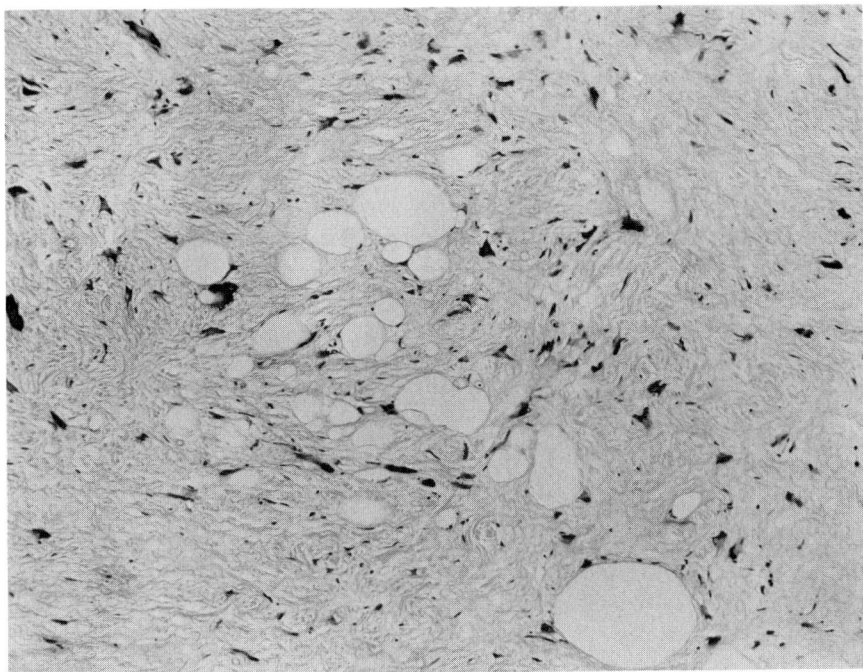

Fig. 6.12   Atypical lipoma: lipoblasts are absent, but the tumour shows variation in adipocyte size, fibrosis and bizarre, hyperchromatic cells in the stroma. H & E × 63.

identified in the majority of pleomorphic (MFH-like) sarcomas. It is also the case that metastatic carcinomas, melanomas or even anaplastic (usually T-cell) lymphomas may closely mimic this pattern.

Inevitably, this whole topic remains a matter of controversy (Dehner 1988) which will take some time to resolve. However, it is worth bearing in mind that it is only by careful subclassification that differences in prognosis or treatment-response will ever be identified in this large group of pleomorphic sarcomas.

With regard to the less common subtypes of MFH, space does not allow a discussion of each. Nevertheless, given that the myxoid, giant cell and inflammatory variants were only so-named because of their focal morphological similarity to pleomorphic 'MFH', then it seems reasonable to suggest that these entities will also be reclassified. There is already some evidence that the angiomatoid variant, which in any case is clinically and morphologically very different (Costa & Weiss 1990), is myoid in origin (Fletcher 1991).

Kaposi's sarcoma

Largely as a consequence of its association with AIDS, this tumour has been the subject of extensive studies in recent years. These have been thoroughly reviewed recently (Bayley & Lucas 1990) but, in view of the significance of changes in our attitude to this lesion, it warrants a brief reappraisal.

It is now increasingly believed that Kaposi's 'sarcoma' is not, in fact, a neoplasm (let alone a sarcoma) but is a multifocal reactive vascular hyperplasia. With one or two notable exceptions (Costa & Rabson 1983, Brooks 1986b), this belief has only become widespread since the introduction of modern investigative technology. Clinicopathological clues had been evident for years and the accumulated evidence is best summarized as follows.

Clinicopathological features

From the clinical point of view, sporadic and, to a lesser extent, endemic Kaposi's sarcoma has long been known to be a fairly indolent disease (Cox & Helwig 1959, Reynolds et al 1965, Hutt 1984), with an unusual pattern of proximal tumour spread and a low mortality except in African children. The cause of death is usually hard to define. Individual lesions in all clinical subgroups frequently undergo spontaneous regression, particularly when the degree of immune competence improves. Furthermore, in all groups, if lesions are excised, they do not recur in the scar, although new lesions may continue to develop elsewhere. The anatomical distribution is distinctive, being largely confined to skin, oral mucosa, lymph nodes, lungs and gastrointestinal tract. The old adage that Kaposi's sarcoma is confined only to tissues in which there are lymphatics may well account for the virtual non-existence of intracerebral lesions, but does not explain the sparing of kidney, prostate and skeletal muscle (Bayley & Lucas 1990). Another unusual clinical feature, seen in AIDS patients, is the tendency for simultaneous development of lesions at many different sites, including the symmetrical involvement of lymph nodes. This is hardly in keeping with the usual progressive metastatic spread of a single primary.

The progression of Kaposi's sarcoma through patch, plaque and nodular stages at all affected sites would also be most odd for a metastasizing lesion. Nuclear pleomorphism or abnormal mitotic activity are not seen at any stage and cases with intravascular spread are exceedingly rare. The usual pattern of lymph node involvement, commencing as a patch-like deposit in the capsule and then spreading along the sinusoidal fibrous architecture to gradually replace the node, is also distinctive and is not shared by other tumours.

Immunohistochemical findings

Arguments have raged over the 'histogenesis' of Kaposi's sarcoma for years. These have largely reflected the variable or disputed expression of a range of different endothelial markers in both the vascular slits and the spindle cells of these lesions. The general consensus now seems to be that Kaposi's

sarcoma displays features of both blood vascular and lymphatic endothelium, which would be in keeping with the clear demonstration of
lymphaticovenous shunts in the tumour (Dictor 1986, Dictor & Andersson
1988) and would also fit better with a mixed reactive rather than a
monoclonal population of cells.

Experimental findings

No strictly comparable lesion to human Kaposi's sarcoma has yet been
devised in an animal model (Bayley & Lucas 1990). When cultured AIDS
Kaposi's cells were injected into nude mice, they did not survive but
stimulated a murine vascular proliferation (Salahuddin et al 1988), which
suggests a reactive angiogenic response. Others have found that cell cultures
from Kaposi's lesions are not tumorigenic in mice (Delli Bovi et al 1986) and
have also shown an entirely normal karyotype in the majority of cases. This
has been further backed up by the demonstration that all cases examined to
date are diploid and have a low S-phase fraction (Fukunaga & Silverberg
1990). Based on data derived from HTLV-II infected lymphocytes
(Nakamura et al 1988), it has been postulated (Bayley & Lucas 1990) that
HIV-infected cells (such as lymphocytes and monocytes/macrophages) may
release angiogenic factors which act directly on endothelial cells. These in
turn may produce cytokines which enhance their own growth (Salahuddin
et al 1988) in an autocrine manner.

Some still cling to the concept of Kaposi's being a true sarcoma (Krigel &
Friedman-Kien 1990) but the weight of evidence is now heavily against this
and a unanimous resolution of this conceptual dilemma is likely to be
achieved in the near future.

Extraskeletal Ewing's sarcoma and peripheral primitive neuroectodermal tumours

The pattern of differentiation (often referred to as histogenesis) manifested
by extraskeletal Ewing's sarcoma and its more common osseous counterpart
has been a source of debate for many years (Yunis 1986). In general, it has
been regarded as an ultrastructurally undifferentiated primitive mesenchymal tumour which usually contains intracytoplasmic glycogen. It has,
however, been demonstrated that at least 50% of cases show immunohistochemical and/or ultrastructural evidence of neuroectodermal differentiation
not only in surgical specimens (Shimada et al 1988, Ushigome et al 1989)
but also in cell lines derived from them (Lipinski et al 1987, Lizard-Nacol
et al 1989). It has also been shown that this neural differentiation can be
switched on and off in tissue culture by the addition of differentiation
inducers or inhibitors (Cavazzana et al 1987, Noguera et al 1990). It has,
therefore, been proposed that Ewing's sarcoma should be reclassified as a
variant of malignant peripheral primitive neuroectodermal tumour (PNET)
(Dehner 1986, 1990).

Further supportive evidence for this concept, which effectively leads us into the impact of new technology, has come from cytogenetic analysis. It has been repeatedly shown that typical examples of PNET, and its distinctive thoracopulmonary subset (Askin tumour) as well as examples of both extra-osseous and osseous Ewing's sarcoma all exhibit a specific chromosome translocation, t(11;22)(q24;q12) (Turc-Carel et al 1983, Aurias et al 1984, Whang-Peng et al 1984, Seemayer et al 1985, Cavazzana et al 1987, Heinemann et al 1989). This adds considerable weight to the proposed close relationship amongst members of this group of tumours, although it remains to be seen whether these translocations are identical at the molecular level. It has been suggested that the eponym, Ewing's sarcoma, be retained for those few cases which show neither immunohisto-chemical, ultrastructural nor cytogenetic evidence of neural differentiation. It should be noted in passing that the demonstration of PAS-positive glycogen has ceased to be of value in differential diagnosis, since glycogen has now been repeatedly demonstrated not only in classical PNET but also in lymphomas.

THE IMPACT OF NEW TECHNOLOGY

Evidence of the close relationship between Ewing's sarcoma and PNET is a good example of the advances that have been made in recent years as a direct result of close collaboration between histopathologists and molecular biologists. Further examples of the benefits of such interaction are now being described at an increasing rate (Cooper & Stratton 1991) and only the more important findings are described below.

Chromosome translocations

It has become considerably easier to undertake cytogenetic analysis of solid tumours (Trent et al 1986, Sandberg & Turc-Carel 1987) and, in no field more so than soft tissue tumours. This has revealed a wide range of tumour-specific karyotypic abnormalities. In addition to the findings in Ewing's sarcoma already discussed, perhaps one of the most significant and clinicopathologically useful translocations, t(X;18)(p11.2;q11.2), has been demonstrated in synovial sarcoma (Turc-Carel et al 1986a, Smith et al 1987, Bridge et al 1988, Noguera et al 1988). This reciprocal translocation is present in both biphasic and monophasic variants of synovial sarcoma, thereby providing further evidence that both are phenotypic expressions of the same tumour, which was long denied by some. The precise breakpoint of this translocation has been recently mapped (Reeves et al 1989) but, as yet, no abnormality of the adjacent genes has been identified.

Among fatty tumours, rather surprisingly given their fairly inert nature, lipomas have proved to show a range of abnormalities, the commonest of which is translocation of the q13–14 region on chromosome 12 and the most frequent pattern is t(3;12)(q27–28;q13–14) (Mandahl et al 1987, 1988, Turc-Carel et al 1988). Taken in conjunction with the findings in many uterine leiomyomas (Heim et al 1988, Nilbert et al 1988, Mark et al 1989), this has demonstrated, contrary to previously held beliefs, that chromosomal abnormalities are not confined to malignant neoplasms. The other fatty tumour with a well characterized translocation, t(12;16)(q13;p11), is myxoid liposarcoma (Turc-Carel et al 1986b, Mertens et al 1987). It is notable that the breakpoint on chromosome 12 is very similar, if not identical, to that in benign lipomas, but again, no rearrangements of the genes located in this region have been identified to date. It will be of interest to see if the poorly differentiated form of this tumour, round cell liposarcoma, shows the same translocation.

A whole range of other karyotypic anomalies have been reported in isolated examples of different soft tissue tumours but the only other consistent reciprocal translocation has been t(2;13)(q37;q14) in alveolar rhabdomyosarcoma (Seidal et al 1982, Turc-Carel et al 1986c, Wang-Wuu et al 1988). This is distinct from the abnormality on chromosome 11 in embryonal rhabdomyosarcoma (Scrable et al 1989).

Oncogenes and anti-oncogenes

Oncogene expression, particularly of the *ras* and *myc* gene families, has been shown to be quite widespread among soft tissue sarcomas (Gupta et al 1988, Cooper & Stratton 1991) but, as yet, has not proved to be of any prognostic relevance, in contrast to neuroblastoma. Point mutations in the *ras* gene family seem especially common in embryonal rhabdomyosarcoma, particularly in those tumours arising in the genitourinary tract (Stratton et al 1989a). Although unexplored as yet, this is potentially of considerable significance since genitourinary lesions are well known to be the most curable of these childhood rhabdomyosarcomas. However, gene amplification, as a mechanism of oncogene activation, seems surprisingly infrequent in soft tissue sarcomas (Cooper & Stratton 1991).

With regard to anti-oncogenes (tumour suppressor genes), interesting and pathogenetically relevant findings have emerged which initially stemmed from the well-known observation that patients with familial retinoblastoma show an increased incidence of both osteosarcoma and soft tissue sarcomas. Both homozygous and heterozygous deletions of the retinoblastoma (RB1) gene have been demonstrated in about a third of sporadic soft tissue sarcomas (Stratton et al 1989b). The same authors (Stratton et al 1990) have gone on to show that mutations within the p53 gene, another well-characterized tumour suppressor gene, are also quite common in sarcomas and are frequently associated with abnormalities of the RB1 gene. This provides support for Knudson's theory that two mutational 'hits' are required for neoplastic transformation.

Growth factors and receptors

Growth factors, which are generally regarded as the normal equivalent of oncogene products, and their receptors are believed to be closely involved in the regulation of normal (and probably neoplastic) cell proliferation and growth. It has been shown that growth factors, particularly nerve growth factor (NGF) and platelet-derived growth factor (PDGF), and growth factor receptors, particulary NGF-R and epidermal growth factor receptor (EGF-R), are widely expressed in both benign and malignant soft tissue tumours. However, expression of more than one growth factor and/or their corresponding receptor(s) is more often seen in sarcomas (Gusterson et al 1985, Perosio & Brooks, 1988, 1989). This provides further evidence that some tumours indulge in auto-stimulation (the autocrine hypothesis).

Differentiation genes

Fascinating new information is beginning to emerge on the identification and expression of genes which determine a specific line of differentiation. An increasing number of such genes of particular relevance to connective tissue differentiation are being identified in experimental animal models but, to date, only the *myf* family (two of which were formerly known as MyoDI and myogenin respectively) have been studied in human tissues. The *myf* gene family encodes factors which determine or programme skeletal muscle differentiation. Their expression has recently been studied in rhabdomyosarcomas and other small round cell tumours (Scrable et al 1989, Dias et al 1990, Navarro et al 1990) and it has been found to be confined to lesions showing true rhabdomyoblastic differentiation. This may prove to be of considerable value in the differential diagnosis of small round cell sarcomas of children and perhaps of other sarcomas in adults as well.

REFERENCES

Arias-Stella J, Lieberman P H, Erlandson R A et al 1986 Histology, immunohistochemistry and ultrastructure of the verruga in Carrion's disease. American Journal of Surgical Pathology 10: 595–610

Arias-Stella J, Lieberman P H, Garcia-Caceres U et al 1987 Verruga peruana mimicking malignant neoplasms. American Journal of Dermatopathology 9: 279–291

Aurias A, Rimbaut C, Buffe D et al 1984 Translocation involving chromosome 22 in Ewing's sarcoma. A cytogenetic study of four fresh tumors. Cancer Genetics and Cytogenetics 12: 21–25

Azumi N, Curtis J, Kempson R L et al 1987 Atypical and malignant neoplasms showing lipomatous differentiation. A study of 111 cases. American Journal of Surgical Pathology 11: 161–183

Bayley A C, Lucas S B 1990 Kaposi's sarcoma or Kaposi's disease? A personal reappraisal. In: Fletcher C D M, McKee P H (eds) Pathobiology of soft tissue tumours. Churchill Livingstone, Edinburgh, pp 141–163

Bittesini L, Dei Tos A, Fletcher C D M 1991 Metastatic malignant melanoma showing a rhabdoid phenotype: further evidence of a non-specific histological pattern. Histopathology (in press)

Bridge J A, Bridge R S, Borek D A et al 1988 Translocation t(X;18) in orofacial synovial sarcoma. Cancer 62: 935–937

Brooks J J 1986a The significance of double phenotypic patterns and markers in human sarcomas. A new model of mesenchymal differentiation. American Journal of Pathology 125: 113–123

Brooks J J 1986b Kaposi's sarcoma: a reversible hyperplasia. Lancet ii: 1309–1311

Carter R L, McCarthy K P, Al-Sam S Z et al 1989 Malignant rhabdoid tumour of the bladder with immunohistochemical and ultrastructural evidence suggesting histiocytic origin. Histopathology 14: 179–190

Cavazzana A D, Miser J S, Jefferson J et al 1987 Experimental evidence for a neural origin of Ewing's sarcoma of bone. American Journal of Pathology 127: 507–518

Chan J K C, Fletcher C D M, Hicklin G A et al 1990 Glomeruloid hemangioma. A distinctive cutaneous lesion of multicentric Castleman's disease associated with POEMS syndrome. American Journal of Surgical Pathology 14: 1036–1046

Cockerell C J, Friedman-Kien A E 1988 Epithelioid angiomatosis and cat scratch bacillus. Lancet i: 1334–1335

Cockerell C J, Webster G F, Whitlow M A et al 1987 Epithelioid angiomatosis: a distinct vascular disorder in patients with the acquired immunodeficiency syndrome or AIDS-related complex. Lancet ii: 654–656

Cooper C S, Stratton M R 1991 Soft tissue tumours: the genetic basis of development. Carcinogenesis 12: 155–165

Costa J, Rabson A S 1983 Generalised Kaposi's sarcoma is not a neoplasm. Lancet ii: 58

Costa M J, Weiss S W 1990 Angiomatoid malignant fibrous histiocytoma. A follow-up study of 108 cases with evaluation of possible histologic predictors of clinical outcome. American Journal of Surgical Pathology 14: 1126–1132

Cox F H, Helwig E B 1959 Kaposi's sarcoma. Cancer 12: 289–298

Dehner L P 1986 Peripheral and central primitive neuroectodermal tumours. A nosologic concept seeking a concensus. Archives of Pathology and Laboratory Medicine 110: 997–1005

Dehner L P 1988 Malignant fibrous histiocytoma. Nonspecific morphological pattern, specific pathologic entity or both. Archives of Pathology and Laboratory Medicine 112: 236–237

Dehner L P 1990 Whence the primitive neuroectodermal tumor? Archives of Pathology and Laboratory Medicine 114: 16–17

Delli Bovi P, Donti E, Knowles I D M et al 1986 Presence of chromosomal abnormalities and lack of AIDS retrovirus DNA sequences in AIDS-associated Kaposi's sarcoma. Cancer Research 46: 6333–6338

Dias P, Parham D M, Shapiro D N, Webber B L, Houghton P J, 1990 Myogenic regulatory protein (myoDI) expression in childhood solid tumours: utility in rhabdomyosarcoma. American Journal of Pathology 137: 1283–1291

Dictor M 1986 Kaposi's sarcoma. Origin and significance of lymphaticovenous connections. Virchow's Archiv A (Pathological Anatomy) 409: 23–35

Dictor M, Andersson C 1988 Lymphaticovenous differentiation in Kaposi's sarcoma. Cellular phenotypes by stage. American Journal of Pathology 130: 411–417

Enzinger F M 1986 Malignant fibrous histiocytoma 20 years after Stout. American Journal of Surgical Pathology 10 (suppl. 1): 43–53

Enzinger F M, Weiss S W 1988 Soft tissue tumors. 2nd Edn. C. V. Mosby, St Louis

Enzinger F M, Zhang R 1988 Plexiform fibrohistiocytic tumor presenting in children and young adults. An analysis of 65 cases. American Journal of Surgical Pathology 12: 818–826

Enzinger F M, Weiss S W, Liang C Y 1989 Ossifying fibromyxoid tumor of soft parts. A clinicopathologic analysis of 59 cases. American Journal of Surgical Pathology 13: 817–827

Evans H L, Soule E H, Winkelmann R K 1979 Atypical lipoma, atypical intramuscular lipoma and well-differentiated retroperitoneal liposarcoma. A reappraisal of 30 cases formerly classified as well-differentiated liposarcoma. Cancer 43: 574–584

Fletcher C D M 1987 Malignant fibrous histiocytoma? Histopathology 11: 433–437

Fletcher C D M 1990 Benign fibrous histiocytoma of subcutaneous and deep soft tissue: a clinicopathologic analysis of 21 cases. American Journal of Surgical Pathology 14: 801–809

Fletcher C D M, McKee P H 1990 Progress in malignant soft tissue tumours. In Fletcher C D M, McKee P H (eds) Pathobiology of soft tissue tumours. Churchill Livingstone, Edinburgh pp 259–318

Fletcher C D M, Stirling R W 1990 Intranodal myofibroblastoma presenting in the submandibular region: evidence of a broader clinical and histological spectrum. Histopathology 16: 287–294

Fletcher C D M 1991 Angiomatoid 'malignant fibrous histiocytoma': an immunohistochemical study indicative of myoid differentiation. Human Pathology 22: 563–568

Fletcher C D M, Beham A, Schmid Ch 1991 Spindle cell haemangioendothelioma: a clinicopathological and immunohistochemical study indicative of a non-neoplastic lesion. Histopathology 18: 291–301

Fukunaga M, Silverberg S G 1990 Kaposi's sarcoma in patients with AIDS. A flow cytometric DNA analysis of 21 patients. Laboratory Investigation 62: 35A (Abstract)

Gonzalez-Crussi F, Goldschmidt R A, Hsueh W et al 1982 Infantile sarcoma with intracytoplasmic filamentous inclusions. Distinctive tumor of possible histiocytic origin. Cancer 49: 2365–2375

Goodlad J R, Fletcher C D M 1991 Malignant peripheral nerve sheath tumour with annulate lamellae mimicking pleomorphic malignant fibrous histiocytoma. Journal of Pathology 164: 23–29

Gupta V, Donner L R, Shin D M et al 1988 Oncogene expression in human tumors of soft tissue and bone. Laboratory Investigation 58: 36A (Abstract)

Gusterson B A, Cowley G, McIlhinney J et al 1985 Evidence for increased epidermal growth factor receptors in human sarcomas. International Journal of Cancer 36: 689–693

Haas J E, Palmer N F, Weinberg A G et al 1981 Ultrastructure of the malignant rhabdoid tumor of the kidney. A distinctive renal tumor of children. Human Pathology 12: 646–657

Heim S, Nilbert M, Vanni R et al 1988 A specific translocation t(12:14)(q14–15;q23–24) characterizes a subgroup of uterine leiomyomas. Cancer Genetics and Cytogenetics 32: 13–17

Heinemann F S, Lladanyi M, Huvos A et al 1989 Ewing's sarcoma and primitive neuroectodermal tumor: a clinicopathologic and cytogenetic study of eight cases. Laboratory Investigation 60: 39a (Abstract)

Hirose T, Kudo E, Hasegawa T et al 1989 Expression of intermediate filaments in malignant fibrous histiocytomas. Human Pathology 20: 871–877

Hutt M S R 1984 Kaposi's sarcoma. British Medical Bulletin 40: 355–358

Jabi M, Jeans D, Dardick I 1987 Ultrastructural heterogeneity in malignant fibrous histiocytoma of soft tissue. Ultrastructural Pathology 11: 583–592

Kempson R L, Kyriakos M 1972 Fibroxanthosarcoma of the soft tissues. A type of malignant fibrous histiocytoma. Cancer 29: 961–976

Kent A L, Mahoney D H, Gresik M V et al 1987 Malignant rhabdoid tumor of the extremity. Cancer 60: 1056–1059

Kindblom L-G, Angervall L, Fassina A S 1982 Atypical lipoma. Acta Pathologica et Microbiologica Scandinavica (A) 90: 27–36

Koehler J E, LeBoit P E, Egbert B M et al 1988 Cutaneous vascular lesions and disseminated cat-scratch disease in patients with the acquired immunodeficiency syndrome (AIDS) and AIDS-related complex. Annals of Internal Medicine 109: 449–455

Krigel R L, Friedman-Kien A E 1990 Epidemic Kaposi's sarcoma. Seminars in Oncology 17: 350–360

Lawson C W, Fisher C, Gatter K C 1987 An immunohistochemical study of differentiation in malignant fibrous histiocytoma. Histopathology 11: 375–383

LeBoit P E, Egbert B M, Stoler M H et al 1988 Epithelioid haemangioma-like vascular proliferation in AIDS: manifestation of cat scratch disease bacillus infection? Lancet i: 960–963

LeBoit P E, Berger T G, Egbert B M et al 1989 Bacillary angiomatosis. The histopathology and differential diagnosis of a pseudoneoplastic infection in patients with human immunodeficiency virus disease. American Journal of Surgical Pathology 13: 909–920

Lipinski M, Braham K, Philip I et al 1987 Neuroectoderm-associated antigens on Ewing's sarcoma cell lines. Cancer Research 47: 183–187

Lizard-Nacol S, Lizard G, Justrabo E et al 1989 Immunologic characterization of Ewing's sarcoma using mesenchymal and neural markers. American Journal of Pathology 135: 847–855

Lynch H T, Shurin S B, Dahms B B et al 1983 Paravertebral malignant rhabdoid tumor in infancy. In vitro studies of a familial tumor. Cancer 52: 290–296

Mandahl N, Heim S, Johansson B et al 1987 Lipomas have characteristic structural chromosomal rearrangements of 12q 13–14. International Journal of Cancer 39: 685–688

Mandahl N, Heim S, Arheden K et al 1988 Three major cytogenetic subgroups can be identified among chromosomally solitary lipomas. Human Genetics 79: 203–208

Mark J, Havel G, Grepp C et al 1989 Cytogenetical observations in human benign uterine leiomyomas. Anticancer Research 8: 621–626

Mertens F, Johansson B, Mandahl N et al 1987 Clonal chromosomal abnormalities in two liposarcomas. Cancer Genetics and Cytogenetics 28: 137–144

Miettinen M, Soini Y 1989 Malignant fibrous histiocytoma. Heterogeneous patterns of intermediate filament proteins by immunohistochemistry. Archives of Pathology and Laboratory Medicine 113: 1363–1366

Molenaar W M, DeJong B, Buist J et al 1989 Chromosomal analysis and the classification of soft tissue sarcomas. Laboratory Investigation 60: 266–274

Nakamura S, Salahuddin S Z, Biberfeld P et al 1988 Kaposi's sarcoma cells: longterm culture with growth factor from retrovirus infected CD4 + T-cells. Science 242: 426–429

Navarro S, Noguera R, D'Orazi G et al 1990 Expression of the MyoDI gene and protein in various myogenous and non-myogenous tumors. Laboratory Investigation 62: 73A (Abstract)

Nilbert M, Heim S, Mandahl N et al 1988 Karyotypic rearrangements in 20 uterine leiomyomas. Cytogenetics and Cell Genetics 49: 300–304

Noguera R, Lopez-Gines C, Gile R et al 1988 Translocation (X;18) in a synovial sarcoma: a new case. Cancer Genetics and Cytogenetics 33: 311–312

Noguera R, Arakawa S, Navarro S et al 1990 Modulation of antigenic expression by Ewing's sarcoma cells with differentiation. Laboratory Investigation 62: 74A (Abstract)

Perosio P M, Brooks J J 1988 Expression of nerve growth factor receptor in paraffin-embedded soft tissue tumors. American Journal of Pathology 132: 152–160

Perosio P M, Brooks J J 1989 Expression of growth factors and growth factor receptors in soft tissue tumors. Implications for the autocrine hypothesis. Laboratory Investigation 60: 245–253

Reeves B R, Smith S, Fisher C et al 1989 Characterisation of the translocation between chromosomes X and 18 in human synovial sarcomas. Oncogene 4: 373–378

Reynolds W A, Winkelmann R K, Soule E H 1965 Kaposi's sarcoma: a clinicopathologic study with particular reference to its relationship to the reticuloendothelial system. Medicine 44: 419–443

Salahuddin S Z, Nakamura S, Biberfeld P et al 1988 Angiogenic properties of Kaposi's sarcoma-derived cells after longterm culture in vitro. Science 242: 430–433

Sandberg A A, Turc-Carel C 1987 The cytogenetics of solid tumors. Relation to diagnosis, classification and pathology. Cancer 59: 387–395

Schinella R A, Greco M A 1990 Bacillary angiomatosis presenting as a soft tissue tumor without skin involvement. Human Pathology 21: 567–569

Scott G A, Rosai J 1988 Spindle cell hemangioendothelioma. Report of seven additional cases of a recently described vascular neoplasm. American Journal of Dermatopathology 10: 281–288

Scrable H, Witte D, Shimada H et al 1989 Molecular differential pathology of rhabdomyosarcoma. Genes, Chromosomes and Cancer 1: 23–35

Seemayer T, Vekamans T, De Chadarevian J-P 1985 Histological and cytogenetic findings in a malignant tumor of the chest wall and lung (Askin tumor). Virchows Archiv A (Pathological Anatomy) 408: 289–296

Seidal T, Mark J, Hagmar B et al 1982 Alveolar rhabdomyosarcoma: a cytogenetic and correlated cytological and histological study. Acta Pathologica et Microbiologica Immunologica Scandinavica (A) 90: 345–354

Shimada H, Newton W A, Soule E H et al 1988 Pathologic features of extraosseous Ewing's sarcoma: a report from the Intergroup Rhabdomyosarcoma Study. Human Pathology 19: 442–453

Skaniawski W K, Don P C, Bitterman S R et al 1990 Epithelioid angiomatosis in patients with AIDS. Journal of the American Academy of Dermatology 23: 41–48

Smith S, Reeves B R, Wong L et al 1987 A consistent chromosomal translocation in synovial sarcoma. Cancer Genetics and Cytogenetics 26: 179–180

Smith S, Fletcher C D M, Smith M A et al 1990 Cytogenetic analysis of a plexiform fibrohistiocytic tumor. Cancer Genetics and Cytogenetics 48: 31–34

Soini Y, Miettinen M 1988 Widespread immunoreactivity for alpha-1-antichymotrypsin in different types of tumors. American Journal of Clinical Pathology 89: 131–136

Soini Y, Miettinen M 1989 Alpha-1-antitrypsin and lysozyme. Their limited significance in fibrohistiocytic tumors. American Journal of Clinical Pathology 91: 515–521

Sotelo-Avila C, Gonzalez-Crussi F, deMello D et al 1986 Renal and extra-renal rhabdoid tumors in children: a clinicopathologic study of 14 patients. Seminars in Diagnostic Pathology 3: 151–163

Stoler M H, Bonfiglio T A, Steigbigel R T et al 1983 An atypical subcutaneous infection associated with acquired immune deficiency syndrome. American Journal of Clinical Pathology 80: 714–718

Stratton M R, Fisher C, Gusterson B A et al 1989a Human embryonal rhabdomyosarcomas: detection of point mutations in N-ras and K-ras genes using oligonucleotide probes and the polymerase chain reaction. Cancer Research 49: 6324–6327

Stratton M R, Williams S, Fisher C et al 1989b Structural alterations of the RB1 gene in human soft tissue tumours. British Journal of Cancer 60: 202–205

Stratton M R, Moss S, Warren W et al 1990 Mutation of the p53 gene in human soft tissue sarcomas: association with abnormalities of the RB1 gene. Oncogene 5: 1297–1301

Suster S, Rosai J 1989 Intranodal hemorrhagic spindle cell tumor with amianthoid fibers. Report of six cases of a distinctive mesenchymal neoplasm of the inguinal region that simulates Kaposi's sarcoma. American Journal of Surgical Pathology 13: 347–357

Trent J, Crickard K, Gibas Z et al 1986 Methodological advances in the cytogenetic analysis of human solid tumors. Cancer Genetics and Cytogenetics 19: 57–66

Tsuneyoshi M, Daimaru Y, Hashimoto H et al 1985 Malignant soft tissue neoplasms with the histologic features of renal rhabdoid tumors: an ultrastructural and immunohistochemical study. Human Pathology 16: 1235–1242

Tsuneyoshi M, Daimaru Y, Hashimoto H et al 1987 The existence of rhabdoid cells in specific soft tissue sarcomas. Histopathological, ultrastructural and immunohistochemical evidence. Virchow's Archiv A (Pathological Anatomy) 411: 509–514

Turc-Carel C, Philip I, Berger M-P et al 1983 Chromosome translocations in Ewing's sarcoma. New England Journal of Medicine 390: 497–498

Turc-Carel C, Dal Cin P, Limon J et al 1986a Translocation X;18 in synovial sarcoma. Cancer Genetics and Cytogenetics 23: 93

Turc-Carel C, Limon J, Dal Cin P et al 1986b Cytogenetic studies of adipose tissue tumors. II. Recurrent reciprocal translocation t(12;16)(q13;p11) in myxoid liposarcomas. Cancer Genetics and Cytogenetics 23: 291–300

Turc-Carel C, Lizard-Nacol S, Justrabo E et al 1986c Consistent chromosomal translocation in alveolar rhabdomyosarcoma. Cancer Genetics and Cytogenetics 19: 361–362

Turc-Carel C, Dal Cin P, Boghosian L et al 1988 Breakpoints in benign lipomas may be at 12q13 or 12q14. Cancer Genetics and Cytogenetics 36: 131–135

Ushigome S, Shimoda T, Takaki K et al 1989 Immunocytochemical and ultrastructural studies of the histogenesis of Ewing's sarcoma and putatively related tumors. Cancer 64: 52–62

Walford N, Van der Wouw P A, Das P K et al 1990 Epithelioid angiomatosis in the acquired immunodeficiency syndrome: morphology and differential diagnosis. Histopathology 16: 83–88

Wang-Wuu S, Soukup S, Ballard E et al 1988 Chromosome analysis of sixteen human rhabdomyosarcomas. Cancer Research 48: 983–987

Weeks D A, Beckwith J B, Mierau G W 1989a Rhabdoid tumor. An entity or a phenotype? Archives of Pathology and Laboratory Medicine 113: 113–114

Weeks D A, Beckwith J B, Mierau G W et al 1989b Rhabdoid tumor of kidney. A report of 111 cases from the National Wilms' Tumor Study Pathology Center. American Journal of Surgical Pathology 13: 439–458

Weiss S W, Enzinger F M 1978 Malignant fibrous histiocytoma. An analysis of 200 cases. Cancer 41: 2250–2266

Weiss S W, Enzinger F M 1986 Spindle cell hemangioendothelioma. A low grade angiosarcoma resembling a cavernous hemangioma and Kaposi's sarcoma. American Journal of Surgical Pathology 10: 521–530

Weiss S W, Gnepp D R, Bratthauer G L 1989 Palisaded myofibroblastoma. A benign mesenchymal tumor of lymph node. American Journal of Surgical Pathology 13: 341–346

Whang-Peng J, Triche T J, Knutsen T et al 1984 Chromosome translocation in peripheral neuroepithelioma. New England Journal of Medicine 311: 584–585
Wood G S, Beckstead J H, Turner R R et al 1986 Malignant fibrous histioctyoma tumor cells resemble fibroblasts. American Journal of Surgery and Pathology 10: 323–335
Yunis E J 1986 Ewing's sarcoma and related small round cell neoplasms in children. American Journal of Surgical Pathology 10 (suppl. 1): 54–62

7

Cystic tumours of the exocrine pancreas

W. V. Bogomoletz

Cystic tumours of the pancreas are rare, compared to the more common ductal adenocarcinoma, and represent about 6% of all exocrine epithelial tumours (Klöppel 1984, Chen & Baithun 1985). The serous and mucinous cystadenomas and cystadenocarcinomas are best known and are the commonest members of this group. Cystic papillary neoplasms and a few other miscellaneous types must also be included. The main feature shared by all the members of this group is their gross and microscopic cystic appearance. They must be differentiated from the non-neoplastic cystic lesions which also arise in the pancreas.

Cystic tumours of the pancreas are generally large, well delineated and multilocular lesions. Their histogenesis is diverse and not entirely resolved, despite recent immunohistochemical and ultrastructural investigations. There is a striking predominance in women, and some variation in age distribution. The prognosis is generally good, even in the malignant forms, and contrasts with the dismal clinical course of ductal adenocarcinoma of the pancreas.

SEROUS AND MUCINOUS CYSTIC TUMOURS (CYSTADENOMAS AND CYSTADENOCARCINOMAS)

In the past, and despite some attempts at classification (Glenner & Mallory 1956, Campbell & Cruickshank 1962), serous and mucinous cystic tumours of the pancreas were generally regarded as a single group and often described as if they were interchangeable. This resulted in much confusion of terminology. Compagno & Oertel (1978a,b) were the first to clearly distinguish two separate groups:

a. Microcystic adenomas (glycogen-rich cystadenomas), considered uniformly benign; and

b. Mucinous cystic neoplasms with latent or overt malignancy (mucinous cystadenomas and cystadenocarcinomas).

This classification has hitherto been accepted by most workers (Hodgkinson et al 1978a,b, Morohoshi et al 1983, Cubilla & Fitzgerald 1984, Klöppel 1984, Shorten et al 1986, Albores-Saavedra et al 1987, Yamaguchi & Enjoji

1987, Alpert et al 1988, Lack 1989). Recently, however, a reappraisal of the biological behaviour of these serous and mucinous cystic tumours has become necessary. This has resulted from an increasing awareness that a much wider spectrum of lesions exists within the two groups (Yamaguchi & Enjoji 1987, George et al 1989, Katoh et al 1989). This spectrum covers a range of benign, borderline and malignant serous and mucinous cystic tumours.

Clinical features

Serous and mucinous cystic tumours account for 1–3.5% of all exocrine tumours (Morohoshi et al 1983, Chen & Baithun 1985) and share several clinical features (Compagno & Oertel 1978a,b, Hodgkinson et al 1978a,b, Katoh et al 1989). The tumours can be symptomatic or asymptomatic, regardless of their serous or mucinous nature and irrespective of benign or malignant features. The mode of presentation depends on the size of the lesion and on its location within the pancreas. Symptoms and signs are those usually associated with a slowly increasing expansile rather than invasive abdominal tumour, namely abdominal pain and a palpable mass. In the past, asymptomatic cases were mostly an incidental finding at autopsy or during abdominal surgery for another cause. In the last ten years, however, an increasing number of asymptomatic cases have been diagnosed on angiography, ultrasonography, computed tomography and endoscopic retrograde pancreatography.

70% to 75% of serous and mucinous cystic tumours occur in women. The median age is about 66 years for serous tumours and about 55 years for mucinous tumours. Serous and mucinous cystic tumours can arise from any part of the pancreas and in our opinion tend to show an even distribution, despite some claims to the contrary. Some tumours may involve both head and body or body and tail and others may involve the gland diffusely.

Serous cystic tumours

Serous cystic tumours have been variably reported in the literature as 'serous cystadenoma', 'microcystic adenoma', 'microcystic cystadenoma', or 'glycogen-rich cystadenoma'. Serous cystic tumours had been considered as uniformly benign lesions, until very recently (George et al 1989).

Gross appearances

Serous cystic tumours are well-circumscribed round to ovoid lesions ranging in size from 1 to 25 cm in diameter with an average of 10 cm. The external aspect is coarsely nodular due to bulging of multiple subcapsular cysts. On section, tumours are multiloculated or 'polycystic' with a honeycombed translucent and at times gritty surface (Fig. 7.1). The colour

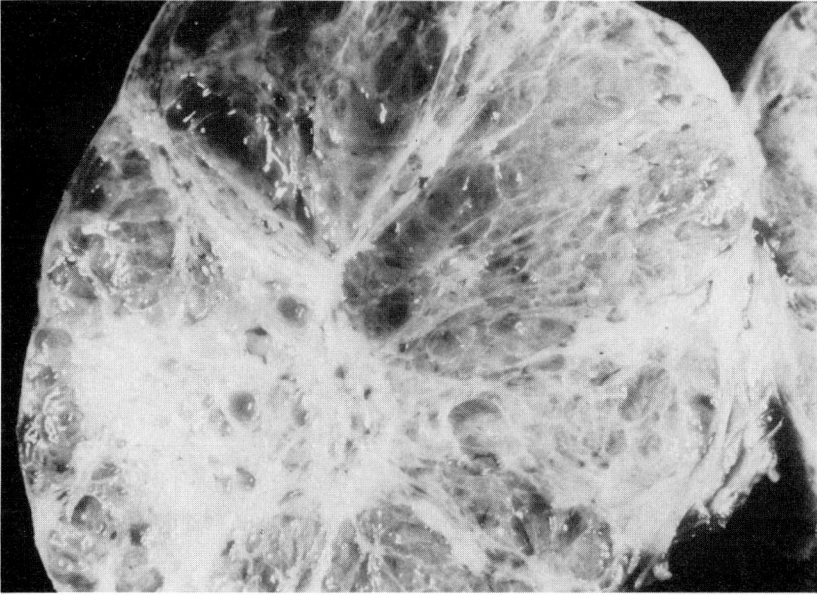

Fig. 7.1 Serous cystadenoma in cross section showing a multicystic pattern with cysts of varying size separated by thin fibrous septa.

is greyish, but may be brown in cases of haemorrhage. The cysts range from a few millimetres to several centimetres in diameter, and are separated by a fibrous stroma. Occasionally, there is a central stellate scar which may be calcified. The cysts tend to have smooth walls and contain thin watery 'serous' fluid. The lesions are usually separated from the adjacent and compressed pancreatic tissue by a layer of fibrous tissue of varying thickness, often providing a plane of cleavage, but rarely forming a distinct wall or a true capsule.

Histological features

Microscopically also, there is considerable variation in the size of the cysts and accordingly, two basic patterns have been described (Bogomoletz et al 1980). The 'porous' pattern consists of very small cysts lined by cuboidal epithelium and embedded in a loose connective tissue stroma (Fig. 7.2). The 'spongy' pattern somewhat resembles the alveolar structure of the lung and consists of larger dilated cysts separated by thin fibrous septa. In the spongy pattern, the cysts are lined by flattened epithelium which may mimic endothelium. Transition zones from porous to spongy patterns can be observed in most cases, although one pattern may be predominant. The fibrous septa separating the cysts are generally acellular and well vascu-

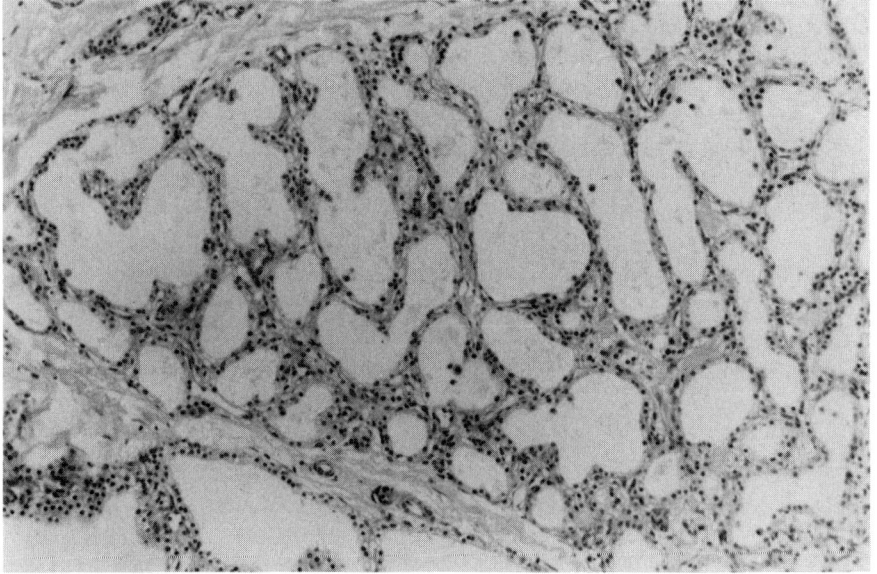

Fig. 7.2   Serous cystadenoma with a porous pattern. Cysts are uniformly small and lined by cuboidal epithelium. H & E × 125.

larized. The septa and the fibrous layer surrounding the tumour may contain lymphoid aggregates and occasional entrapped pancreatic structures e.g. ducts, acini or islets. Haemorrhage, leaving haemosiderin deposition, can occur but necrosis is not a feature.

The characteristic epithelial cells with vacuolated cytoplasm are best seen in the smallest cysts of the porous pattern. The cells are cuboidal or polygonal and usually arranged in a single row. Nuclear pleomorphism and mitotic figures are rare. The cell vacuolation is due to glycogen and stains with the periodic acid–Schiff reaction before diastase or with Best's carmine. Mucin stains are negative; goblet cells and argentaffin or argyrophil granules are absent.

The presence of papillae in serous cystic tumours has been a contentious issue. Whilst some authors have not found any (Hodgkinson et al 1978a, Shorten et al 1986, Corbally et al 1989), papillae have been recorded and illustrated by others (Glenner & Mallory 1956, Compagno & Oertel 1978a, Bogomoletz et al 1980, Yamaguchi & Enjoji 1987). Moreover, the significance of such papillae has not been resolved. Glenner & Mallory (1956) felt that the presence of papillae carried a worse prognosis but, given adequate tissue sampling, small papillae are often present in otherwise benign serous cystic tumours. These papillae consist of small tufts resulting from the infolding of the cuboidal epithelial and true papillae with fibrovascular cores are rare (Fig. 7.3). The epithelium covering papillae is cytologically bland.

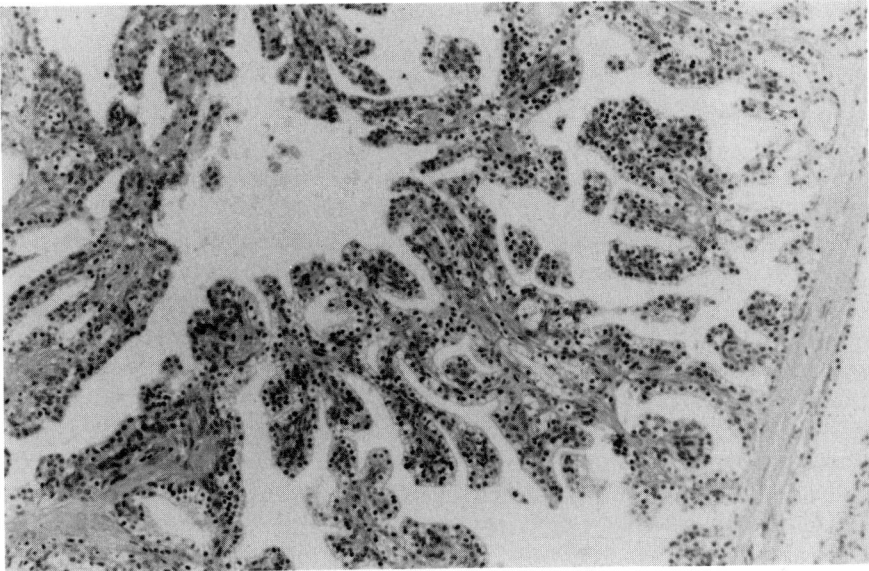

Fig. 7.3 Serous cystadenoma with papillary projections. Papillae are covered by bland cuboidal epithelial cells with vacuolated cytoplasm. H & E × 125.

Electron microscopy and immunohistochemistry

The ultrastructural features of serous cystic tumours have been reported by several authors (Compagno & Oertel 1978a, Bogomoletz et al 1980, Nyongo & Huntrakoon 1985, Shorten et al 1986, Alpert et al 1988, Kim et al 1990). The cuboidal epithelial cells lining the cysts have poorly developed apical microvilli and contain variable amounts of glycogen and occasional small lipid droplets. Two reports have mentioned the presence of small apical secretory vacuoles (Bogomoletz et al 1980, Shorten et al 1986). Zymogen granules or neurosecretory granules have not been found. These ultrastructural features resemble those found in the centroacinar cells seen in the duct system of the developing fetal human pancreas (Bogomoletz et al 1980) and suggest a possible histogenesis for these tumours.

Immunohistochemical studies have shown that the epithelial cytoplasm expresses cytokeratin and epithelial membrane antigen (Shorten et al 1986, Yamaguchi & Enjoji 1987, Alpert et al 1988, Helpap & Vogel 1989). No immunoreactivity for carcinoembryonic antigen (Shorten et al 1986, Helpap & Vogel 1989) or endocrine peptide markers (Helpap & Vogel 1989) have been demonstrated.

Occasional myoepithelial cells in close proximity to the cuboidal epithelium have been reported on electron microscopy (Nyongo & Huntrakoon 1987) and using immunohistochemical markers (Yamaguchi & Enjoji 1989).

However, Shorten et al (1986) and Alpert et al (1988) did not observe myoepithelial cells in their ultrastructural studies.

Malignant potential

The low morbidity and mortality recorded in serous cystic tumours have resulted from rare instances of bile duct obstruction, pancreatic insufficiency, duodenal ulceration, vascular rupture and operative complications. All previous reports of serous cystic tumours have stressed the uniformly benign behaviour of these tumours (Compagno & Oertel 1978a, Hodgkinson et al 1978a, Shorten et al 1986, Alpert et al 1988). However, this has been challenged recently by George et al (1989) who reported the first convincing case of serous cystadenocarcinoma of the pancreas with metastases occurring in a 70-year-old man. The primary pancreatic tumour as well as the metastatic deposits found in the stomach and liver were histologically indistinguishable from an otherwise benign serous cystic tumour.

Associated conditions

These have included extrapancreatic malignant neoplasms, diabetes and renal or liver cysts (Compagno & Oertel 1978a). Montag et al (1990) have reported two cases of coexisting pancreatic serous cystic tumour and ductal adenocarcinoma. These associated conditions seem likely to be coincidental findings in an elderly population.

Mucinous cystic tumours

These include mucinous cystadenomas and mucinous cystadenocarcinomas. Some authors have reported mucinous cystadenomas together with serous cystadenomas under the general term of 'pancreatic cystadenoma' and they considered both to be benign (Hodgkinson et al 1978b, Corbally et al 1989, Katoh et al 1989). Others have reported mucinous cystadenomas and cystadenocarcinomas as a single group, on the basis that all mucinous cystic tumours are either malignant or potentially malignant, irrespective of their histological features (Compagno & Oertel 1978b, Santini et al 1988).

Gross appearances

Mucinous cystic tumours are round well-circumscribed lesions, ranging in size from 2 to 30 cm with an average of 10 cm. Their external surface may be smooth or irregular, due to invasive tumour tissue. On section, the tumours are either unilocular or multilocular and contain abundant thick mucus (Fig. 7.4). The multilocular variety is characterized by several large cysts, lacking the peculiar 'honeycombing' pattern seen in the serous type. The

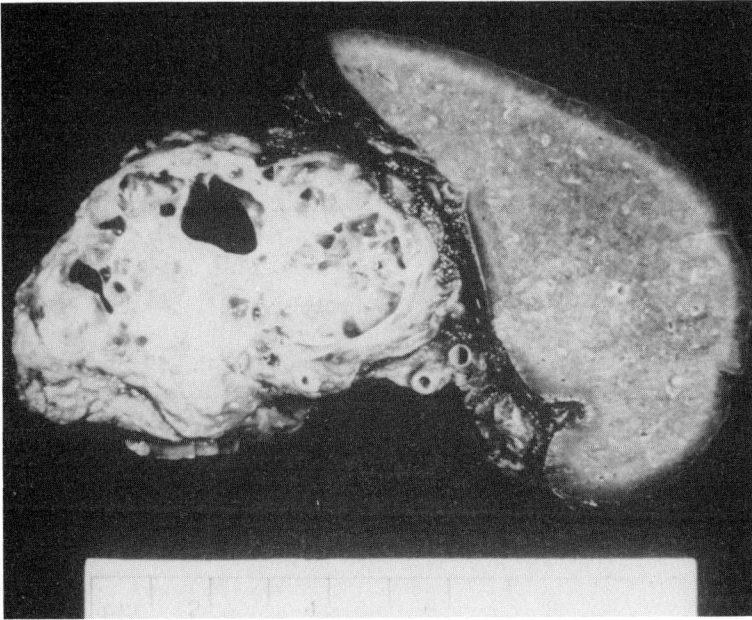

Fig. 7.4   Mucinous cystadenoma, cross section of gross specimen with attached spleen. Multicystic pattern, with some fairly large cysts and incomplete fibrous septa.

inner surface of the cysts may be smooth or show shaggy papillary projections. The tumours are surrounded by dense fibrous tissue which may be focally calcified. Fibrous adhesions to adjacent structures may also be present.

Histological features

The epithelial lining consists predominantly of mucus-secreting tall columnar cells with varying numbers of goblet cells. The epithelium is usually arranged in a single row, but may show a range of growth patterns: stratification, glandular formation, crypt-like invagination and papillary projections (Fig. 7.5). The mucus producing cells predominantly secrete acidic mucins, with variable proportions of sulphomucins and sialomucins, and some neutral mucins (Bogomoletz et al 1980, Santini et al 1988). Glycogen is not found. Scattered argyrophil cells and a few Paneth cells can be identified by appropriate special stains or immunohistochemistry.

   In mucinous cystadenoma, the histological and cytological features are benign. Conversely, in mucinous cystadenocarcinoma, the growth patterns and cellular features in most areas are obviously those of a malignant neoplasm. Diagnostic difficulties may arise when the histopathologist is

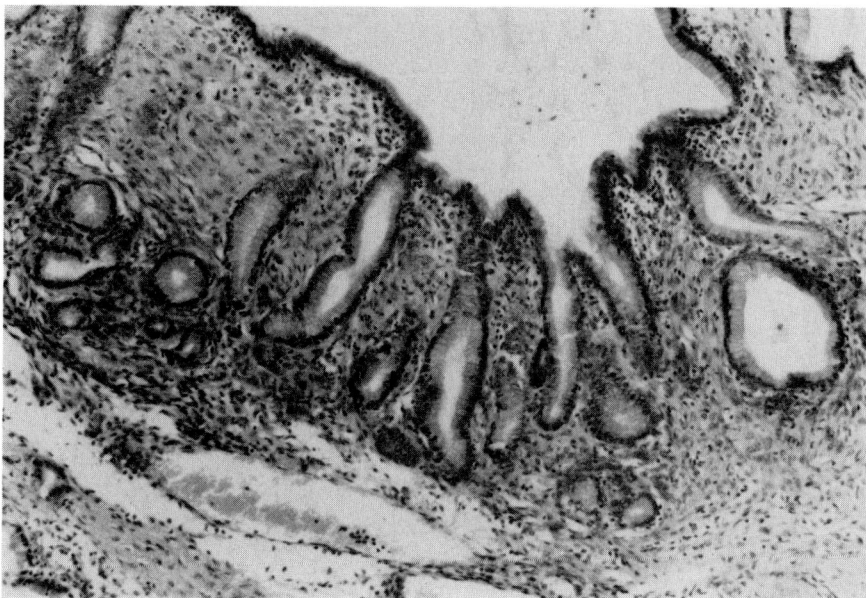

Fig. 7.5 Mucinous cystadenoma lined by mucus-secreting columnar epithelium. Numerous crypt-like glandular invaginations are present. The stroma is dense and cellular. H & E × 125.

confronted with focal atypical or malignant change in an otherwise benign-looking mucinous cystadenoma.

Underlying the mucus-secreting columnar epithelium there is a dense and cellular connective tissue stroma, somewhat resembling that found in the ovary. There may be stromal haemorrhage and necrosis. The fibrous tissue surrounding the tumour contains occasional lymphoid aggregates and adjacent pancreatic tissue is compressed. In cystadenocarcinoma, stromal and capsular invasion may be seen.

Electron microscopy and immunohistochemistry

The few reports on ultrastructure have confirmed the presence of mucous vacuoles within the cytoplasm of the columnar cells; they also display well developed apical microvilli (Albores-Saavedra et al 1987).

Immunohistochemical studies have shown strong immunostaining for carcinoembryonic antigen in addition to immunoreactivity with conventional epithelial markers (Yu & Shetty 1985, Helpap & Vogel 1989). The presence of serotonin, neuron specific enolase, chromogranin and pancreatic polypeptides has occasionally been demonstrated in columnar cells (Albores-Saavedra et al 1987, Helpap & Vogel 1989).

Malignancy and malignant potential

A proportion of mucinous cystic tumours are malignant when first discovered, with invasion of adjacent organs or metastatic spread. These are clearly mucinous cystadenocarcinomas and carry a correspondingly high mortality (Hodgkinson et al 1978b, Katoh et al 1989).

Several authors have claimed however that a clear distinction, in pathological and biological terms, between benign and malignant mucinous cystic tumours is difficult and unwarranted (Hodgkinson et al 1978b, Compagno & Oertel 1978b, Klöppel 1984). There are well-documented cases of apparently histologically benign mucinous cystadenomas which have recurred as invasive cystadenocarcinomas, and it has even been suggested that most mucinous cystadenocarcinomas probably arise from a pre-existing benign tumour (Campbell & Cruickshank 1962, Hodgkinson et al 1978b). Some mucinous cystic tumours, if sampled exhaustively, are found to contain a range of coexisting benign, atypical borderline and frankly malignant epithelia in varying proportions (Compagno & Oertel 1978b, Albores-Saavedra et al 1987). On the other hand, there are also examples of patients who have had histologically benign mucinous cystadenomas removed and who survived for many years without recurrence or malignant transformation (Yamaguchi & Enjoji 1987, Corbally et al 1989). Yamaguchi & Enjoji (1987) have tried to resolve these difficulties by subdividing mucinous cystic tumours into three histological groups: benign mucinous cystic tumour, borderline mucinous cystic tumour and mucinous cystadenocarcinoma. Clearly, the finding of a benign-looking mucinous cystic tumour should prompt the histopathologist to take multiple blocks from the specimen and examine numerous sections in order to exclude unequivocal malignancy. For these reasons, needle biopsy or fine needle aspiration are probably contraindicated in the diagnosis and management of mucinous cystic tumours.

Mucinous cystadenocarcinoma must be differentiated from mucinous or colloid adenocarcinoma of the pancreas. This is a variant of the common ductal adenocarcinoma and shows a similar behaviour with early spread to lymph nodes and the liver.

Pathogenesis

Pancreatic mucinous cystic tumours have been induced in Syrian hamsters using nitrosamine derivatives (Klöppel 1984). Albores-Saavedra et al (1987) have recently stressed the intestinal features often displayed by mucinous cystic tumours, irrespective of their benign or malignant course, and have suggested that these tumours could arise from an endodermal stem cell with subsequent differentiation towards an intestinal phenotype. It is of interest that biliary cystadenoma and cystadenocarcinoma show a female preponderence similar to that of serous and mucinous cystic tumours of the pancreas (Compagno & Oertel 1978b).

PAPILLARY CYSTIC TUMOUR

Papillary cystic tumour of the pancreas has been described under a variety of synonyms including 'papillary and solid epithelial neoplasm', 'solid and cystic acinar cell tumour', reflecting the variegated gross and microscopic features as well as the uncertain pathogenesis. More than 100 cases of this rare tumour have now been reported (Pezzi et al 1988, Hernandez-Maldonado et al 1989, Matsunou & Konishi 1990).

Clinical features

The tumour occurs predominantly in adolescent girls and young women with a median age of 22 years and a range of 2 to 44 years (Hernandez-Maldonado et al 1989). Patients present with an enlarging abdominal mass and often complain of upper abdominal pain or discomfort (Morrison et al 1984, Lieber et al 1987). Older patients may be asymptomatic (Morrison et al 1984, Matsunou & Konishi 1990). The tumours are more common in the head and tail of the pancreas (Hernandez-Maldonado et al 1989). The tumours are highly vascular and this may cause haemoperitoneum or intraoperative haemorrhage in some patients. No glandular differentiation is seen. The fibrous layer surrounding the tumour may contain atrophic pancreatic structures. Staining for argyrophil cells has produced conflicting results (Learmonth et al 1985, Lieber et al 1987, Matsunou & Konishi 1990).

Gross appearances

Papillary cystic tumours are round and well demarcated by a fibrous layer from the surrounding pancreatic tissue. They have an average diameter of 10 cm (range 2 cm to 20 cm). On section, the lesions are lobulated and solid areas at the periphery surround a central cystic zone of necrosis and haemorrhage.

Histological features

Microscopically, the solid areas consist of sheets of uniform, small polygonal cells, with dark nuclei and moderate amounts of eosinophilic cytoplasm. Some tumour cells may show a clear vacuolated cytoplasm, which occasionally contains PAS-positive hyaline granules resistant to diastase digestion. Mitotic figures are few. There are widespread foci of degenerative changes with cystic necrosis, haemorrhage, cholesterol clefts or granulomas and hyalinization. The central cystic zone may contain papillary projections covered by one or more layers of cells similar to those present in the solid areas. These structures are considered by some to represent pseudopapillae resulting from the degenerative changes (Klöppel

1984, Lieber et al 1987). No glandular differentiation is seen. Staining for argyrophil cells has produced conflicting results (Learmonth et al 1985, Lieber et al 1987, Matsunou & Konishi 1990).

The solid areas contain a rich, delicate vascular network which often imparts an organoid pattern to the tumour and this may cause diagnostic confusion with an endocrine neoplasm. Papillary cystic tumour must be differentiated from pancreatic neuroendocrine or islet-cell tumours.

Electron microscopy and immunohistochemistry

Studies on the ultrastructure and the immunoreactivity of papillary cystic tumour have produced some conflicting findings. This may reflect differences in tissue sampling and processing. Ultrastructurally, most reports describe closely packed polygonal cells with a clear cytoplasm, rounded or indented nuclei and eccentric nucleoli. Mitochondria are numerous, whilst Golgi apparatus and rough endoplasmic reticulum are sparse. The cells often contain numerous membrane-bound electron-dense granules, which have been variously interpreted as mucigen (Miettinen et al 1987) or zymogen granules (Lieber et al 1987, Matsunou & Konishi 1990). There is general agreement on the absence of glycogen, mucous granules and neurosecretory granules.

Immunohistochemical findings include positive results for alpha-1-antitrypsin, considered by some workers to be a specific marker for pancreatic acinar cell tumours (Learmonth et al 1985, Miettinen et al 1987, Morohoshi et al 1987, Matsunou & Konishi 1990). Immunostaining for pancreatic enzymes, pancreatic hormones and pancreatic polypeptides and neuron specific enolase has not produced consistent findings (Morrison et al 1984, Learmonth et al 1985, Lieber et al 1987, Miettinen et al 1987, Morohoshi et al 1987, Matsunou & Konishi 1990).

Malignant potential

It seems that papillary cystic tumour has a low-grade malignant potential. Most patients have had a favourable course following surgery, with long survival periods. A few patients have shown local tumour recurrences or metastatic spread.

Aetiology and histogenesis

The sex and age distribution suggests that hormonal factors may be important in the pathogenesis of papillary cystic tumour (Cubilla & Fitzgerald 1984). Miettinen et al (1987), however, could not demonstrate oestrogen receptors in two cases examined.

There is no general agreement on either a pancreatic duct or acinar cell origin. It has been suggested that papillary cystic tumour is a neoplasm of totipotential epithelial stem cells which can show either exocrine or endocrine differentiation or both (Miettinen et al 1987, Matsunou & Konishi 1990).

MISCELLANEOUS CYSTIC TUMOURS

A few cases of so-called '*ductectatic*' *mucinous cystadenomas and cystadeno-carcinomas* have been described in Japan in both male and female patients who were in their sixties (Itai et al 1986). The lesions were detected by endoscopic retrograde pancreatography or postoperative pancreatography. The pathological features were those of well-defined unilocular or multi-locular masses (average diameter 3 cm), with cluster-like cysts containing thick mucus. The cysts were lined by mucus-secreting columnar epithelium which showed either benign or malignant histological appearances. Itai et al (1986) claimed that such 'ductectatic' mucinous cystadenomas and cystadeno-carcinomas resulted from cystic dilatation of a collateral branch of the main pancreatic duct and that the lesions were different from conventional serous and mucinous cystic tumours. This concept is interesting, but requires further confirmatory studies.

Acinar cell cystadenocarcinoma is a rare multicystic variant of acinar cell carcinoma (Lack 1989), of which two cases have been reported in males (Cantrell et al 1981, Stamm et al 1987). One patient developed a liver metastasis 16 months after operation (Stamm et al 1987). The two resected lesions were large (25 cm and 35 cm in diameter) appeared encapsulated and involved the body and tail of the pancreas. The cysts were of varying size and lined by cuboidal to columnar epithelium. Tubular or cribriform structures were present. Glycogen and mucins were not detected. Electron microscopy showed abundant zymogen granules suggesting an acinar cell origin. This was confirmed by positive staining for trypsin in one case (Cantrell et al 1981) and for alpha-1-antitrypsin in the other (Stamm et al 1987). It is possible, as suggested by Cantrell et al (1981), that some cases previously diagnosed as serous or mucinous cystic tumours, might have demonstrated acinar cell differentiation if electron microscopic or immuno-histochemical examination had been carried out.

Two single case reports further emphasize the variety of lesions which present as cystic tumours of the pancreas. These are included here for the sake of completeness.

Warfel et al (1988) reported an unusual multilocular cystadenoma (10 cm in diameter), involving the body and the tail of the pancreas in a 4-month-old infant. The cysts were lined by non-mucin secreting and non glycogen-producing cuboidal cells. Warfel et al (1988) considered the lesion was a hamartoma.

Friedman (1990) reported an encapsulated, multilocular cystadeno-carcinoma of the pancreas, as a postmortem finding in a 74-year-old female patient which measured 19 cm in diameter. The tumour had metastasized widely to various organs and lymph nodes. The lesion consisted of multiple cysts, lined by a single layer of cuboidal or columnar epithelium, but with some pseudostratified papillary projections. Benign, atypical and overt malignant areas coexisted. The tumour cells expressed carcinoembryonic antigen, but were negative for endocrine markers. Traces of cytoplasmic glycogen were present but mucins were not detected. The ultrastructural features were consistent with a ductal or centroacinar derivation.

CONCLUSION

Cystic tumours of the exocrine pancreas are unusual. They occur predominantly in females. Grossly they are well-delineated and have a characteristic multiloculated appearance. These tumours show a broad histological range of benign, borderline and malignant features. Their histogenesis is uncertain. The best treatment is wide surgical resection, irrespective of histological type. Their progress is relatively good.

ADDENDUM

In a comprehensive review of the subject, Albores-Saavedra et al (1990) have stressed the need for the subdivision of mucinous cystic tumours into benign, borderline and malignant categories. A case report of mucinous cystadenocarcinoma with stromal pseudosarcomatous features has re-emphasized morphological similarities with ovarian tumours (Garcia Rego et al 1991). An ultrastructural and immunohistochemical study of 10 cases of papillary cystic (solid) tumour has favoured a dual exocrine and endocrine differentiation for this peculiar neoplasm (Stömmer et al 1991). Finally, the hitherto undescribed occurrence of papillary cystic (solid) tumour in male patients has been reported (Klöppel et al 1991).

REFERENCES

Albores-Saavedra J, Angeles-Angeles A, Nadji M et al 1987 Mucinous cystadenocarcinomas of the pancreas. Morphologic and immunocytochemical observations. American Journal of Surgical Pathology 11: 11–20
Albores-Saavedra J, Gould E W, Angeles-Angeles A et al 1990 Cystic tumors of the pancreas. In: Rosen P P, Fechner R E (eds) Pathology Annual, vol 25, part 2. Appleton & Lange, East Norwalk, pp 19–50
Alpert L C, Truong L D, Bossart M I et al 1988 Microcystic adenoma (serous cystadenoma) of the pancreas. A study of 14 cases with immunohistochemical and electron-microscopic correlation. American Journal of Surgical Pathology 12: 251–263
Bogomoletz W V, Adnet J J, Widgren S et al 1980 Cystadenoma of the pancreas: a histological, histochemical and ultrastructural study of seven cases. Histopathology 4: 309–320
Campbell J A, Cruickshank A H 1962 Cystadenoma and cystadenocarcinoma of the pancreas. Journal of Clinical Pathology 15: 432–437
Cantrell B B, Cubilla A L, Erlandson R A et al 1981 Acinar cell cystadenocarcinoma of human pancreas. Cancer 47: 410–416

Chen J, Baithun S I 1985 Morphological study of 391 cases of exocrine pancreatic tumours with special reference to the classification of exocrine pancreatic carcinoma. Journal of Pathology 146: 17–29

Compagno J, Oertel J E 1978a Microcystic adenomas of the pancreas (glycogen-rich cystadenomas). A clinicopathologic study of 34 cases. American Journal of Clinical Pathology 69: 289–298

Compagno J, Oertel J E 1978b Mucinous cystic neoplasms of the pancreas with overt and latent malignancy (cystadenocarcinoma and cystadenoma). A clinicopathologic study of 41 cases. American Journal of Clinical Pathology 69: 573–580

Corbally M T, McAnema O J, Urmacher C et al 1989 Pancreatic cystadenoma. A clinicopathologic study. Archives of Surgery 124: 1271–1274

Cubilla A L, Fitzgerald P J 1984 Tumors of the exocrine pancreas. Armed Forces Institute of Pathology, Washington

Friedman H D 1990 Nonmucinous, glycogen-poor cystadenocarcinoma of the pancreas. Archives of Pathology and Laboratory Medicine 114: 888–891

Garcia-Rego J A, Valbuena Ruvira L, Alvarez Garcia A et al 1991 Pancreatic mucinous cystadenocarcinoma with pseudosarcomatous mural nodules. A report of a case with immunohistochemical study. Cancer 67: 494–498

George D H, Murphy F, Michalki R et al 1989 Serous cystadenocarcinoma of the pancreas: a new entity? American Journal of Surgical Pathology 13: 61–66

Glenner G G, Mallory G K 1956 The cystadenoma and related nonfunctional tumors of the pancreas. Pathogenesis, classification, and significance. Cancer 9: 980–996

Helpap B, Vogel J 1989 Immunohistochemical studies on cystic pancreatic neoplasms. Pathology, Research and Practice 184: 39–45

Hernandez-Maldonado J J, Rodriguez-Bigas M A, Gonzalez de Pesante A et al 1989 Papillary cystic neoplasm of the pancreas. A report of a case presenting with carcinomatosis. Annals of Surgery 55: 552–559

Hodgkinson D J, ReMine W H, Weiland L H 1978a Pancreatic cystadenoma. A clinicopathologic study of 45 cases. Archives of Surgery 113: 512–519

Hodgkinson D J, ReMine W H, Weiland L H 1978b A clinicopathologic study of 21 cases of pancreas cystadenocarcinoma. Annals of Surgery 188: 679–684

Itai Y, Ohhashi K, Nagai H et al 1986 "Ductectatic" mucinous cystadenoma and cystadenocarcinoma of the pancreas. Radiology 161: 697–700

Katoh H, Rossi R L, Braasch J W et al 1989 Cystadenoma and cystadenocarcinoma of the pancreas. Hepato-gastroenteroly 36: 424–430

Kim Y I, Seo J W, Suh J S et al 1990 Microcystic adenomas of the pancreas. Report of three cases with two of multicentric origin. American Journal of Clinical Pathology 94: 150–156

Klöppel G 1984 Pancreatic, non-endocrine tumours. In: Klöppel G, Heitz P U (eds) Pancreatic pathology. Churchill Livingstone, Edinburgh, pp 79–113

Klöppel G, Maurer R, Hofman E et al 1991 Solid-cystic (papillary-cystic) tumours within and outside the pancreas in men: report of two patients. Virchow's Archiv A (Pathological Anatomy) 418: 179–183

Lack E E 1989 Primary tumors of the exocrine pancreas. Classification, overview and recent contributions by immunochemistry and electron microscopy. American Journal of Surgical Pathology 13 (suppl. 1): 68–88

Learmonth G M, Price S K, Visser A E et al 1985 Papillary and cystic neoplasm of the pancreas—an acinar cell tumour? Histopathology 9: 63–79

Lieber M R, Lack E E, Roberto J R et al 1987 Solid and papillary epithelial neoplasms of the pancreas. An ultrastructural and immunocytochemical study of six cases. American Journal of Surgical Pathology 11: 85–93

Matsunou H, Konishi F 1990 Papillary-cystic neoplasm of the pancreas. A clinicopathologic study concerning the tumor aging and malignancy in nine cases. Cancer 65: 283–291

Miettinen M, Partanen S, Fräki O, Kivilaakso E 1987 Papillary cystic tumor of the pancreas. An analysis of cellular differentiation by electron microscopy and immunohistochemistry. American Journal of Surgical Pathology 11: 855–865

Montag A G, Fossati N, Michelassi F 1990 Pancreatic microcystic adenoma coexistent with pancreatic ductal carcinoma. A report of two cases. American Journal of Surgical Pathology 14: 352–355

Morohoshi T, Held G, Klöppel G 1983 Exocrine pancreatic tumours and their histological classification. A study based on 167 autopsy and 97 surgical cases. Histopathology 7: 645–661

Morohoshi T, Kanda M, Horie A et al 1987 Immunocytochemical markers of uncommon pancreatic tumors. Acinar-cell carcinoma, pancreatoblastoma, a solid cystic (papillary-cystic) tumor. Cancer 59: 739–747

Morrison D M, Jewel L D, McCaughey W T et al 1984 Papillary cystic tumor of the pancreas. Archives of Pathology and Laboratory Medicine 108: 723–727

Nyongo A, Huntrakoon M 1985 Microcystic adenoma of the pancreas with myoepithelial cells. A hitherto undescribed morphologic feature. American Journal of Clinical Pathology 84: 114–120

Pezzi C M, Schuerch C, Erlandson R A et al 1988 Papillary-cystic neoplasm of the pancreas. Journal of Surgical Oncology 37: 278–285

Santini D, Bazzocchi F, Ricci M et al 1988 Mucinous cystic tumour of the pancreas. A histological and histochemical study. Pathology, Research and Practice 183: 767–770

Shorten S D, Hart W R, Petras R E 1986 Microcystic adenomas (serous cystadenomas) of pancreas. A clinicopathologic investigation of eight cases with immunohistochemical and ultrastructural studies. American Journal of Surgical Pathology 10: 365–372

Stamm B, Burger H, Hollinger A 1987 Acinar cell cystadenocarcinoma of the pancreas. Cancer 60: 2542–2547

Stömmer P, Kraus J, Stole M et al 1991 Solid and cystic pancreatic tumors. Clinical, histochemical and electron microscopic features in ten cases. Cancer 67: 1635–1641

Warfel K A, Faught P R, Hull M T 1988 Pancreatic cystadenoma in an infant: ultrastructural study. Pediatric Pathology 8: 559–565

Yamaguchi K, Enjoji M 1987 Cystic neoplasms of the pancreas. Gastroenterology 92: 1934–1943

Yu H C, Shetty J 1985 Mucinous cystic neoplasm of the pancreas with high carcinoembryonic antigen. Archives of Pathology and Laboratory Medicine 109: 375–377

8

Aspects of tumours of the urinary bladder and prostate gland

J. N. Webb

The purpose of this chapter is to discuss aspects of tumours of the urinary bladder and prostate, which give rise to diagnostic problems in the routine practice of surgical histopathology.

LOW GRADE PAPILLARY TRANSITIONAL CELL TUMOURS

The great majority of bladder tumours are of transitional cell type—and most of these are papillary tumours. As currently defined in the WHO classification, a transitional cell papilloma (Grade 0) is a rare neoplasm—certainly accounting for no more than about 2% of papillary tumours (Fig. 8.1). For this reason the diagnosis of papilloma is virtually never made. Other authorities take a different view in that papillary transitional cell carcinoma Grade 1 (Fig. 8.2) is considered to be a benign neoplasm and is

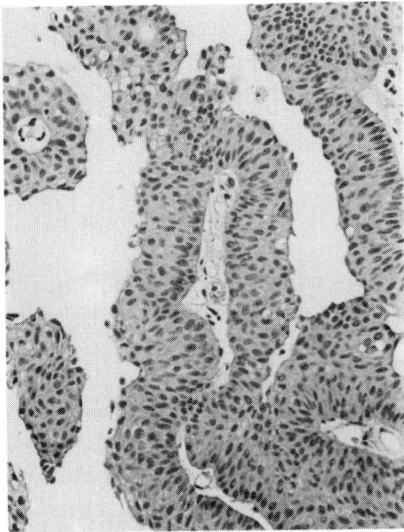

Fig. 8.1 Transitional cell papilloma of bladder, Grade 0, as defined in WHO classification of bladder tumours. H & E × 55.

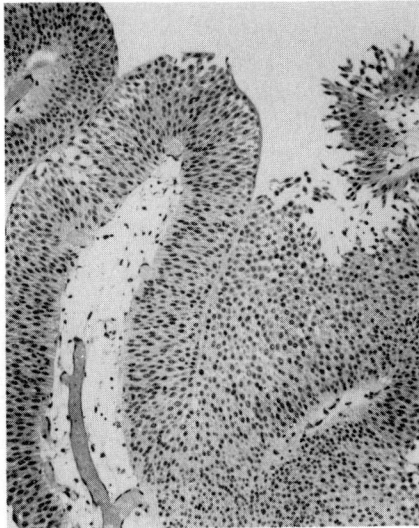

Fig. 8.2 Papillary transitional cell carcinoma—Grade 1. H & E × 50.

described as a papilloma (Bergqvist et al 1965, Jordan et al 1987, Eagan 1989, Murphy 1989). The reasoning is that this very well-differentiated tumour is rarely—some would say never—invasive. On this basis perhaps 30% of transitional cell tumours of the bladder would be called papillomas. If one takes this view, then the current Grade 2 tumour would be considered a low grade, and a Grade 3 tumour a high grade transitional cell carcinoma (Murphy 1989).

However, urologists have been reluctant to view Grade 1 papillary tumours in this light. The principal reasons for this are that patients presenting with superficial papillary tumours of the bladder have an unpredictable course and there is no certain means of knowing which patients will develop recurrent tumours or show progression of their disease. Gilbert et al (1978) showed that 60% of 155 unselected patients with Grade 1 papillary tumour of the bladder developed recurrences, and also that 13% of the total went on to develop tumours of higher grade. A large series from the Mayo Clinic showed an even higher percentage (73%) of cases of Grade 1 tumours which recurred and 22% developed tumours of higher grade (Greene et al 1973). However, it is possible to look at it from another standpoint, that few patients presenting initially with Grade 1 tumours will die of their disease (Bergqvist et al 1965, Gilbert et al 1978, Jordan et al 1987).

The problem with bladder cancer is that it is a disease which may affect much of the urothelium of the urinary tract, and so the initial superficial tumour may not be the most significant event (Brawn 1982). The development of neoplastic change in the urothelium elsewhere in the bladder may be—in terms of morbidity and mortality—of greater significance. The term recurrence in this context is used rather loosely. It can be taken to mean the recurrence at the same site of an incompletely excised neoplasm, but is also taken in a clinical sense to mean the subsequent development of new tumours elsewhere in the bladder.

CARCINOMA IN-SITU, DYSPLASIA AND HYPERPLASIA OF THE UROTHELIUM

The unpredictable behaviour of superficial transitional cell tumours of the bladder has led to the standard practice of taking random mucosal biopsies in addition to the biopsy or resection of any visible bladder tumour. These may be quadrant biopsies or samples taken close to and distant from the tumour itself. The histological assessment of these mucosal biopsies is subject to considerable observer variation. Part of the problem is that a number of terms have been applied to abnormalities of the urothelium which many have assumed to be premalignant lesions. These terms include carcinoma-in-situ (CIS grades 1, 2 and 3); dysplasia—often categorized as mild, moderate or severe, atypia and atypical hyperplasia.

Carcinoma-in-situ of the urothelium should not usually present major diagnostic problems. Our knowledge of the subject extends back to the pioneering work of Melicow (1952) and Melamed et al (1966) who mapped the field changes in the urothelium of the bladder. Subsequently, this topic has been discussed by Koss (1979), Farrow et al (1976), Soto et al (1977), Soloway et al (1978) and Wallace et al (1979).

Carcinoma-in-situ is defined as a *flat* epithelial lesion of the urothelial layer composed of neoplastic transitional cells which cytologically correspond to a Grade 3 transitional carcinoma, i.e. are always poorly differentiated (Fig. 8.3). The number of cell layers may or may not be increased, and may even be reduced, and in places the mucosa may appear denuded with an absent epithelial layer. This is due to the fact that the neoplastic cells of CIS lack cohesion so that gaps or slits occur between them or else the entire layer becomes detached from the subepithelial stroma. A less usual pattern is where the neoplastic cells infiltrate pre-existing urothelium imparting a Pagetoid appearance.

The clinical significance of finding CIS in a random biopsy in the presence of concurrent superficial transitional cell carcinoma is a matter of debate, but the commonly held view is that its presence indicates a greater likelihood of disease progression (Althausen et al 1976, Koss 1979, Smith et al 1983, Wolf et al 1985). It must be remembered that the presence of widespread flat CIS of the bladder in the absence of a macroscopic tumour is known to carry a high risk of invasion (Koss et al 1969). However, modern methods of treating superficial bladder cancer by means of intra-vesical instillations of chemotherapeutic agents, e.g. mitomycin, BCG, appear to modify considerably the course of the disease (Cumming et al 1989), with high response rates and a reduced likelihood of progression to invasive carcinoma.

It is possible to recognize atypical changes in the urothelium which fall short of those seen in CIS. These changes may be referred to as dysplasia and, in common with similar lesions in the gastrointestinal and the female genital tracts, they have been graded into mild, moderate and severe forms. In such a classification, severe dysplasia merges with the changes of CIS as it does in the cervix. Moreover, it is doubtful whether one can consistently identify three degrees of dysplasia in the urothelium. It is best to define it as a flat epithelial lesion in which the cells show abnormalities that fall short of those seen in CIS. There is some enlargement of cells, disturbance but not loss of polarity, slight nuclear pleomorphism and mitoses that are not confined to the basal layer. In contradistinction to CIS, there is no loss of cellular cohesion and splits or gaps in the epithelial layer are not observed (Fig. 8.4). Urothelial dysplasia as so defined probably corresponds to the term atypical hyperplasia (Koss 1975).

A third form of abnormality in the urothelium is hyperplasia, sometimes referred to as simple hyperplasia, to distinguish it from atypical hyperplasia or dysplasia. Simple hyperplasia is seen at sites of mucosal inflammation and is presumed to be a reactive process. However, hyperplasia otherwise

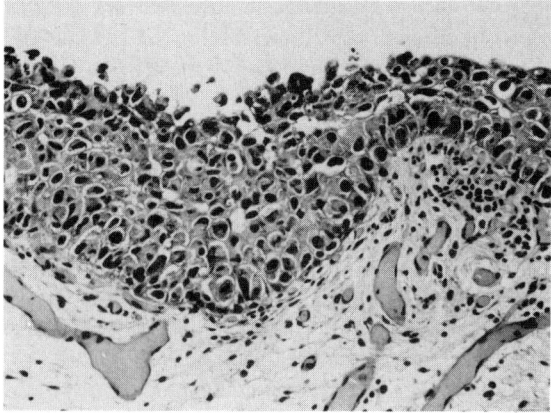

Fig. 8.3   Flat Carcinoma-in-situ (CIS) of bladder mucosa, composed solely of poorly differentiated cells. H & E × 130.

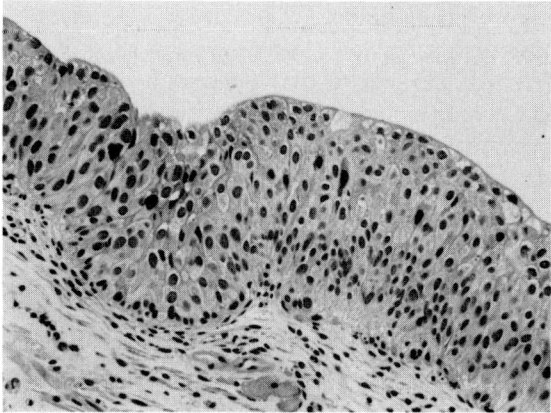

Fig. 8.4   Bladder mucosa showing urothelial dysplasia with disturbed polarity, cellular enlargement and some nuclear pleomorphism. H & E × 130.

indistinguishable from this reactive type, can also be seen in the absence of any obvious stimulus, such as chronic irritation or inflammation. It may be defined as a state in which the number of cell layers is increased beyond the normal but without any cellular atypia. A practical, even if somewhat arbitrary, definition is where the urothelium is seven or more cell layers thick (Fig. 8.5). Whether urothelial hyperplasia, in the absence of obvious inflammation, has any clinical significance is not known at the present time. Uncommonly, the hyperplastic urothelium forms a corrugated or un-dulating profile, but without true papillae. This appearance has been described as papillary hyperplasia. It is unclear whether this represents the very earliest changes of a low grade papillary tumour.

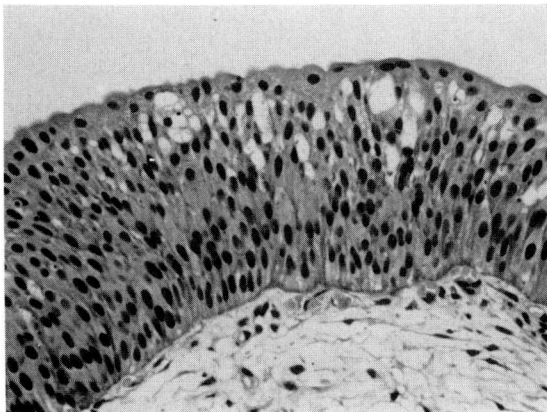

Fig. 8.5 Urothelial hyperplasia of bladder mucosa: the cells are arranged in many layers but there is no atypia. H & E × 208.

In summary, therefore, it is recommended to categorize the urothelium in random mucosal biopsies as normal or abnormal, i.e. simple hyperplasia, dysplasia or carcinoma-in-situ.

ASSESSMENT OF INVASION OF BLADDER CARCINOMA

The proper management of patients with bladder carcinoma is dependent upon an accurate assessment of the grade and stage. It is often difficult in transurethral resection specimens to establish whether invasion has taken place, and to what extent. The majority of high grade transitional cell carcinomas are found to be invasive when first diagnosed. If there is invasion of the muscularis propria, there is no means of knowing whether it is a T2 or a T3 tumour, that is to say, whether it invades the superficial half of the muscularis propria or has extended deeper. All that can be said is that when muscle invasion is present the tumour is at least a T2 tumour.

The subepithelial stroma or lamina propria of the bladder mucosa may contain strands of smooth muscle fibres and these should not be confused with the muscularis propria. Ro et al (1987) have drawn attention to the presence of these smooth muscle fibres (Fig. 8.6), and refer to it as a muscularis mucosae, with the implication that there is a submucosa between it and the muscularis propria. They studied 100 cystectomy specimens and found a continuous smooth muscle layer between the epithelium and the muscularis propria in only three cases. In 20 other cases this layer was discontinuous, while in 71 cases smooth muscle fibres were dispersed or scattered within the lamina propria. It was noted that these muscle fibres were closely related to large blood vessels. However, it hardly seems justified to refer to such an irregular and inconstant feature as a muscularis mucosae, especially since in no case could the bladder be considered normal.

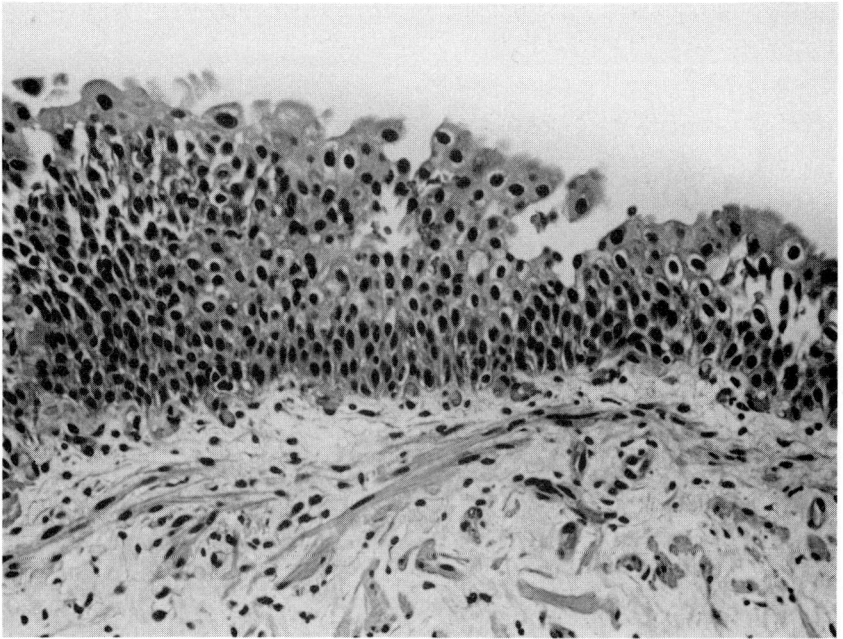

Fig. 8.6   Bladder mucosa. Note thin strands of smooth muscle in the subepithelial stroma. These may extend close to the epithelial layer as shown. H & E × 200.

The development of muscle fibres within the lamina propria probably occurs as a response to inflammation, previous surgery, irradiation and so forth, and the close association with large blood vessels may indicate that muscle fibres have grown out from these vessels. All the structures between the luminal surface of the bladder and the muscularis propria are best referred to as the mucosa of the bladder whether or not muscle fibres can be found in that layer.

UNCOMMON EPITHELIAL TUMOURS OF THE BLADDER

Squamous carcinoma

The great majority of epithelial tumours of the urinary bladder are of transitional cell type. However, in areas of the world where infestation with *Schistosoma haematobium* (bilharziasis) is endemic, there is a high incidence of vesical squamous carcinoma. This tumour accounts for only about 5% of bladder carcinomas in Europe and North America where it may be associated with bladder calculi or long-standing urinary tract infection. Squamous carcinomas are nearly always invasive when first diagnosed and nearly all have penetrated the muscularis propria and are stage T2 or more. The five year survival is correspondingly poor. Grading these tumours offers little prognostic information, in contradistinction to transitional cell carcinomas, and does not influence management.

Undifferentiated carcinomas

Undifferentiated carcinomas of the bladder are also uncommon. Three types are recognized.

Undifferentiated carcinoma NOS (not otherwise specified)

Bergqvist et al (1965) regarded this tumour as the undifferentiated end of transitional cell carcinoma and designated it a Grade 4 tumour—Grade 3 carcinomas being poorly differentiated but still recognizably of transitional cell type. Undifferentiated carcinomas consist of sheets of anaplastic carcinoma cells with large vesicular nuclei and prominent nucleoli. Mitotic figures are plentiful. These tumours may contain multinucleated giant cells which resemble syncytiotrophoblast. Immunohistochemical studies have shown that they, and some high grade transitional cell carcinomas, produce human chorionic gonadotrophin (Fig. 8.7) and in a few cases, increased amounts of hormone have been demonstrated in the blood (Kawamura et al 1978). This is probably an example of ectopic hormone production by the tumour rather than evidence of germ cell differentiation (Ainsworth & Gresham 1960, Civantos & Rywlin 1972). Their behaviour and prognosis is similar to high grade transitional cell carcinoma of similar stage.

Spindle cell carcinoma (carcinoma of sarcomatoid type)

Histologically these uncommon tumours closely resemble sarcomas and the distinction can be difficult to achieve (Fig. 8.8). They are often large tumours and appear polypoid or ulcerated. They consist of interlacing fascicles of spindle cells which tend to have abundant cytoplasm. They may also show a myxoid pattern in which the spindle cells are set in an abundant pale-staining stroma. Nuclear pleomorphism may be prominent and mitotic figures are numerous. Where the biopsy includes foci of epithelial differentiation the nature of the tumour is revealed. In the absence of such foci, however, it may be difficult or impossible to distinguish it from a sarcoma.

Immunohistochemistry is helpful in difficult cases. Spindle cell carcinomas are nearly always positive for cytokeratins and epithelial membrane antigen. They may also be positive for vimentin, generally considered to be a marker of mesenchymal differentiation, but they are negative for other soft tissue markers (Wick et al 1988). The main differential diagnosis is from a leiomyosarcoma of the bladder. These latter tumours are negative for epithelial markers and are likely to be positive for muscle markers, e.g. desmin or muscle specific actin (Mills et al 1989).

Spindle cell carcinomas are high grade, widely invasive tumours with a

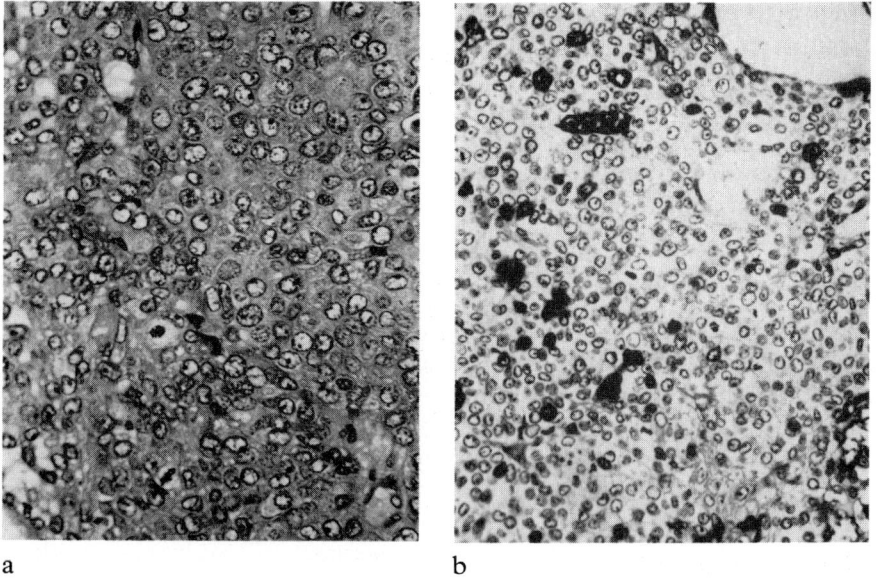

a   b

Fig. 8.7   **(a)** Undifferentiated carcinoma of bladder. NOS. H & E × 130. **(b)** Same tumour with some cells immunoreactive for HCG. H & E × 32.

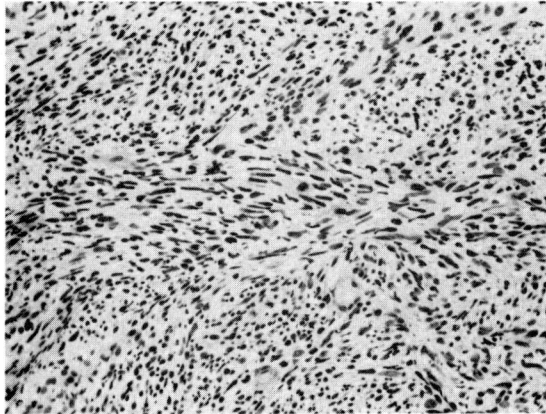

Fig. 8.8   Spindle cell carcinoma (carcinoma of sarcomatoid type). H & E × 32.

poor prognosis. Their management is similar to other high grade invasive bladder carcinomas. In contrast, many sarcomas at this site are less aggressive in their behaviour and are in consequence more amenable to surgical resection (Mills et al 1989). Rarely, carcinosarcomas with chondroid or rhabdomyoblastic differentiation can arise in the bladder (Young 1987).

Small cell undifferentiated carcinoma

This is rare in the bladder but histologically resembles similar tumours of the bronchopulmonary system and other sites. It occurs predominantly in the elderly. The tumour usually presents as a large polypoid mass and is extensively invasive at the time of diagnosis. It consists of sheets, clumps and cords of cells with small, round, oval or irregular nuclei and inconspicuous cytoplasm. The nuclei are hyperchromatic and may show a distinct stippled chromatin pattern. Nuclear 'moulding' may be seen. In the majority of cases a minor component of the tumour has a different histological pattern and may be of transitional cell, glandular or squamous type and there may be evidence of carcinoma-in-situ of the urothelium. These tumours may be positive for both epithelial (cytokeratins, EMA) and neuro-endocrine (NSE, chromogranin, VIP or serotonin) markers or show dense core granules on electron microscopy, but the diagnosis ultimately depends on the characteristic histological appearance (Mills et al 1987). The prognosis is poor with most patients dead in a few months, but longer survival has been reported (Davies et al 1983, Reyes & Soneru 1985, Williams et al 1986).

Adenocarcinoma of the bladder

Most adenocarcinomas, which account for 1% or less of all bladder tumours, do not have any distinctive histological appearance. It may therefore be impossible to distinguish between a primary vesical adenocarcinoma and a secondary adenocarcinoma from, say, a primary tumour of colon or ovary. The exclusion of an origin outside the bladder is mandatory before a diagnosis of adenocarcinoma of the bladder is made. It has been reported that some vesical adenocarcinomas are positive for prostate specific acid phosphatase (Epstein et al 1986) and this has been demonstrated in female, as well as in male patients.

Adenocarcinoma of the bladder is often associated with, and may arise at sites of, glandular metaplasia (Fig. 8.9). The term glandular metaplasia refers to a glandular mucosa that resembles colonic epithelium and it should not be confused with cystitis glandularis which is not truly metaplastic but represents a normal variant of bladder mucosa (Wiener et al 1979). Adenocarcinoma has been particularly associated with extrophy of the bladder where glandular metaplasia is extensive and more than 80 such cases have been reported in adults between 40 and 60 years of age (Nielsen & Nielsen 1983). It seems possible, however, that early reconstructive surgery will greatly reduce or even eliminate the development of this complication.

There is also a significant incidence of glandular metaplasia and adenocarcinoma in bilharziasis, in addition to the commoner squamous carcinoma. This is shown in Table 8.1, the data for which are derived from five major series totalling 916 cases of bladder cancer. Both squamous and glandular

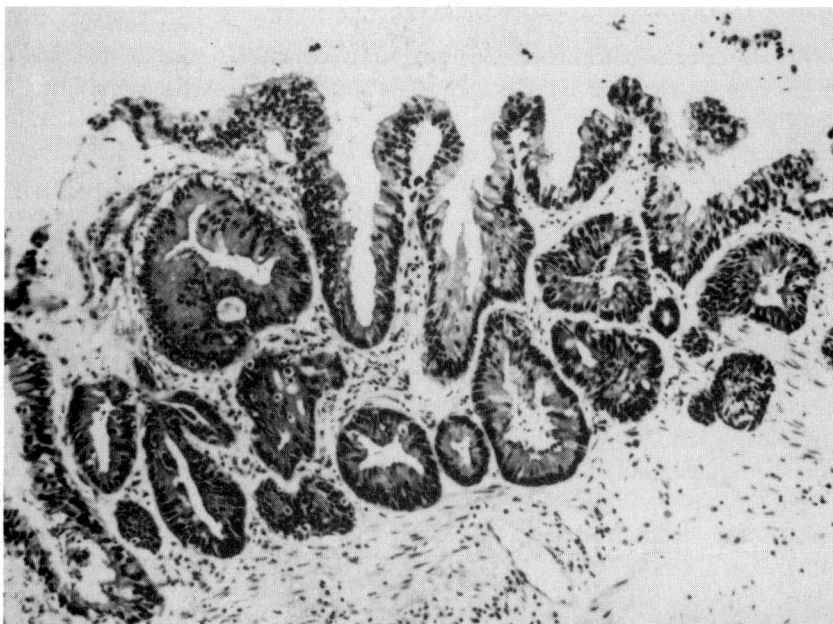

Fig. 8.9   Glandular metaplasia of bladder. Note resemblance to colonic mucosa. H & E × 80.

metaplasia of the bladder mucosa is extremely common in bilharzia-associated cancer and may determine the tumour type (Table 8.2).

Many adenocarcinomas of the bladder are assumed to be of urachal derivation but proof of this may be difficult to establish. Features include an origin in the bladder vault, an intra-mural location (perhaps with an intact overlying mucosa), and the presence of residual urachal elements.

A few cases of signet ring adenocarcinoma of the bladder have been described (De Filipo et al 1987). These diffusely infiltrating tumours consist of cells with mucin-filled cytoplasm arranged singly and in clumps. Tumours of similar type commonly arise in the stomach and colon so it is important to exclude a primary carcinoma at either of these two sites. Based on the few acceptable cases in the literature, the prognosis appears to be poor (Choi et al 1984).

Table 8.1   Tumour type in bilharzia-infected bladders (see Webb 1985 for references)

No. of cases	Tumour type			
	Squamous	Transitional	Adenocarcinoma	Other
916	603	211	67	35

Table 8.2 Mucosal lesions in relation to bilharzia-associated bladder cancer (after Khagafy et al 1972)

Tumour	No. of cases	Squamous metaplasia	Glandular metaplasia
Squamous ca.	66	54	35
Transitional cell ca.	18	3	8
Adenocarcinoma	2	—	2

Clear cell adenocarcinoma is a very rare tumour of bladder or urethra but resembles histologically its much commoner counterparts in the ovary and uterus. They occur in middle-aged or elderly subjects and most cases have been in females (Young & Scully 1985). Tubular, glandular, cystic or papillary structures may be seen and these patterns are often admixed in the same tumour. Solid masses are often present in which mitoses are usually evident. The tumour cells have abundant clear cytoplasm which is rich in glycogen, and the nuclei are pleomorphic and hyperchromatic. Eosinophilic mucinous secretions are present within the glandular lumina and the prominent nuclei may impart a hobnail pattern to the glands.

The principal differential diagnosis, apart from secondary tumour, is nephrogenic adenoma. Young & Scully (1986) have reviewed the diagnostic problems associated with this lesion, mainly from the point of view of distinguishing it from clear cell adenocarcinoma. Nephrogenic adenoma occurs predominantly in males and there is a wide age range. In contrast, the majority of cases of clear cell carcinoma of the urinary tract have been in middle-aged or elderly females. In nephrogenic adenoma there is often a history of preceding trauma or damage to the urinary tract, calculus formation or recent operative procedure. Grossly, nephrogenic adenoma is usually a small lesion, whereas clear cell adenocarcinoma is likely to present as a large tumour. Microscopically, both may have a tubular, glandular, cystic or papillary structure but clear cell carcinoma may also form solid masses of tumour cells. The cytoplasm of the cells in clear cell carcinoma is abundant and rich in glycogen, whereas glycogen is scanty or absent in nephrogenic adenoma. The nuclei of clear cell carcinoma tend to be pleomorphic and mitotic figures can usually be readily identified. Nuclear pleomorphism is not a feature of nephrogenic adenoma and mitotic figures are rare.

SPINDLE CELL LESIONS OF THE LOWER URINARY TRACT AND THEIR DIFFERENTIAL DIAGNOSIS

A number of sarcomas and lesions that may mimic them arise in the bladder in addition to spindle cell carcinoma which has been discussed already.

Sarcomas of the bladder

Rhabdomyosarcoma

Rhabdomyosarcomas can be divided into embryonal and adult or pleomorphic types. Embryonal rhabdomyosarcomas of the urogenital tract are
an important group of tumours occurring in infancy and childhood, but do
not enter into the diagnostic problems under discussion. Adult pleomorphic
rhabdomyosarcomas (Fig. 8.10) may arise in the bladder but are rare.
Immunohistochemically, these may be desmin positive but this is not
specific for rhabdomyoblastic differentiation. The better differentiated
tumours may be positive for myoglobin, but in such cases cross-striations
can usually be demonstrated in the abundant eosinophilic strap-like
cytoplasm or else the characteristic myofibrils can be demonstrated on
electron microscopy.

Leiomyosarcoma

The diagnosis of a leiomyosarcoma of the bladder may present difficulties
on two counts: one, in distinguishing it from spindle cell carcinoma and two,
in assessing its malignant potential (Fig. 8.11).

Leiomyosarcoma is the commonest sarcoma of the bladder. Mills et al
(1989) reviewed 15 cases of which nine were males and six females. There

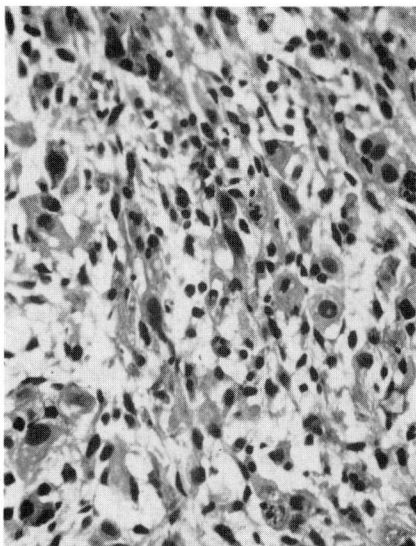

Fig. 8.10 Pleomorphic rhabdomyosarcoma
of bladder. This tumour was positive for
desmin and myoglobin. H & E × 130.

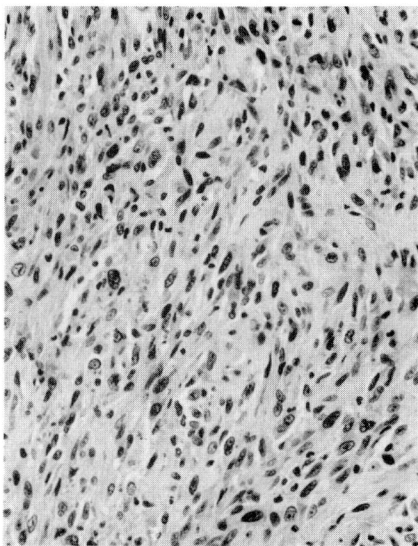

Fig. 8.11 Leiomyosarcoma of bladder: a
moderately pleomorphic example with a low
mitotic count. H & E × 130.

was a wide age range, 16 to 72 years. These tumours form solid, fleshy, often polypoid masses, which are focally haemorrhagic or necrotic. They may measure up to 10 cm in diameter. The degree of differentiation and nuclear pleomorphism are variable. A characteristic pattern is that of interlacing bundles of spindle cells, but prominent myxoid areas with scattered stellate or spindle cells within an abundant pale-staining stroma, is a feature of many tumours. Similar myxoid areas may be seen in spindle cell carcinomas also. Establishing the smooth muscle nature of the tumour may ultimately depend on immunohistochemical or electron microscopic studies. All of 12 cases studied immunohistochemically by Mills et al (1989) were negative for cytokeratin and epithelial membrane antigen but were positive for vimentin and muscle specific actin. Four of the 12 were negative for desmin and one of these four was only faintly positive for actin. However, one or both muscle markers are likely to be positive in a smooth muscle tumour.

Assessing the malignancy of a smooth muscle tumour is a problem not confined to the vesical tumours. Of the 15 cases reviewed by Mills et al (1989), two had metastasized and these had five and 10 mitotic figures/10 HPF respectively, but the follow-up in most of their cases was too short to draw definite conclusions about the significance of mitotic activity. More-over, where a tumour has a prominent myxoid pattern, mitotic counts may be misleading because of the relatively sparsely cellular character of the tumour in such areas. Bearing in mind these considerations, it is best to regard smooth muscle tumours with an infiltrative pattern of growth but with a low mitotic index as low grade leiomyosarcomas.

Post-operative spindle cell nodule

This lesion may readily be misinterpreted as a sarcoma and can present considerable diagnostic difficulties. It is a benign reactive process which may arise in the lower genito-urinary tract following an operative pro-cedure. The clinical and histopathological features have been reviewed by Proppe et al (1984) who described eight cases—four from the vagina following a vaginal hysterectomy, and four from the bladder and prostatic urethra.

The lesion presents as a yellowish or tan coloured nodule usually with an ulcerated surface. The largest nodule described was 4 cm in diameter. Histologically, they consist of interlacing fascicles of spindle cells. Where the margin of the lesion can be identified, it has an infiltrative pattern of growth. A characteristic feature is the presence of a network of blood vessels. Collagen is usually not conspicuous but there is a prominent reticulin pattern. The ulcerated surface is covered by an inflammatory exudate. Within the nodule there may be a prominent chronic inflammatory cell infiltrate as well as oedema and haemorrhage. The nuclear chromatin is finely dispersed and the nucleoli are small. Mitotic figures may be numerous but no atypical forms are seen. The few electron microscopic studies undertaken suggest that the spindle cells are of fibroblastic type (Proppe et al 1984).

Spindle cell carcinoma and leiomyosarcoma enter into the differential diagnosis. However, the clinical setting with a recent operative procedure at the site is distinctive. Immunohistochemical data are limited, but in one report the spindle cells were positive for cytokeratin and negative for epithelial membrane antigen (Wick et al 1988). This contrasts with spindle cell carcinoma which is nearly always positive for both epithelial markers. Postoperative spindle cell nodule may be positive for vimentin, desmin and actin, and therefore similar to leiomyosarcoma or rhabdomyosarcoma in this respect. Markers, such as S-100 protein and α-1-anti-chymotrypsin are too nonspecific to be diagnostically helpful. Table 8.3 summarizes the immunohistochemical findings in spindle cell lesions of the lower urinary tract.

Pseudosarcomatous lesion of bladder

It is not clear whether non-neoplastic spindle cell lesions referred to as pseudosarcoma (Roth 1980), inflammatory pseudotumour (Nochomovitz & Orenstein 1985) and pseudosarcomatous lesion (Young & Scully 1987) are related. It has been suggested that they are analogous to nodular fasciitis of soft tissues (Hughes et al 1991) but since the true nature of these soft tissue lesions has not been elucidated, this hardly resolves the problem.

Hughes et al (1991) have recently reviewed five cases of this condition and their paper may be briefly summarized as follows.

Clinically, they present with haematuria or cystitis. Macroscopically they appear as mucoid polypoid masses—in one case the lesion was as much as 50 g in weight. All were similar on histological examination, consisting of

Table 8.3   Immunohistochemistry of spindle cell lesions of the lower urinary tract (data derived from: Wick et al 1988, Mills et al 1989, Hughes et al 1991)

Diagnosis	CK	EMA	VIM	DES	MSA
Spindle cell carcinoma	+	+	+/0	0	0
Leiomyosarcoma	0	0	+	+/0	+
Rhabdomyosarcoma	0	0	+	+	+
Other sarcomas	0	0	+	0	0
PSCN*	+	0	+	+	+
Pseudosarcomatous lesion†	0	–	+	0	0

CK = cytokeratin; EMA = epithelial membrane antigen;
VIM = vimentin; DES = desmin; MSA = muscle specific actin;
PSCN = postoperative spindle cell nodule.
* Few immunohistochemical studies available but reports suggest that spindle cells may be positive for muscle specific markers and cytokeratins.
† In one case the spindle cells were reported as cytokeratin positive.

spindle cells with prominent eosinophilic cytoplasm with a myxoid matrix rich in acid mucopolysaccharides. They showed an 'infiltrative' growth pattern. The lesions were also highly vascular. Cellular areas had features suggestive of granulation tissue. There was often an inflammatory cell infiltrate. There are, therefore, a number of features which suggest a link with postoperative spindle cell nodule but the spindle cells of pseudo-sarcomatous lesions are negative for desmin and only one case was positive for cytokeratins. All were positive for vimentin.

PSEUDOMALIGNANT LESIONS OF THE PROSTATE

In routine histological sections of the prostate the basal cells are inconspicuous and hard to identify. They form a layer of flattened cells surrounding or enveloping the ductular and acinar epithelium of the gland, and are interposed between the epithelium and the basement membrane. Identification of this basal layer can, however, be helpful in distinguishing benign conditions of the prostate from well differentiated carcinoma which they might resemble (Ronnett & Epstein 1989, Hedrick & Epstein 1989). A cytokeratin monoclonal antibody reactive with prostatic basal cells allows their identification in frozen sections and in paraffin sections pre-treated with pronase.

The monoclonal antibody cytokeratin 34β E12 (Enzo Diagnostics) raised against human stratum corneum (Gown & Vogel 1984) and reacting with cytokeratins of molecular weight 49, 51, 57 and 66 kDa also reacts with the basal cells of the prostate (Brawer et al 1985, Hedrick & Epstein 1989). In frozen sections a continuous or uninterrupted layer of basal cells is demonstrated, whereas in paraffin sections there may be focal disruption of the staining pattern and some glands show large areas which show no staining. Hedrick & Epstein (1989) have also found that, in adenocarcinoma of the prostate, no basal layer can be demonstrated around neoplastic glands or acini.

Intraduct carcinoma, dysplasia and atypical hyperplasia

A variety of terms have been used to describe disordered growth patterns in the prostate which are not carcinomatous. These may be subdivided into glandular proliferations showing cytological atypia or dysplasia and those which show architectural atypia but lacking cytological atypia.

Cytological atypia or dysplasia has been categorized as mild, moderate or severe, the latter being synonymous with intraduct carcinoma (Bostwick & Brawer 1987). The cells have large vesicular nuclei with prominent nucleoli and the cytoplasm appears basophilic. The finding of milder degrees of dysplasia is of doubtful clinical significance, but in severe dysplasia there is a close association with invasive prostatic adenocarcinoma. Severe dysplasia is usually associated with architectural abnormality of the glands including the formation of papillary tufts, transluminal bridging and a cribriform pattern. A basal cell layer can be demonstrated around these dysplastic glands. As a sole finding in a needle biopsy, it indicates a likelihood that there is an associated carcinoma in the gland which was missed in the sample.

Architectural atypia of the micro-acinar type in the absence of cytological atypia is often referred to as adenosis and represents a benign glandular abnormality which may be hard to distinguish from a low grade adenocarcinoma (Brawn 1982, Kovi 1985). Adenosis consists of a circumscribed proliferation of prostatic glands, the cells of which have clear or pale cytoplasm; some of the glands may appear elongated or convoluted and branched. The glands tend to merge with normal prostatic glands. The identification of basal cells within this lesion is helpful in distinguishing it from an adenocarcinoma (Hedrick & Epstein 1989). However, only some of the glands in adenosis may have an identifiable basal cell layer. A rare variant of adenosis is that associated with a prominent sclerosing stroma—sclerosing adenosis. In this form, the glandular cords may readily be misinterpreted as carcinomatous. However, a basal cell layer is prominent in this lesion (Ronnett & Epstein 1989).

Basal cell hyperplasia

Hyperplasia of the basal cells of the prostatic acini is a common finding in

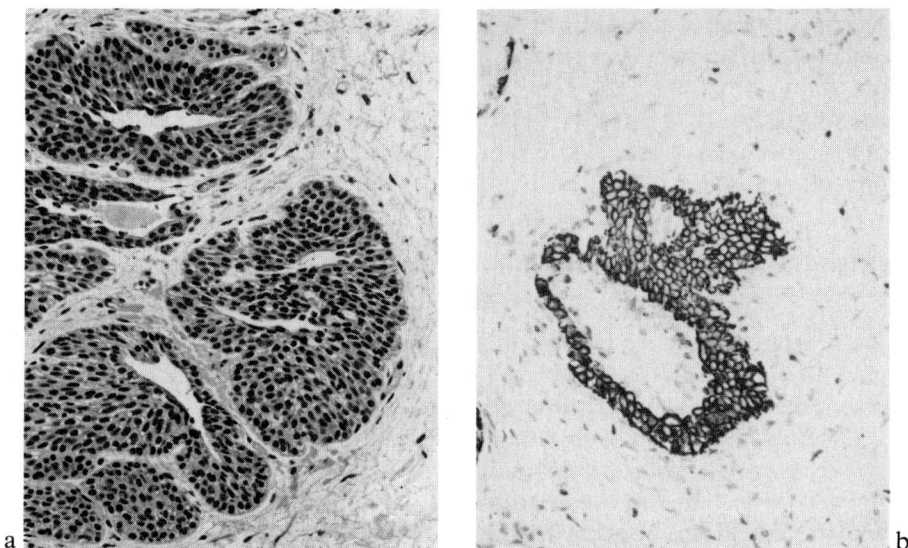

Fig. 8.12   (a) Focus of basal cell hyperplasia in the prostate gland. H & E × 130.
(b) Prostate gland showing basal cell hyperplasia. Immunohistochemical reaction demonstrates multilayered basal cells. Monoclonal antibody 34β E12. H & E × 130.

prostatic biopsies and resections. Histologically, this consists of solid nests of basal cells and/or proliferation of multilayered basal cells surrounding a central acinar lumen, with or without an identifiable epithelial lining (Fig. 8.12). In more florid examples large basaloid nests or nodules, sometimes with an adenoid cystic pattern, may be seen (adenoid basal cell hyperplasia). Larger nodules have been referred to as basal cell adenomas (Lin et al 1978, Grignon et al 1988). All these lesions are strongly positive for cytokeratin 34β E12.

Adenoid cystic and basal cell carcinoma

The great majority of neoplasms of the prostate are carcinomas derived from the glands and acini. Other forms include ductal adenocarcinomas, which may be of endometrioid type, mucinous adenocarcinoma, neuroendocrine carcinoma, transitional and squamous carcinoma, the last two being rare in the absence of an associated bladder carcinoma. Some prostatic carcinomas have an adenoid cystic pattern and this has been compared to the salivary gland counterpart. The origin of adenoid cystic carcinoma of the prostate has remained controversial but several reports emphasized the basaloid character of these tumours (Young et al 1988). This is illustrated in Figure 8.13. More recent reports have shown positive immunoreactivity with the basal cell keratin antibody reinforcing the view that these carcinomas are derived from basal cells (Grignon et al 1988). Follow-up studies have been limited, but there is as yet no case on record which has metastasized.

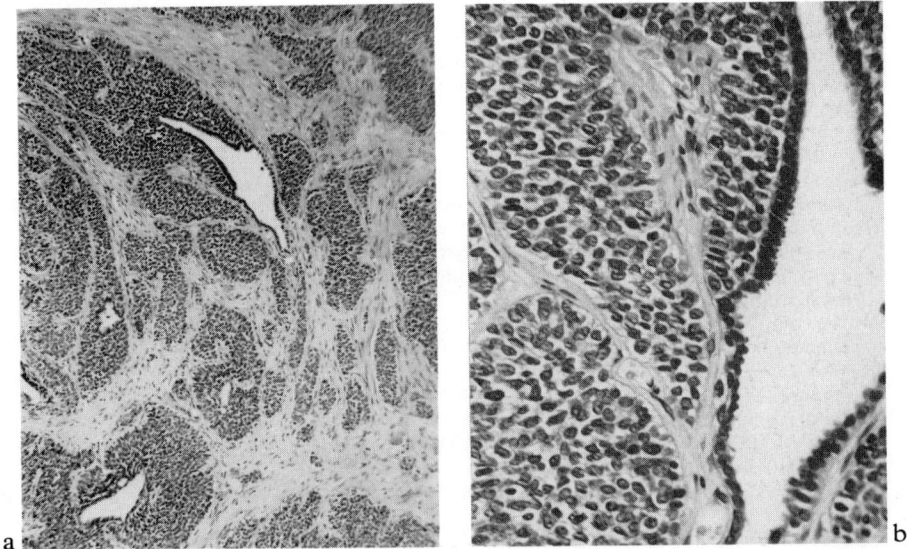

Fig. 8.13 Basaloid carcinoma of prostate gland. **(a)** H & E × 20 **(b)** H & E × 210.

REFERENCES

Ainsworth R W, Gresham G A 1960 Primary choriocarcinoma of the urinary bladder in a male. Journal of Pathology and Bacteriology 79: 185–192

Althausen A F, Prout G R, Daly J J 1976 Non-invasive papillary carcinoma of bladder associated with carcinoma-in-situ. Journal of Urology 116: 575–580

Bergqvist A, Ljungqvist A, Moberger G 1965 Classification of bladder tumours based on the cellular pattern. Preliminary report of a clinical-pathological study of 300 cases with a minimum follow-up of 8 years. Acta Chirurgica Scandinavica 130: 371–378

Bostwick D G, Brawer M K 1987 Prostatic intra-epithelial neoplasia and early invasion in prostate cancer. Cancer 59: 788–794

Brawer M K, Peehl D M, Stamey T A et al 1985 Keratin immunoreactivity in the benign and neoplastic human prostate. Cancer Research 45: 3663–3667

Brawn P N 1982 The origin of invasive carcinoma of the bladder. Cancer 50: 515–519

Brown D C, Theaker J M, Banks P M et al 1987 Cytokeratin expression in smooth muscle and smooth muscle tumours. Histopathology 11: 477–486

Choi H, Lamb S, Pintar K et al 1984 Primary signet ring cell carcinoma of the urinary bladder. Cancer 53: 1985–1990

Civantos F, Rywlin A M 1972 Carcinomas with trophoblastic differentiation and secretion of chorionic gonadotrophin. Cancer 29: 789–797

Cumming J A, Hargreave T B, Webb J N et al 1989 Intravesical Evans B.C.G. in the treatment of carcinoma in-situ. British Journal of Urology 63: 259–263

Davies B H, Ludwig M E, Cole S R et al 1983 Small cell neuro-endocrine carcinoma of the urinary bladder. Report of 3 cases with ultrastructural analysis. Ultrastructural Pathology 4: 197–204

De Filipo N, Blute R, Klein L A 1987 Signet ring cell carcinoma of bladder: evaluation of 3 cases with review of literature. Urology 29: 479–483

Eagan J W 1989 Urothelial neoplasms. Pathologic anatomy. In: Hill G S (ed) Uropathology. Vol 2, Chapter 17, Churchill Livingstone, Edinburgh

Epstein J I, Kuhajda F P, Weberman P H 1986 Prostate specific acid phosphatase immunoreactivity in adenocarcinomas of the urinary bladder. Human Pathology 17: 939–942

Farrow G M, Utz D C, Rife C C 1976 Morphological and clinical observations of patients with early bladder cancer treated with total cystectomy. Cancer Research 36: 2495–2501

Gilbert H A, Logan J L, Kagan A R et al 1978 The natural history of papillary transitional cell carcinoma of the bladder and its treatment in an unselected population on the basis of histological grading. Journal of Urology 119: 488–492

Gown A M, Vogel A R 1984 Monoclonal antibodies to human intermediate filament proteins. II. Distribution of filament proteins in normal tissues. American Journal of Pathology 114: 309–321

Greene L F, Hanash K A, Farrow G M 1973 Benign papilloma or papillary carcinoma of the bladder. Journal of Urology 110: 205–207

Grignon D J, Ro J Y, Ordonez N G et al 1988 Basal cell hyperplasia, adenoid basal cell tumour and adenoid cystic carcinoma of the prostate gland. Human Pathology 19:1425–1433

Hedrick L, Epstein J I 1989 Use of keratin 903 as an adjunct in the diagnosis of prostate carcinoma. American Journal of Surgical Pathology 13: 389–396

Hughes D F, Biggart J D, Hayes D 1991 Pseudosarcomatous lesions of the urinary bladder. Histopathology 18: 67–71

Jordan A M, Weingarten J, Murphy W M 1987 Transitional cell neoplasms of the urinary bladder. Can biologic potential be predicted from histologic grading? Cancer 60: 2766–2774

Kawamura J, Machida S, Yoshida O et al 1978 Bladder carcinoma associated with ectopic production of gonadotrophin. Cancer 42: 2773–2780

Khagafy M, El Bolkainy M N, Mansour M A 1972 Carcinoma of the bilharzial urinary bladder. A study of the associated mucosal lesions in 86 cases. Cancer 30: 2773–2780

Koss L G 1975 Tumours of the urinary bladder. Atlas of Tumour Pathology. Fasc 11, Second series, AFIP, Washington DC

Koss L G 1979 Mapping of the urinary bladder. Its impact on the concepts of bladder cancer. Human Pathology 10: 533–548

Koss L G, Melamed M R, Kelly R E 1969 Further cytologic and histologic studies of bladder lesions in workers exposed to para-aminodiphenyl. Journal of the National Cancer Institute 43: 233

Koss L G, Tiamson E M, Robbins M A 1974 Mapping cancerous and precancerous bladder changes: a study of the urothelium in 10 surgically removed bladders. Journal of the American Medical Association 227–281

Kovi J 1985 Microscopic differential diagnosis of small acinar adenocarcinoma of prostate. Pathology Annual 20: 157–196

Lin J I, Cohen E L, Villacin A B et al 1978 Basal cell adenoma of prostate. Urology 11: 409–410

Melamed M R, Grabstald H, Whitmore W F 1966 Carcinoma-in-situ of bladder. Clinicopathologic study of case with suggested approach to detection. Journal of Urology 96: 466

Melicow M M 1952 Histological study of vesical urothelium intervening between gross tumours in total cystectomy. Journal of Urology 68: 261–269

Mills E, Wolfe J T, Weiss M A et al 1987 Small cell undifferentiated carcinoma of the urinary bladder. A light-microscopic, immunocytochemical, and ultrastructural study of 12 cases. American Journal of Surgical Pathology 11: 606–617

Mills E, Bova G S, Wick M R et al 1989 Leiomyosarcoma of the urinary bladder. A clinicopathologic and immunohistochemical study of 15 cases. American Journal of Surgical Pathology 13: 480–489

Murphy W M 1989 Diseases of the urinary bladder, urethra, ureters and renal pelves. In: Murphy W M (ed) Urological Pathology. Chap 2, Saunders, Philadelphia

Nielsen K, Nielsen K K 1983 Adenocarcinoma in extrophy of the bladder. Journal of Urology 130: 1180–1182

Nochomovitz L E, Orenstein J M 1985 Inflammatory pseudotumour of the urinary bladder— possible relationship to nodular fasciitis. American Journal of Surgical Pathology 9: 366–373

Norton A J, Thomas J A, Isaacson P G 1987 Cytokeratin-specific monoclonal antibodies are reactive with tumours of smooth muscle derivation. Immunocytochemical and biochemical studies using antibodies to intermediate filament cytoskeletal protein. Histopathology 11: 487–499

Proppe K H, Scully R E, Rosai J et al 1984 Post-operative spindle cell nodules of genito-urinary tract resembling sarcomas. A report of 8 cases. American Journal of Surgical Pathology 8: 101–108

Reyes C V, Soneru I 1985 Small cell carcinoma of urinary bladder with hypercalcaemia. Cancer 56: 2530–2533

Ro J Y, Ayala A G, Ordonez N G et al 1986 Pseudosarcomatous fibromyoid tumour of the urinary bladder. American Journal of Clinical Pathology 86: 583–590

Ro J Y, Ayala A G, El Naggar A 1987 Muscularis mucosa of urinary bladder. Importance for staging and treatment. American Journal of Surgical Pathology 11: 668–673

Ronnett M, Epstein J I 1989 A case showing sclerosing adenosis and an unusual form of basal cell hyperplasia of the prostate. American Journal of Surgical Pathology 13: 866–872

Roth J A 1980 Reactive pseudosarcomatous response in the urinary bladder. Urology 16: 635–637

Smith G, Elton R A, Beynon L L et al 1983 Prognostic significance of biopsy results of normal looking mucosa in cases of superficial bladder cancer. British Journal of Urology 55: 665–669

Soloway M S, Murphy W M, Rav M K et al 1978 Serial multiple site biopsies in patients with bladder cancer. Journal of Urology 120: 57–59

Soto E A, Friedell G H, Tiltman A J 1977 Bladder cancer as seen in giant histologic sections. Cancer 39: 447–455

Wallace D M A, Hindmarsh J R, Webb J N et al 1979 The role of multiple biopsies in the management of patients with bladder cancer. British Journal of Urology 51: 535–540

Webb J N 1985 Histopathology of bladder cancer. In: Zingg E J, Wallace D M A (eds) Bladder cancer. Springer Verlag, Heidelberg, pp 23–51

Wick M R, Brown B A, Young R H et al 1988 Spindle-cell proliferations of the urinary tract. An immunohistochemical study. American Journal of Surgical Pathology 12: 379–389

Wiener D P, Koss I G, Sablay B et al 1979 The prevalence and significance of Brunn's nests, cystitis cystica and squamous metaplasia in normal bladders. Journal of Urology 122: 317–321

Williams M R, Dunn M, Ansell I D 1986 Primary oat cell carcinoma of the urinary bladder. British Journal of Urology 58: 225

Wolf H, Olsen P R, Hojgaard K 1985 Urothelial dysplasia concomitant with bladder tumours. A determinant for future new occurrences in patients treated by full course radiotherapy. Lancet i: 1005–1008

Young R H 1987 Carcinosarcoma of the urinary bladder. Report of 3 cases and review of the literature. Cancer 59: 1333–1339

Young R H, Scully R E 1985 Clear cell adenocarcinoma of the bladder and urethra. American Journal of Surgical Pathology 9: 816–826

Young R H, Scully R E 1986 Nephrogenic adenoma. A report of 15 cases, review of the literature, and comparison with clear cell adenocarcinoma of the urinary tract. American Journal of Surgical Pathology 10: 268–275

Young R H, Scully R E 1987 Pseudosarcomatous lesions of the urinary bladder. Archives of Pathology and Laboratory Medicine 111: 354–358

Young R H, Frierson H F, Mills S E et al 1988 Adenoid cystic-like tumour of the prostate gland. A report of 2 cases and review of the literature on adenoid cystic carcinoma of the prostate. American Journal of Clinical Pathology 89: 49–56

9

Germ cell tumours of the testis

K. M. Grigor

Testicular germ cell tumours are not common, but are increasing in incidence (Grigor 1990a). They are now curable in the vast majority of cases although they were associated with a high mortality rate until relatively recently.

In the 1970s two major classifications of testicular tumours were published, which reflected the thinking of British and American pathologists at that time (Mostofi & Price 1973, Pugh 1976). However, Beilby (1978) was unhappy with both classifications and proposed an alternative which was published in a previous edition of *Recent Advances in Histopathology*. Neither Pugh nor Mostofi & Price gave full credit to the work of Teilum (1976) who had clearly demonstrated that many germ cell tumours contained yolk sac elements, and little attention was paid subsequently to yolk sac differentiation in adult testicular tumours. Beilby, on the other hand, went much further than Teilum and suggested that a tumour described as malignant teratoma undifferentiated (MTU) by British pathologists, or embryonal carcinoma (EC) by American pathologists, was mostly yolk sac in nature.

The 1980s saw little progress in the classification of testicular tumours and the two conflicting approaches by Pugh and Mostofi & Price continued to have support in different parts of the world which was largely determined by geography, and Beilby's contribution was virtually ignored. There is no doubt that many histopathologists and clinicians have difficulty in under-standing germ cell tumours because of the two different classifications, and because the same term is used for tumours at the opposite extremes of the prognostic spectrum: in the British classification 'teratoma' describes a tumour which usually has a highly aggressive course, whereas an American 'teratoma' is considered to be almost benign.

Recent advances in our understanding of testicular germ cell tumours have come from a number of studies which have examined, (a) the relationship between testicular carcinoma in situ (CIS) and invasive tumour; (b) the similarities between the cells of CIS and gonocytes, or primordial germ cells; (c) the immunohistochemical phenotype of malignant germ cells; (d) the significance of serum markers in tumour classification; (e) the recognition that spermatocytic seminoma is distinct from all other germ cell tumours; (f) the histological differences between the primary tumour and its metastases; (g) the acceptance of a borderline tumour lying between seminoma and teratoma; (h) the features of prognostic significance when modern therapy is used; and (i) the response of these tumours to modern therapeutic regimens.

All these different facets will be discussed, but first, the classification used in this paper must be defined or else some terms will be meaningless.

CLASSIFICATION OF GERM CELL TUMOURS

The terminology used in this chapter is based on the British classification (Pugh 1976) because it is easier to understand and is more relevant to clinical behaviour. Pugh describes the various components found in germ cell tumours, and they are classified into a small number of groups depending on the combination of individual components which are present. The prognostic significance of these groups has been determined by clinical follow-up. In the American system (Mostofi & Price 1973) tumours are classified according to the individual components present, and less information on clinical outcome is presented. This classification was sub-

Table 9.1 Comparison of British (Pugh 1976) and WHO (Mostofi & Sobin 1977) classifications of testicular germ cell tumours

British Testicular Tumour Panel and Registry	WHO	
	A Tumours of one histological type	B Tumours of more than one histological type
Seminoma (SEM)	1. Seminoma	
Spermatocytic seminoma	2. Spermatocytic seminoma	
Teratoma (TER)	No specific group name*	
Teratoma differentiated (TD)	7. Teratoma (a) mature (b) immature	
Malignant teratoma intermediate (MTI)	(c) with malignant transformation	1. Embryonal carcinoma and teratoma (teratocarcinoma)
Malignant teratoma undifferentiated (MTU)	3. Embryonal carcinoma 4. Yolk sac tumour (embryonal carcinoma infantile type) 5. Polyembryoma	
Malignant teratoma trophoblastic (MTT)	6. Choriocarcinoma	2. Choriocarcinoma with any other type (specify)
Yolk sac tumour (YST)	4. Yolk sac tumour	
Combined tumour (CT) SEM + TER		No specific category
Miscellaneous category not required†		3. Other combinations (specify)

* WHO does not identify this as a specific group of germ cell tumours. By common usage the literature refers to these as NSGCT (non-seminomatous germ cell tumours).
† All possible combinations can be classified in the above groups.

sequently adopted by the World Health Organisation (Mostofi & Sobin 1977). A comparison of terms used in existing classifications is shown in Table 9.1.

Testicular germ cell tumours are subdivided into seminomas and teratomas (Pugh 1976) although both may be found in the same testis. Seminoma tumour cells resemble germ cells whereas teratomas are derived from multipotent or totipotent stem cells capable of producing any embryonic or extra-embryonic tissue. In the American system, fully differentiated teratoma (TD) is called simply 'teratoma' whereas malignant teratoma undifferentiated (MTU) is termed 'embryonal carcinoma'. The British malignant teratoma intermediate (MTI) contains a mixture of differentiated and undifferentiated teratoma in any proportion and is equivalent to the American 'teratocarcinoma' or 'embryonal carcinoma with teratoma'. Extra-embryonic differentiation produces either yolk sac tumour (YST) or malignant teratoma trophoblastic (MTT). The American classification as adopted by WHO (Mostofi & Sobin 1977) accepts yolk sac tumour, but trophoblastic differentiation is known as 'choriocarcinoma' (CC) and the diagnostic criteria for identifying MTT and CC are slightly different.

CARCINOMA IN SITU

The understanding of the histogenesis of germ cell tumours has been greatly enhanced by the work of Skakkebaek (1972) who demonstrated that pre-invasive germ cell malignancy can be identified in seminiferous tubules, and that such carcinoma-in-situ (CIS) is the precursor of all germ cell tumours with the exception of spermatocytic seminoma (Skakkebaek & Berthelsen 1981).

Examination of the residual testis adjacent to virtually every testicular germ cell tumour reveals CIS in at least some of the seminiferous tubules. The cells are large and vacuolated with irregular nuclei and nucleoli (Fig. 9.1). It is rare to see spermatogenesis in a tubule containing CIS although in the early stages Sertoli cells may still be present. Sooner or later these are replaced and the entire tubule is filled with CIS.

Carcinoma-in-situ is most commonly seen in testes which harbour a germ cell tumour (Jacobsen et al 1981) although it may also be identified in testes containing a scar or 'burnt out' testicular cancer (Azzopardi et al 1961). However, CIS has been detected in testicular biopsies from many patients with no clinical suspicion of malignancy (Giwercman et al 1987), the majority of whom were investigated for infertility (Skakkebaek 1978). Other groups with a high incidence of CIS are patients with undescended testes (Krabbe et al 1979); or showing somatosexual ambiguity such as testicular feminization/androgen insensitivity syndrome (Müller & Skakkebaek 1984); and those who have had a previous orchidectomy for germ cell tumour (von der Maase et al 1986, 1987).

A single biopsy is usually sufficient to detect CIS if it is present in a testis

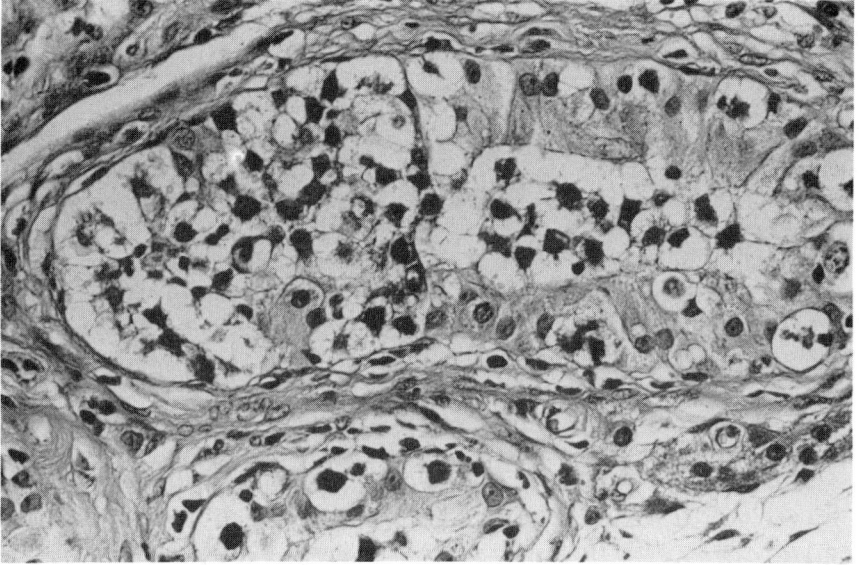

Fig. 9.1 Carcinoma in situ. The seminiferous tubule is devoid of spermatogenic cells. The vacuolated malignant cells have expanded to fill the tubule although residual Sertoli cells are still evident. H & E × 105.

(Berthelsen & Skakkebaek 1981), although an occasional false negative may result from a small biopsy. Patients with CIS have a 50% chance of developing invasive germ cell tumour within 5 years (Skakkebaek et al 1981), and the incidence of testicular cancer increases further with follow up. The invasive tumour which develops is either a seminoma or a teratoma, but not a spermatocytic seminoma. It is therefore important to recognize CIS and to be aware of its clinical significance.

Patients known to have CIS must either be treated or kept under close surveillance. A 'wait and see' policy is common in the UK, but definitive therapy, e.g. orchidectomy or low dose radiotherapy is applied in many other countries (von der Maase et al 1987). Initial hopes that CIS could be eradicated by chemotherapy have not been realized and some patients who received such therapy after unilateral orchidectomy for testicular cancer subsequently developed a second germ cell malignancy in the contralateral testis.

It is now generally accepted that germ cell tumours develop from CIS but it is not clear whether CIS is present from the time of early gonadal development or neoplastic change occurs in mature spermatogonia. In the series from Denmark (Skakkebaek et al 1982) there was only one case of a germ cell tumour developing in a testis which had no evidence of CIS in a previous biopsy. CIS may have developed subsequent to the biopsy in this patient, but a more likely explanation is that this was a rare example of a false negative biopsy resulting from sampling error. This is the only documented case of testicular germ cell tumour subsequent to a negative biopsy, but it must be borne in mind that the large majority of testicular tumour patients have not had a previous biopsy.

Müller et al (1984, 1985) discovered CIS in prepubertal testes from a very early age which suggests that in some cases at least it is present at birth and does not develop as a result of neoplastic change in mature spermatogonia later in life. It can be concluded therefore that an individual who has had a negative testicular biopsy can be reassured that he has only a very small chance of developing testicular cancer.

Most cases of CIS detected prior to tumour development have been found in testicular biopsies taken in the course of investigation of infertility. Such biopsies are now being performed less frequently because of greater reliance on hormone studies. It is now time to consider if biopsies should be taken specifically to look for CIS, which is the policy in some centres.

Intra-abdominal testes associated with somatosexual ambiguity, and high cryptorchid testes should be removed for reasons other than diagnosis of CIS and prior biopsy is not required. Although many instances of CIS have been found in infertile patients, only a small proportion of infertile men have CIS and these patients often have a 'poor quality' testis on physical examination. These are small and soft, with an associated low sperm count, and such findings should be an indication for biopsy.

Patients who have had a previous testicular tumour removed have a higher incidence of CIS in the remaining testis and are also at greater risk of subsequent tumour development. Testicular tumour patients should have a biopsy of the contralateral testis, especially if it is of 'poor quality'. Examination of the semen either by cytology or flow cytometry has not been found to be an accurate indicator of CIS and therefore cannot be used to exclude its presence.

DNA analysis of CIS indicates hyperdiploid and aneuploid nuclei (Müller & Skakkebaek 1981). In addition, these cells have many features in common with primordial germ cells, or gonocytes (Skakkebaek et al 1987). In the embryo, gonocytes are first identified in the region of the yolk sac. After the yolk sac is incorporated into the abdomen to become the precursor of the foregut, gonocytes migrate up the dorsal mesentery and along the posterior abdominal wall to the site of the developing gonad. Gonocytes and cells of CIS are both large vacuolated cells with stainable cytoplasmic glycogen and placental alkaline phosphatase. Similarities between gonocytes and CIS are also seen by electron microscopy (Gondos 1986, Holstein et al 1987). These comparative studies have prompted the suggestion that all germ cell tumours derived from testicular CIS should be called *gonocytomas*, namely all germ cell tumours except spermatocytic seminoma (Skakkebaek et al 1987).

Although formalin fixation is not ideal for the preservation of the morphological features of CIS, it is usually detectable in routinely fixed and stained histological sections (Fig. 9.1). Tubules with CIS are devoid of normal germ cells and spermatogenesis although this may be evident in adjacent tubules. The cells of CIS are large and pleomorphic with large irregular hyperchromatic nuclei and abundant clear cytoplasm with distinct cell boundaries. Initially these malignant cells form a monolayer along the basement membrane at the periphery of the tubule and further proliferation results in the tubule being filled with neoplastic cells. When invasion ensues, similar cells are present in the interstitium surrounding the tubules. Occasionally, intratubular differentiation towards various different germ cell tumour components can be identified (Mostofi 1980).

CIS is better demonstrated by immunocytochemical staining for placental alkaline phosphatase (PLAP) (Jacobsen & Nørgaard-Pedersen 1984) which is highly sensitive and specific and demonstrates the extent of the disease. Giwercman et al (1990) have described a new monoclonal antibody, 43-9F, which is also a sensitive marker for CIS. The malignant cells do not normally stain for cytokeratins although CAM 5.2 positivity may rarely occur (Grigor, unpublished) and the author has seen HCG staining. In tubules with CIS, but not normal tubules, Sertoli cells may also stain for CAM 5.2.

Cytokeratins are normally detected in epithelial tissues. Therefore, the lack of cytokeratin staining in testicular CIS may render the designation 'carcinoma' inappropriate although it is the most widely used term. Other suggestions such as 'intratubular germ cell neoplasia', 'testicular intra-tubular neoplasia' or 'gonocytoma in situ' have been considered. However,

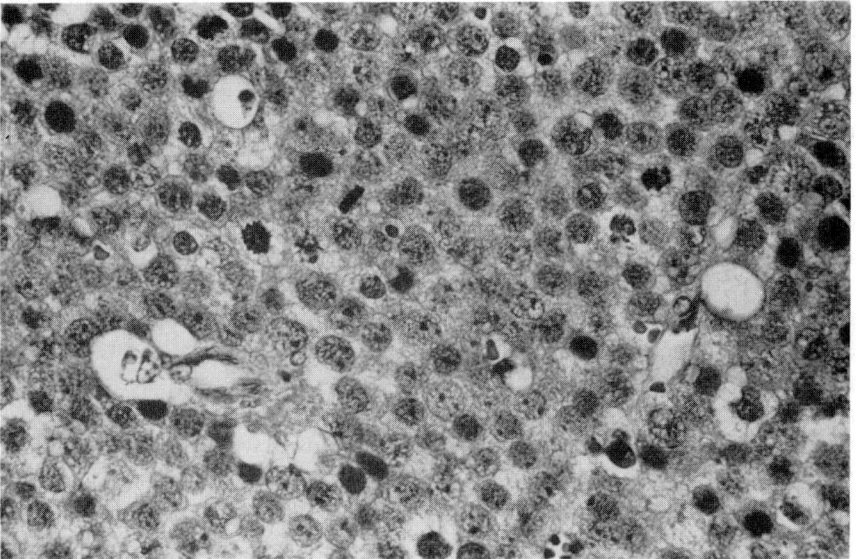

Fig. 9.2   Spermatocytic seminoma (spermatocytoma). This solid tumour shows cellular pleomorphism and mitotic activity. The nuclear chromatin pattern of many of the cells resembles that of spermatocytes. H & E × 105.

there is no clear consensus that the term 'carcinoma in situ' should be abandoned (Mostofi et al 1990).

SPERMATOCYTIC SEMINOMA

Classical and spermatocytic seminomas differ in many respects, the spermatocytic type usually, but not always, occurring in an older age group. Metastases are rare and orchidectomy should be considered curative with no further therapy indicated. It has an excellent prognosis. Macroscopically it is often large and is grey, gelatinous and cystic on the cut surface.

Histologically, this tumour may occasionally resemble a classical seminoma but there are certain features (Fig. 9.2) which make it recognizable as being of the spermatocytic type and therefore having a much better prognosis. The tumour cells are arranged in large sheets with a sparsity of lymphocytic infiltrate and lack of fibrous trabecula. There is marked cellular and nuclear pleomorphism, mitotic activity is high and the mitotic figures are frequently atypical. Many tumour cells have a plasmacytoid appearance, and small multinucleate cells with up to four nuclei are common. The characteristic nucleus has a thread-like pattern of chromatin material resembling that of a meiotically active spermatocyte. The favourable prognosis is rather surprising considering the pleomorphism and mitotic activity.

The differential diagnosis from an anaplastic seminoma is more difficult because this latter tumour also exhibits pleomorphism, mitotic activity and minimal lymphocytic stroma. Well preserved and optimally prepared histological material is essential so that the plasmacytoid cells, thread-like chromatin and small multinucleate cells of spermatocytic seminoma can be identified. The most reliable differentiating feature is placental alkaline phosphatase staining. Tumour cells of classical and anaplastic seminoma stain for PLAP whereas spermatocytic seminoma cells do not. Another important difference is the frequent finding of CIS in the tubules of the surrounding testis in association with classical and anaplastic seminoma but not with the spermatocytic variety.

Spermatocytic seminoma is quite unlike all other germ cell tumours being presumably derived from spermatocytes rather than gonocytes and never being associated with CIS or other germ cell elements. It is therefore inappropriate to classify it along with other seminomas in spite of the superficial resemblance, and a more acceptable and appropriate term is 'spermatocytoma' (Skakkebaek et al 1987) which was ratified at a recent testicular tumour consensus conference (Mostofi et al 1990).

ANAPLASTIC SEMINOMA

Seminomas with many mitotic figures were classified as being 'anaplastic' by Mostofi & Price (1973). Lymphocytes are less numerous and cellular pleomorphism is greater. Classical and anaplastic seminomas have a similar prognosis for a given stage with modern therapy. However, patients with anaplastic seminoma tend to present at a more advanced stage and these tumours must be considered as being inherently more aggressive. There is a good case for continuing to recognize this anaplastic variant of seminoma.

BORDERLINE SEMINOMA/TERATOMA: ANAPLASTIC GERM CELL TUMOUR

All major classifications of testicular tumours subdivide germ cell tumours into seminomas and teratomas (or equivalent terminology) and although these two may co-exist they are considered to be separate and distinct entities. However, it has been suggested that some teratomas may arise from seminoma (Raghavan et al 1982, Grigor 1986, Oliver 1987). Raghavan et al (1982) described an apparently pure seminoma metastasizing as teratoma. Grigor (1986) postulated that some seminoma giant cells have a blastocyst appearance and therefore may contain multipotent cells. Analysis of tumour cell ploidy by Oliver (1987) suggested a progression from seminoma to teratoma. If seminoma and teratoma are at the opposite ends of a continuous spectrum rather than being distinct entities, then a borderline tumour should be identifiable.

Pugh (1976) did not specifically refer to a borderline tumour between

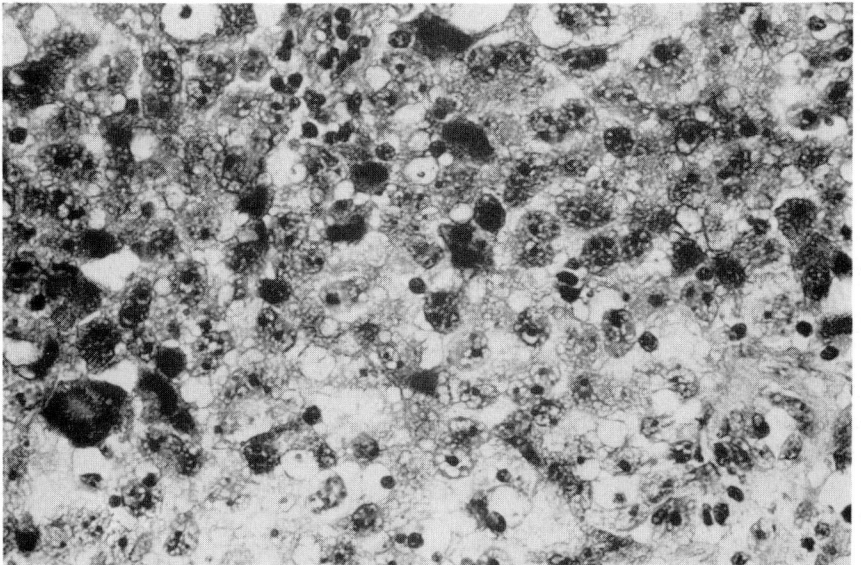

Fig. 9.3   Anaplastic germ cell tumour. Considerable nuclear and cellular pleomorphism is evident and prominent nucleoli are present. The architecture is similar to seminoma but the cells are anaplastic. H & E × 105.

seminoma and teratoma, but he did state that it may be difficult to differentiate between the two on occasions. Features in favour of undifferentiated teratoma include overlapping of nuclei and multiplicity of nucleoli, whereas the lack of these features and the presence of lymphocytes in the stroma favour seminoma.

It is perhaps now time to reappraise the classification of testicular germ cell tumours when there is difficulty in differentiation between seminoma and undifferentiated teratoma. Such tumours have the solid architecture characteristic of seminoma, but with fewer lymphocytes, and the tumour cells stain for PLAP. Cellular details are more reminiscent of undifferentiated teratoma with marked pleomorphism, overlapping nuclei and multiple nucleoli (Fig. 9.3). The author has found that these tumours contain occasional cells which stain for CAM 5.2 (cytokeratin), and rather than attempting to classify them as either seminoma or teratoma, the term 'anaplastic germ cell tumour' has been used (Grigor 1990a,b,c).

Little is known about the behaviour of the borderline tumour at the interface of seminoma and teratoma because it is not included in the major classifications and therefore does not appear in published data. However, preliminary impressions suggest that it is highly aggressive.

EXTRA-EMBRYONIC ELEMENTS

Yolk sac tumour

Teilum's description of yolk sac tumour (YST), or endodermal sinus tumour (EST), is still the definitive account (Teilum 1976), and routine H & E stained material remains best for diagnosis. YST resembles normal embryonic yolk sac in its capacity to secrete alpha-fetoprotein (AFP) and many other serum proteins such as α_1 antitrypsin, ferritin etc., and these can be demonstrated by immunocytochemistry. AFP is the most useful tumour marker for yolk sac differentiation although it does lack sensitivity and specificity (Grigor 1981). Most yolk sac tumours stain for AFP but in a patchy distribution with large areas of tumour remaining unstained. Localization is better after Bouin's fixation because AFP is soluble in formalin.

Tumour elements other than YST frequently stain for AFP, for example undifferentiated teratoma and differentiated structures such as mature epidermis, nerve bundles and tubular epithelial structures. Some teratomas contain tissue resembling liver and this stains for AFP as does normal fetal liver, hepatoblastoma and hepatocellular carcinoma. It must be concluded, therefore, that AFP is not specific for YST, nor does negative staining exclude the diagnosis.

The incidence of YST in testicular tumours is difficult to ascertain. Pugh (1976) was reluctant to accept its occurrence in testicular teratomas in adults, and although the WHO classification (Mostofi & Sobin 1977) recognizes yolk sac differentiation, the incidence is not stated. It frequently occurs in pure form in childhood (Pugh 1976) but in adults it is usually associated with other germ cell elements. In the author's experience, YST is recognized histologically as a component part of two-thirds to three-quarters of adult teratomas (Grigor 1981).

Trophoblastic differentiation

Trophoblastic tissue in germ cell tumours is recognizable in three different forms.

(i) *Isolated syncytiotrophoblastic giant cells which are unaccompanied by cytotrophoblast.* These are frequently seen in association with different types of teratomatous tissues especially yolk sac tumour and undifferentiated teratoma (embryonal carcinoma). They stain for human chorionic gonotrophic (HCG) and their presence does not influence the clinical behaviour of the tumour. Up to 20% of seminomas may contain these giant cells and an elevated serum HCG may be detected in such patients. Grigor (1986) has suggested that syncytiotrophoblastic cells in seminoma may develop into teratomatous elements. Seminomas with or without such cells respond equally well to modern therapy. However, retrospective studies suggested that their presence was associated with diminished survival in untreated individuals (Pugh 1976).

(ii) *Syncytiotrophoblast in association with cytotrophoblast.* This appearance is sufficient to make a diagnosis of choriocarcinoma (CC) according to WHO criteria. However, Mostofi & Sobin (1977) insisted that pure choriocarcinoma, which is very rare, must be differentiated from choriocarcinoma mixed with other germ cell elements.

(iii) *Syncytiotrophoblast and cytotrophoblast forming a villous or papillary pattern.* The villous pattern is required before malignant teratoma trophoblastic (MTT) can be diagnosed according to the British criteria (Pugh 1976). This tumour often exists as a thin rim surrounding a large central haemorrhagic area.

The clinical significance of CC and MTT is their marked propensity for early widespread haematogenous dissemination. This is hardly surprising as one of the functions of normal syncytiotrophoblast is to erode uterine blood vessels in order to allow a pool of maternal blood to percolate over the chorionic villi of the placental tissue. These tumours are frequently haemorrhagic and are associated with high levels of serum HCG. They are highly aggressive but respond well to modern multiagent chemotherapy.

UNDIFFERENTIATED TERATOMA

A malignant germ cell tumour which is neither a seminoma nor shows differentiation towards organoid structures is called 'malignant teratoma undifferentiated' (MTU) (Pugh 1976) or 'embryonal carcinoma' (EC)

(Mostofi & Sobin 1977). However, neither name is ideal; indeed, both are inaccurate, confusing and inappropriate!

A teratoma is a neoplasm containing differentiated structures derived from all three germ layers, namely ectoderm, mesoderm and endoderm. The term 'undifferentiated teratoma' therefore appears to be self-contradictory. The rationale for its use is that MTU has the *potential* for differentiating along totipotential lines although this is not manifest (Pugh 1976).

The word 'teratoma' is used in both the British and American classifications, but unfortunately its prognostic connotations are diametrically opposite in the two. In the American classification, 'teratoma' is equivalent to the British teratoma differentiated (TD) and has a good prognosis. On the other hand, in the British classification, 'teratoma' includes all non-seminomatous germ cell tumours and is an aggressive tumour except in the relatively rare instance when it is composed entirely of differentiated structures with no frankly malignant tissue. Many authors are indiscriminate in their use of the term 'teratoma' and may oscillate between the British and American usages thereby adding to confusion. A strict definition of 'teratoma' should be included in all papers describing testicular tumours.

'Embryonal carcinoma' (EC) as a descriptive term is no better than MTU, and in many respects is less appropriate. Although it is now used to classify a subtype of non-seminomatous tumour, Ewing (1911) first used 'embryonal carcinoma' for tumours which we now classify as seminoma. EC cells are considered to be totipotent or multipotent cells analogous to the pre-gastrulation embryo and therefore 'carcinoma', implying epithelial differentiation, is hardly appropriate. The multipotent stem cell of undifferentiated teratoma is analogous to the multipotent cells of the post-blastocyst early embryo which are found in the epiblast of the inner cell mass. The terminology of germ cell tumours consisting of cells analogous to the epiblast should reflect this similarity.

TUMOUR MARKERS AND IMMUNOCYTOCHEMISTRY

All patients with a definite or suspected testicular tumour must have serum assayed for AFP and HCG, neither of which should be detectable in post-infancy males (AFP < 2.5 ng/ml; HCG < 1 IU/l). Both are excellent tumour markers for malignant germ cell tumours and both must be measured because they are produced by different cell types, fluctuate independently of each other, and frequently only one is elevated. Any testicular germ cell tumour may secrete HCG although high levels are not produced by seminoma. Serum AFP is not elevated in association with pure MTT or seminoma. AFP levels greater than 1000 ng/ml and/or HCG levels greater than 50 000 IU/l are indicative of bulky malignant teratoma and suggest a poor prognosis unless radical therapy is implemented. A patient with an apparently pure seminoma but who has an elevated serum AFP must be

Table 9.2   Immunocytochemical localization of antigens in different tumour subtypes: common findings

	AFP	HCG	PLAP	CK*
Seminoma: classical	−	+/−	+	−
anaplastic	−	+/−	+	−
Spermatocytoma (spermatocytic seminoma)	−	−	−	−
Anaplastic germ cell tumour	−	+/−	+	+/−
Undifferentiated teratoma (MTU/EC)	+/−	+/−	+/−	+
Yolk sac tumour	+	+/−	+/−	+
Trophoblastic tumour (choriocarcinoma)	−	+	+/−	−
Carcinoma in situ	−	−	+	−

CK = cytokeratin (CAM 5.2); + = normally stains positively; − = normally does not stain; +/− = variable staining pattern.

considered as having undiagnosed teratoma in addition, and must be treated accordingly, as the tumour will behave aggressively.

Immunocytochemistry is important in the assessment of germ cell tumours (Table 9.2), but interpretation of results requires caution because staining is not always specific. Tumours with trophoblastic differentiation stain for HCG, but positivity can also be found in undifferentiated teratoma. YST stains for AFP, but not invariably and often patchily: non-yolk sac elements may also stain for AFP, but seminoma does not. Seminoma, whether classical or anaplastic, stains for placental alkaline phosphatase. The borderline anaplastic germ cell tumour also stains strongly and uniformly for PLAP but MTU shows a variable staining pattern and this is often focal. PLAP is an excellent stain for CIS with high sensitivity and specificity. Cytokeratin (CAM 5.2) normally stains MTU and YST but not seminoma. However anaplastic seminoma or anaplastic germ cell tumour may contain CAM 5.2 positive cells and such a finding in a seminoma should suggest a more aggressive tumour.

Spermatocytic seminoma (spermatocytoma) does not stain for any of the common antigens.

PROGNOSTIC INDICATORS AND RESPONSE TO THERAPY

The most comprehensive study of the inherent prognosis of different histological subtypes was that of the British Testicular Tumour Panel described by Pugh (1976). This was set up in 1958 and consisted of eight histopathologists from five different cities in the UK with a central organization at St Paul's Hospital, London. Almost 3000 testicular and paratesticular tumours were examined and follow-up studies performed. No other study has examined as many testicular tumours, and in such great detail. The results of the study must be considered the definitive assessment of prognostic features prior to the introduction of modern chemotherapeutic agents which include cisplatinum.

Patients with seminoma or differentiated teratoma fared well whereas MTU was associated with a poor prognosis. The outlook of malignant teratoma intermediate (MTI) was better, but not as good as that of TD or seminoma. MTT had the worst prognosis.

The prognosis of germ cell tumours was revolutionized by the introduction of cisplatinum (Cis P) as a chemotherapeutic agent in the mid-1970s (Einhorn & Donohue 1977). Prior to Cis P, seminoma had a good prognosis because of its marked radiosensitivity, and differentiated teratoma had a good prognosis because of its low inherent aggressiveness. Other malignant teratomas carried a poor prognosis.

Malignant germ cell tumours including those of a histological type previously considered to have a poor prognosis respond well to CIS P-based chemotherapeutic regimes. Up to 95% of all testicular tumours are now completely curable (Einhorn 1987), a remarkable advance in medical management. The poorly differentiated elements respond better to chemotherapy and the differentiated teratomatous structures are more resistant. Paradoxically, therefore, the advent of effective chemotherapy has almost reversed the prognostic significance of differentiated and undifferentiated components.

Patients with a testicular tumour can be subdivided into a good prognosis group and a poor prognosis group depending on

a. clinical status (on a sliding scale ranging from fit to moribund)
b. whether the tumour is pure seminoma, or combined with malignant teratomatous elements
c. the extent of the tumour, using the Royal Marsden Hospital staging system (Peckham 1981) viz:
   Stage I   : tumour confined to the testis
   Stage II : involvement of lymph nodes below the diaphragm
   Stage III: involvement of nodes above and below the diaphragm
   Stage IV : extranodal metastases

Each stage can be subdivided according to bulk and number of metastatic deposits.

d. the serum level of tumour markers. Very high AFP (>1000 ng/ml) or HCG ($>50\,000$ IU/l) levels indicate a worse prognosis.

Clearly, in certain respects, the role of the histopathologist in the assessment of prognosis is now complementary. However, it is important to have a thorough assessment of metastatic tumour especially in the detection of subdiaphragmatic nodal metastases. Some centres perform retroperitoneal lymph node dissection routinely after orchidectomy and in expert hands this is an effective therapeutic procedure. A few centres, especially in the USA, specialize in this operation but it is not commonly performed in the UK.

The management of stage I teratoma patients is either conservative (surveillance) or by immediate active therapy which may be surgery, chemotherapy, or radiotherapy to pelvic and para-aortic nodes. 70% to

80% of stage I patients are cured by orchidectomy alone whereas 20–30% will develop recurrent disease in the absence of further therapy (Peckham 1981). Those who advocate a surveillance policy argue that recurrent disease can be detected early by careful follow-up and it can be treated effectively thus making active treatment unnecessary in the majority. The proponents of immediate active therapy for all patients say that it is too risky to leave patients when it is known that up to 30% will relapse. Attempts are now being made to identify features of prognostic significance in the primary tumour so that the patients with a greater chance of relapse can be identified.

The MRC testicular tumour working party examined testicular tumours retrospectively and determined the histopathological features associated with relapse (Freedman et al 1987). Predictably, undifferentiated teratoma and invasion of blood vessels and lymphatics were indicators of a worse prognosis; however, the presence of yolk sac tumour was an indication of a more favourable outcome. This latter finding was unexpected because YST is related to AFP secretion, and a very high level of serum AFP is an indication of poor prognosis in patients with metastatic disease.

The MRC working party, having identified the independently variable factors of prognostic significance in stage I teratomas, proposed a scheme to quantify prognosis. A score of one (1) is given to each of the following:

Presence of undifferentiated teratoma
Absence of yolk sac tumour
Presence of blood vessel invasion
Presence of lymphatic vessel invasion.

Otherwise each feature is scored zero (0). A tumour with a total score of 0 is much less likely to recur than a tumour with a score of 3 or 4. Therefore, low scoring (0, 1 and 2) stage I teratomas may be followed by surveillance whereas the high scoring (3 and 4) tumours should receive further immediate therapy without waiting for recurrent disease to become manifest. Patients on surveillance are followed very closely, and any evidence of subsequent recurrence is treated without delay.

METASTASES

Spermatocytic seminoma (spermatocytoma) is unlikely to metastasize. Classical seminoma is less likely to metastasize than teratoma containing undifferentiated or extra-embryonic elements, and extranodal spread is uncommon for seminoma.

Prior to cisplatinum-based chemotherapy, metastatic deposits resembled the primary disease morphologically. However, differentiated teratoma is more resistant to chemotherapy than histologically malignant elements, and it may persist in metastatic deposits. Secondary tumours detected radiographically usually shrink dramatically as therapy commences. However, on numerous occasions residual masses persist and are refractory to further drug treatment. Histological examination usually reveals necrotic tumour, dense fibrous tissue or differentiated teratoma but without evidence of other viable tumour elements (Whillis et al 1991). It is important to remove any residual tumour because even innocuous-looking differentiated teratoma will continue to grow and may spread further (Newlands et al 1987).

The most sinister finding in a residual mass after chemotherapy is the presence of sarcomatous elements, especially undifferentiated spindle cell tumour. Such elements are of germ cell origin, are highly malignant and are resistant to further therapy. They account for a substantial proportion of the small number of testicular tumour patients who succumb to their disease in spite of advanced therapy.

A NEW APPROACH TO CLASSIFICATION OF GERM CELL TUMOURS

Existing classifications of testicular tumours have their deficiencies as outlined in the early part of this chapter. There is no doubt that Pugh (1976) and his colleagues in the Testicular Tumour Panel and Registry added greatly to the understanding of teratomas and his classification is practical, easy to understand and clinically relevant. However, their concepts must now be updated in view of advances made in the understanding of the histogenesis of germ cell malignancies.

The classification of Mostofi & Price (1973) continues to hold sway in the USA and it has been adopted with minimal changes by the WHO (Mostofi & Sobin 1977). In the author's view, this classification simply describes individual components within tumours, which is useful, but it does not categorize whole tumours into meaningful entities.

A new approach is now required which would allow international communication between centres dealing with testicular tumours. The following suggestions have been presented in abstract form (Grigor 1990b,c), and will soon be published in detail. A brief outline is given below.

Spermatocytic seminoma is a germ cell tumour but it is unrelated to all other tumours of germ cell origin and should be called 'spermatocytoma'. All other germ cell tumours are derived from carcinoma-in-situ which has characteristics of gonocytes (primordial germ cells) and the generic name for this entire group should be 'gonocytoma'. They can be subdivided into 'seminoma', 'anaplastic germ cell tumour' and 'teratogenic gonocytoma'. Seminoma, classical or anaplastic, is well described and is uncontroversial. Anaplastic germ cell tumour is the borderline tumour between seminoma and teratoma. Teratogenic gonocytoma is equivalent to teratoma in the British classification, but avoids the confusion associated with this term. The WHO classification does not have a generic term equivalent to teratoma and, by common usage, the phrase non-seminomatous germ cell tumour has evolved. This is a clumsy and negative term for a well-defined

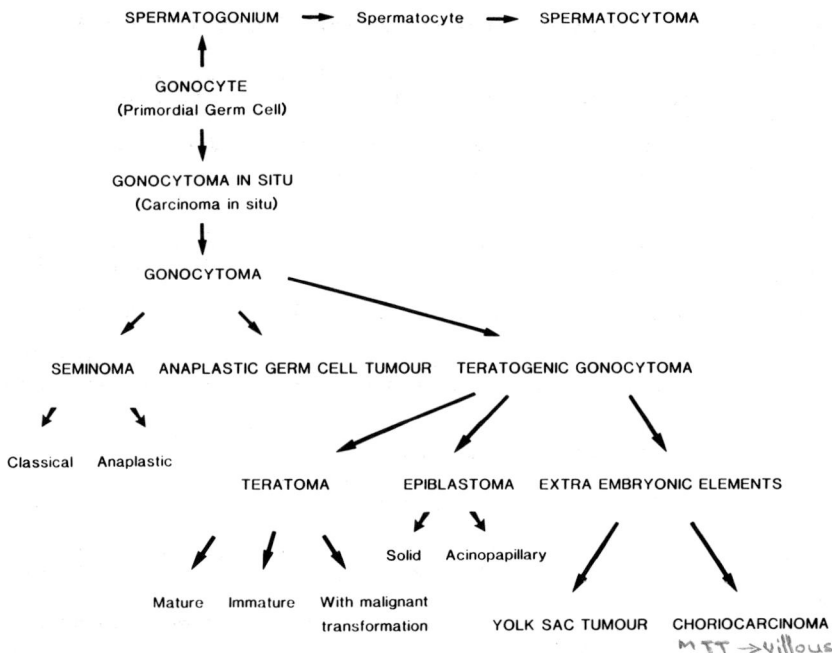

Fig. 9.4   The new approach to testicular germ cell tumour classification: flow diagram showing histogenesis of different tumour types. 'Gonocytoma in situ' is an alternative name for 'carcinoma in situ'.

group of tumours, and teratogenic gonocytoma is considered more meaningful.

The term 'teratoma' should only be used if organized structures are identified, and should be qualified depending on whether the structures are mature or immature. Malignant change in a differentiated tumour should also be indicated.

'Malignant teratoma undifferentiated' (MTU) and 'embryonal carcinoma' (EC) are both poor terms. The component cells are similar to the epiblast and a suitable term is 'epiblastoma'.

Extra-embryonic elements, namely yolk sac tumour and choriocarcinoma, must be recognized. 'Choriocarcinoma' could be used for tumours without a villous pattern and 'malignant trophoblastic tumour' for those with villous structures.

A flow diagram of this new classification is shown in Figure 9.4 which has been constructed with the collaboration of Professor Niels E. Skakkebaek.

REFERENCES

Azzopardi J G, Mostofi F K, Theiss E A 1961 Lesions of testes observed in certain patients with wide-spread choriocarcinoma and related tumors. The significance and genesis of

hematoxylin-staining bodies in the human testis. American Journal of Pathology 38:
    207–225
Beilby J O W 1978 Germ cell and sex cord-mesenchymal tumours of the gonads. In: Anthony
    P P, Woolf N (eds) Recent advances in histopathology No 10, Churchill Livingstone,
    Edinburgh, pp 259–274
Berthelsen J G, Skakkebaek N E 1981 Distribution of carcinoma-in-situ in testes from
    infertile men. International Journal of Andrology (suppl. 4) 172–183
Einhorn L H 1987 Treatment strategies of testicular cancer in the United States.
    International Journal of Andrology 10: 399–407
Einhorn L H, Donohue J P 1977 Cis-diamminedichloroplatinum, vinblastine and bleomycin
    combination chemotherapy in disseminated testicular cancer. Annals of Internal Medicine
    87: 293–298
Ewing J 1911 Teratoma testis and its derivatives. Surgery, Gynecology and Obstetrics 12:
    230–261
Freedman L S, Parkinson M C, Jones W G et al 1987 Histopathology in the prediction of
    relapse of patients with stage I testicular teratoma treated by orchidectomy alone. Lancet ii:
    294–298
Giwercman A, Berthelsen J G, Müller J et al 1987 Screening for carcinoma-in-situ of the
    testis. International Journal of Andrology 10: 173–180
Giwercman A, Lindenberg S, Kimber S J et al 1990 Monoclonal antibody 43-9F as a
    sensitive immunohistochemical marker of carcinoma in situ of human testis. Cancer 65:
    1135–1142
Gondos B 1986 Intratubular germ cell neoplasia: ultrastructure and pathogenesis. In:
    Talerman A (ed) Pathology of the testis and its adnexa. Churchill Livingstone, Edinburgh,
    pp 11–28
Grigor K M 1981 Extra embryonic elements in testicular tumours. International Journal of
    Andrology (suppl. 4) 35–49
Grigor K M 1986 The role of histopathology in germ cell tumours: a review. In: Jones W G,
    Milford Ward A, Anderson C K (eds) Germ cell tumours II. Advances in the Biosciences,
    Vol 55, Pergamon, Oxford, pp 37–43
Grigor K M 1990a Pathology of testicular tumours. In: Chisholm G D, Fair W R (eds)
    Scientific foundations of urology. 3rd edn. Heinemann, Oxford, pp 632–641
Grigor K M 1990b Classification of gonadal germ cell tumours. Bulletin Royal College of
    Pathologists 71: iii
Grigor K M 1990c The relationship of germ cell cancer to gonocytes. Journal of Cancer
    Research and Clinical Oncology 116: 1208
Holstein A F, Schütte B, Becker H et al 1987 Morphology of normal and malignant germ
    cells. International Journal of Andrology 10: 1–18
Jacobsen G K, Nørgaard-Pedersen B 1984 Placental alkaline phosphatase in testicular germ
    cell tumours and in carcinoma-in-situ of the testis. Acta Pathologica Microbiologica
    Immunologica Scandinavica A 92: 323–329
Jacobsen G K, Henriksen O B, von der Maase H 1981 Carcinoma in situ of testicular tissue
    adjacent to malignant germ-cell tumors: a study of 105 cases. Cancer 47: 2660–2662
Krabbe S, Berthelsen J G, Volsted P et al 1979 High incidence of undetected neoplasia in
    maldescended testes. Lancet i: 999–1000
Mostofi F K 1980 Pathology of germ cell tumors of the testis. Cancer 45: 1735–1754
Mostofi F K, Price E B 1973 Tumors of the male genital system. Atlas of tumor pathology
    2nd series, Fasc 8. Armed Forces Institute of Pathology, Washington, DC
Mostofi F K, Sobin L H 1977 Histological typing of testis tumours, International histological
    classification of tumours No. 16. World Health Organisation, Geneva
Mostofi F K et al 1990 In: Newling D W W, Jones W G EORTC Genitourinary Group
    Monograph 7. Prostate cancer and Testicular Cancer. Progress in Clinical and Biological
    Research 357: Wiley-Liss
Müller J, Skakkebaek N E 1981 Microspectrophotometric DNA measurements of
    carcinoma-in-situ germ cells in the testis. International Journal of Andrology (suppl. 4)
    211–221
Müller J, Skakkebaek N E 1984 Testicular carcinoma in situ in children with the androgen
    insensitivity (testicular feminisation) syndrome. British Medical Journal 288: 1419–1420
Müller J, Skakkebaek N E, Nielsen O H et al 1984 Cryptorchidism and testis cancer:

atypical infantile germ cells followed by carcinoma in situ and invasive carcinoma in adulthood. Cancer 54: 629–634

Müller J, Skakkebaek N E, Ritzen M et al 1985 Carcinoma in situ of the testis in children with 45,X/46,XY gonadal dysgenesis. Journal of Paediatrics 106: 431–436

Newlands E S, Bagshawe K D, Begent R H J et al 1987 Treatment of patients with poor prognosis anaplastic germ cell tumours (AGCT) of the testis and other sites. International Journal of Andrology 10: 301–309

Oliver R T D 1987 HLA phenotype and clinicopathological behaviour of germ cell tumours: possible evidence for clonal evolution from seminomas to nonseminomas. International Journal of Andrology 10: 85–93

Peckham M J 1981 Investigation and staging: general aspects and staging classification. In: Peckham M J (ed) The management of testicular tumours. Edward Arnold, London, pp 89–101

Pugh R C B 1976 Pathology of the testis. Blackwell, Oxford

Raghavan D, Sullivan A L, Peckham M J et al 1982 Elevated serum alphafetoprotein and seminoma: clinical evidence for a histological continuum. Cancer 50: 982–989

Skakkebaek N E 1972 Possible carcinoma-in-situ of the testis. Lancet ii: 516–517

Skakkebaek N E 1978 Carcinoma-in-situ of the testis: frequency and relationship to invasive germ cell tumours in infertile men. Histopathology 2: 157–170

Skakkebaek N E, Berthelsen J G 1981 Carcinoma-in-situ of the testis and invasive growth of different types of germ cell tumour. A revised germ cell theory. International Journal of Andrology (suppl. 4) 26–33

Skakkebaek N E, Berthelsen J G, Visfeldt J 1981 Clinical aspects of testicular carcinoma-in-situ. International Journal of Andrology (suppl. 4) 153–162

Skakkebaek N E, Berthelsen J G, Müller J 1982 Carcinoma-in-situ of the undescended testis. Urologic Clinics of North America 9: 377–385

Skakkebaek N E, Berthelsen J, Giwercman A et al 1987 Carcinoma in situ of the testis: possible origin from gonocytes and precursor of all types of germ cell tumours except spermatocytoma. International Journal of Andrology 10: 19–28

Teilum G 1976 Special tumors of ovary and testis. Comparative pathology and histological identification. 2nd edn. Munksgaard, Copenhagen

von der Maase H, Rørth M, Walbom-Jorgensen S et al 1986 Carcinoma in situ of the contralateral testis in patients with testicular germ cell cancer. A study of 27 cases in 500 patients. British Medical Journal 293: 1398–1401

von der Maase H, Giwercman A, Muller J et al 1987 Management of carcinoma-in-situ of the testis. International Journal of Andrology 10: 209–220

Whillis D, Coleman R E, Lessells A M et al 1991 Surgery following chemotherapy for metastatic testicular teratoma. British Journal of Urology (in press)

10

Aspects of ovarian pathology

T. P. Rollason

This review attempts to outline some areas of ovarian pathology where opinions are changing and new entities have recently been described; some of the conditions discussed are rare but they enter into the differential diagnosis of common diseases.

BORDERLINE OVARIAN TUMOURS AND RELATED ENTITIES

The concept of borderline epithelial ovarian tumours has been well reviewed by Fox (1989). The least objectionable definition of these tumours is that of the Ovarian Tumour Panel of the Royal College of Obstetricians and Gynaecologists (1983) which defines a borderline tumour as 'one which shows some, or all, of the characteristics of malignancy but in which there is no stromal invasion'. The presence of extra-ovarian spread does not alter the primary diagnosis.

Variants of mucinous borderline tumour

Serous borderline tumours usually maintain the same histological pattern throughout, i.e. fine, complex papillae overlying branching, broad cores, with no coexistent benign or overtly malignant elements being seen. By contrast, mucinous borderline tumours often show coexistent mucinous cystadenoma, and mucinous carcinomas may have adjacent borderline or benign areas. It has, however, recently been shown that three major types of mucinous borderline tumour exist (Rutgers & Scully 1988a,b).

The first type has Müllerian (endocervical) mucinous epithelium and shows a fine papillary pattern. Patchy acute inflammation is a typical feature (Fig. 10.1) and there is coexistent endometriosis in 30% of cases. This tumour probably behaves like a serous borderline tumour, with a good overall prognosis even in the presence of peritoneal spread, but is bilateral in 40% of cases.

The second type shows the variable pattern referred to previously, with coexistent benign areas, multilocular masses showing epithelial budding, attempts at rudimentary crypt formation and intestinal type (goblet cell)

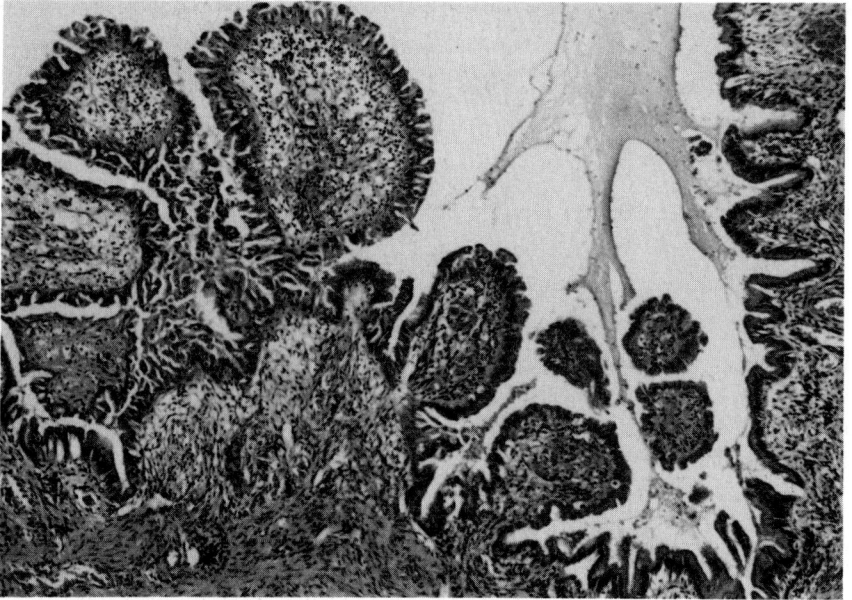

Fig. 10.1   To the left of the photograph the typical lace-like, papillary pattern of a Müllerian-type mucinous borderline tumour is evident. The typical inflammatory infiltrate is also seen. The mucinous differentiation is more clearly seen on the right. H & E × 60.

epithelium in the most atypical areas (Fig. 10.2). It has a lower incidence of bilaterality (perhaps 6%) and is the tumour associated with pseudomyxoma peritonei. Whilst some workers have recently argued that this is a form of metastasis (Michael et al 1987) most would accept it as part of the spectrum of peritoneal Müllerian metaplasia and neoplasia.

The third type of borderline tumour shows Müllerian-type mucinous epithelium but with significant areas of endometrioid, squamous or serous differentiation (Rutgers & Scully 1988b). Pelvic endometriosis is seen in 50% of cases. This tumour behaves in a manner similar to the pure Müllerian type.

Borderline endometrioid and clear cell tumours

There are two main variants of borderline endometrioid ovarian tumour. The first has an adenofibromatous pattern with endometrioid epithelium showing multilayering, budding and nuclear atypia (Bell & Scully 1985). These are unilateral, usually solid tumours with abundant, dense, fibrous stroma. The second variant resembles atypical hyperplasia of the endometrium but arises in ovarian endometriosis (Czernobilsky & Morris 1979, Fox 1989). Similar epithelium to that in the 'endometriotic' variant may also occur rarely in cysts lined by endometrioid epithelium without stroma (Fox 1989).

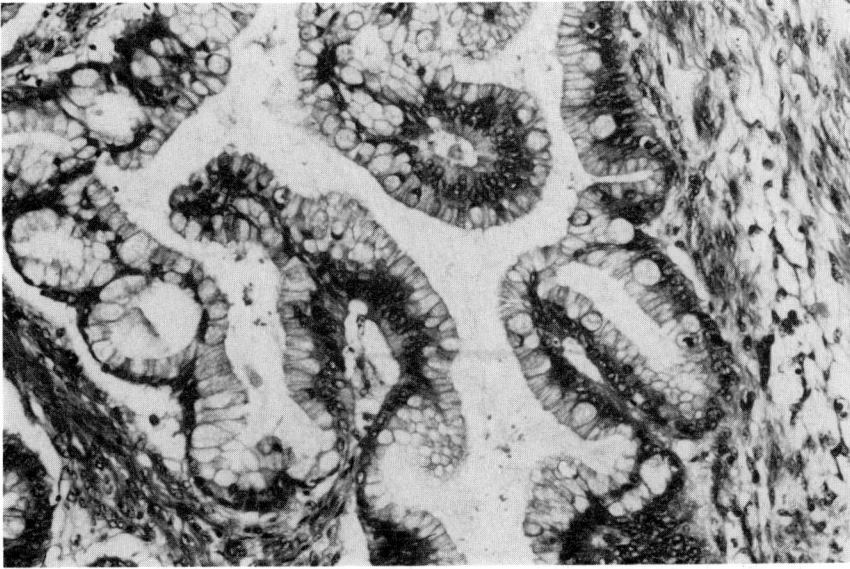

Fig. 10.2 'Intestinal' type mucinous borderline tumour showing goblet cells. H & E × 135.

The nomenclature of these tumours is unsettled. Some divide them into 'proliferative' and 'low malignant potential' categories on the basis of size of solid cellular aggregates and cellular atypicality (Snyder et al 1988) whilst others divide them into 'atypical' and 'borderline' on the basis of cribriform areas, degree of glandular crowding and degree of atypia (Bell & Scully 1985). As only two cases have had extra-ovarian tumour (Russell 1979, Snyder et al 1988) there is little reason at present for subdivision beyond the borderline category.

Borderline clear cell tumours are rare and take the form of adenofibromas with increased cellular pleomorphism and epithelial proliferation (Russell 1979, Roth et al 1984); none of the tumours have behaved in a malignant fashion.

Borderline and malignant Brenner tumours and transitional cell tumours of the ovary

Borderline Brenner tumours form large, unilateral, partly cystic masses. The solid areas often show coexistent benign Brenner tumour. The cyst lining is composed of masses of epithelium, closely resembling papillary transitional cell carcinoma of the bladder. Stromal invasion is absent (Fig. 10.3).

Roth et al (1985a) further subdivided Brenner tumours into benign, metaplastic, proliferating, low malignant potential and frankly malignant. The proliferating and low malignant potential groups were separated

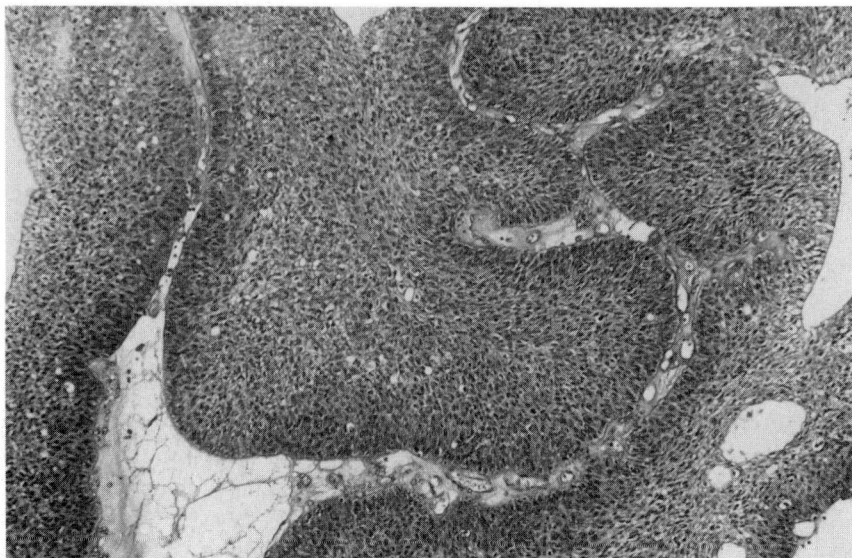

Fig. 10.3   The typical clear demarcation of transitional epithelium and stroma seen in borderline Brenner tumours is shown. H & E × 70.

according to the degree of cellular and nuclear atypia and lack of differentiation. Neither proliferating nor low malignant potential tumours recurred and this subdivision has no clinical significance (Fox, 1989).

Malignant Brenner tumours are rare and again closely resemble transitional cell carcinoma of the bladder though squamous and undifferentiated variants exist. Transitional cell carcinomas, however, may also occur as primary tumours of the ovary and only the presence or absence of a benign or borderline Brenner tumour differentiates the two (Austin & Norris 1987). Recognition is important as, stage for stage, pure transitional cell carcinoma appears to have a considerably poorer prognosis after surgery alone (Austin & Norris 1987), but responds well to chemotherapy. Foci of transitional cell differentiation may be seen in up to 10% of ovarian carcinomas and when this pattern predominates in the primary tumour or in metastases this confers an improvement in survival with chemotherapy (Silva et al 1990).

Ovarian metastases from transitional cell carcinoma of the bladder are well described and their differentiation from ovarian primaries is difficult, if not impossible (Young & Scully 1988). Features favouring metastasis are a deeply invasive urothelial primary, bilateral ovarian tumours and distant metastases.

Serosal involvement in borderline ovarian tumours

Some patients with borderline ovarian tumours do die of their disease but the time course is often long. Colgan & Norris (1983) found that although survival at 5 years was 95%, this fell to less than 75% at 10 years. Death is due to extra-ovarian tumour but the nature and site of origin of such deposits are debated. Extra-ovarian intraperitoneal deposits are present at the time of primary surgery in 30% to 50% of cases (Bell & Scully 1990a). Historically, these have been termed 'implants' but it is difficult to conceive how they could have arisen from a tumour which was, by definition, non-invasive. Recent studies offer evidence that these deposits are examples of multifocal tumour development in the so-called 'secondary Müllerian system' of the pelvic peritoneum, under the same stimulus that produced the primary ovarian tumour. This is supported by similarities between ovarian serosal and mesothelial cells (Blaustein 1984), and the occurrence of entirely, or largely, extra-ovarian borderline and malignant serosal tumours of ovarian type (Bell & Scully 1990a). Mortality in borderline tumours might therefore be due to late development of independent carcinomatosis of the peritoneum (Lauchlan 1990).

It has been suggested that the tumour pattern in these serosal deposits is prognostically important (McCaughey et al 1984, Russell 1984, Bell et al 1988), thus borderline ovarian serous tumour with invasive peritoneal foci would be expected to have the prognosis of serous adenocarcinoma involving the peritoneum. Although there is good evidence that serous borderline tumours with non-invasive deposits do have a progress similar to serous borderline tumours confined to the ovary (Aslani et al 1988, Gershenson & Silva 1990) considerable debate still surrounds the invasive 'implants'. Whilst these may not have the poor prognosis associated with serous surface carcinoma of the peritoneum (Truong et al 1990), outcome is highly variable, with survivals between 0 and 100% in different studies (Gershenson & Silva 1990). This undoubtedly relates to the small size of some series and the variability in histological criteria. Care should be taken to avoid misdiagnosis of benign peritoneal and ovarian serosal papillary mesotheliomas as serous papillary tumour deposits (Goepel 1981, Addis & Fox 1983). The papillary mesotheliomas have a slightly folded nucleus with an inconspicuous nucleolus and a more orderly tubulo-papillary pattern. Hyaluronic acid is present but not neutral mucin (Goepel 1981) and ultrastructural differences have been demonstrated (Addis & Fox 1983). Immunohistochemistry has been stated to be of little use in the past (Dienemann & Pickartz 1987) but recently CEA, Leu-M1 and B72–3 (TAG-72) antibodies have been found to be useful (Khoury et al 1990).

'Microinvasive' ovarian carcinoma

Recently, ovarian serous borderline tumours with stromal microinvasion have been defined as a specific entity (Bell & Scully 1990b). These tumours show the typical appearances of serous borderline tumours but with foci of stromal invasion less than 3 mm in maximum diameter and without significant stromal reaction. The prognosis is similar to that of borderline serous tumour without invasion.

PROGNOSTIC FACTORS IN OVARIAN CANCER

The most important prognostic factor in ovarian carcinoma is stage of disease utilizing the FIGO system (Adcock & Dehner 1989). Interpretation of the results of grading and typing these tumours is fraught with difficulties (Silverberg 1989). The great majority of early studies showed cell type to be important, with mucinous and endometrioid tumours having a better prognosis than serous tumours, and undifferentiated tumours the worst (Bjorkholm et al 1982). The outlook for clear cell tumours has varied greatly between studies. Most series utilizing multivariate analysis find histological type to be of less importance than other features or even of no importance at all (Silverberg 1989). It should nonetheless be borne in mind that tumour type may carry indirectly useful prognostic information e.g. risk of bilaterality and prediction of response to chemotherapy.

Most studies on ovarian carcinoma have found histological grade to be more important than histological type. Since the introduction of chemotherapy however, particularly with cis-platin, the importance of grading is much less clear. Stage I tumours excepted (Sevelda et al 1990), it is probable that only division into borderline, differentiated and anaplastic groups in patients not treated with cis-platin will be of practical importance (Silverberg 1989). High inter-observer variability makes its position even less certain, an argument that can also be used against histological typing (Cramer et al 1987).

Grading in this generally accepted sense should not be confused with the grading *indices* used by some workers (Bichel & Jakobsen 1989) which incorporate multiple, predominantly semi-quantitative, features and do appear to have prognostic value.

Morphometric methods to predict prognosis have been encouraging. Baak et al (1985) showed high accuracy in predicting outcome in borderline ovarian tumours by the use of mitotic rate, volume percentage of tumour epithelium and nuclear shape factor. However, morphometric studies on invasive ovarian cancer are bedevilled by the lack of standardization for stage and therapy. In stage I tumours morphometric techniques do appear to offer useful prognostic information (Baak et al 1987, Haapasalo 1989). Few studies have been performed in advanced ovarian cancer and these were of limited value (Baak et al 1988, Ludescher et al 1990).

Static and flow cytometry have been widely used in ovarian cancer. Most borderline tumours are diploid and all such cases in one study survived (Erhardt et al 1984). Friedlander et al (1984) suggested that aneuploidy in borderline tumours implies aggressive behaviour. Rodenburg et al (1987) showed that, in advanced ovarian carcinoma, ploidy and the presence of ascites were of prognostic importance and diploid tumours had a better response to chemotherapy. Aneuploidy has also correlated with advanced stage and high proliferative index (Friedlander et al 1983, Feichter et al 1985, Kallioniemi et al 1988a) but other studies found that proliferative index was more useful in prognosis than ploidy (Barnabei et al 1990). Kallioniemi et al (1988b) demonstrated that DNA multiploid, especially hypertetraploid, tumours had a very poor prognosis compared to diploid carcinomas. Estimates of S-phase fraction appeared to be particularly of benefit in prognosis in diploid carcinomas.

The value of DNA studies in nonepithelial ovarian tumours, e.g. dysgerminoma (Oud et al 1988) and granulosa cell tumours (Klemi et al 1990, Kwang-Sun et al 1990), is unclear at present.

Progesterone receptor status has correlated with survival in some studies, receptor positive tumours having the better prognosis (Slotman et al 1990) but this has not been found by others (Rose et al 1990). Oestrogen receptor status may be of some use in high stage tumours.

AgNOR measurements in mucinous tumours were found not to be useful in prognosis (Mauri et al 1990); data on other ovarian tumours is lacking.

MISCELLANEOUS OVARIAN TUMOURS

Ovarian tumours with a 'hepatoid' pattern

The differential diagnosis of oxyphilic epithelial tumours of the ovary has been recently clarified by the definition of three apparently distinct entities, hepatoid yolk sac tumour (Prat et al 1982a), hepatoid carcinoma (Ishikura & Scully 1987) and oxyphilic clear cell carcinoma (Young & Scully 1987a).

Hepatoid yolk sac tumour is predominantly solid, with masses of eosinophilic cells resembling hepatocellular carcinoma being seen in a proportion of cases, in a setting of classical yolk sac elements. Recently, small foci of hepatoid differentiation have been found in 22% to 48% of yolk sac tumours (Ulbright et al 1986, Nakashima et al 1987). Hyaline, PAS positive, diastase resistant, intracellular droplets may be prominent. Spaces of varying size divide the cell aggregates and these also contain droplets. Bile is not seen but extra- and intracellular mucin is often present. Alpha-fetoprotein (AFP) and alpha-1-antitrypsin (A1AT) staining is positive in a minority of cells and anti-A1AT also stains the hyaline bodies. The absence of bile and the presence of mucin are the major features differentiating the tumour from metastatic hepatocellular carcinoma. The prognosis is poor. A further yolk sac tumour variant has also been described which, although often containing foci of hepatoid differentiation and classical yolk sac elements, shows prominent endometrioid-like areas (Clement et al 1987).

Hepatoid carcinoma is similar in appearance to hepatoid yolk sac tumour but it consists purely of cells resembling hepatocellular carcinoma. The other major differentiating feature is the age of the patient. Hepatoid yolk sac tumour is seen in children and young women and hepatoid carcinoma in middle to old age. The prognosis is again poor.

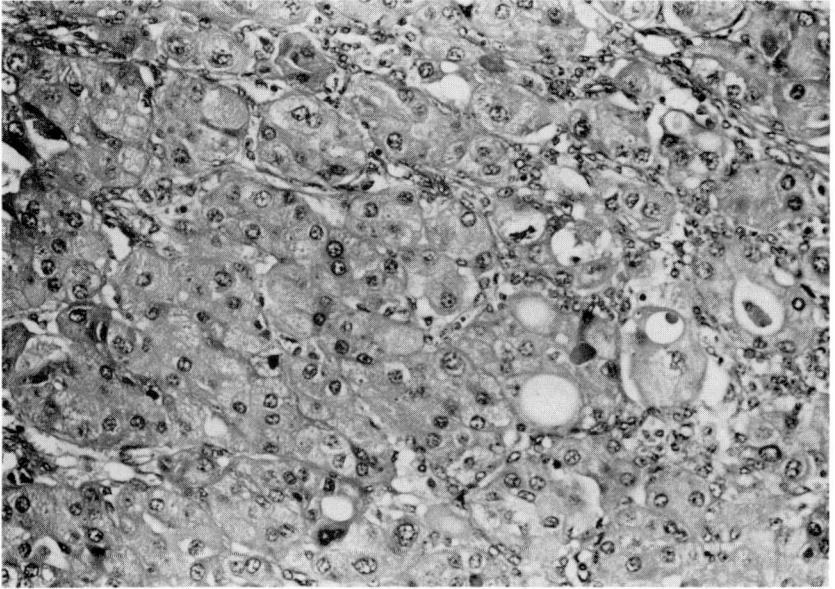

Fig. 10.4   In this oxyphilic clear cell carcinoma the polyhedral, large, pale cells, acinar pattern and nuclear pleomorphism are well illustrated. Typical tubulopapillary clear cell carcinoma was evident elsewhere (courtesy of Prof. R E. Scully, Boston, USA). H & E × 165.

An eosinophilic cell pattern of differentiation in ovarian clear cell carcinoma has been recognized for many years. Young & Scully (1987a) have described a variant where the 'oxyphilic' pattern is prominent producing a tumour composed of large, pale, eosinophilic cells (Fig. 10.4). The cells contain intracytoplasmic glycogen and, in some cases, mucin. Some have an adjacent adenofibromatous component. The age range and clinical features are similar to 'typical' clear cell carcinoma. The key to the diagnosis is the focal presence of a typical tubulopapillary clear cell pattern, though extensive sampling may be necessary to locate this.

Small cell carcinoma

The true nature of these ovarian tumours remains unclear. They are highly malignant with a 5-year survival of approximately 10% (Dickersin et al 1982, Patsner et al 1985, Young et al 1987). They almost always occur before the age of 40. Two-thirds of cases are associated with hypercalcaemia (Young et al 1987). They may be variants of yolk sac tumour (Ulbright et al 1987) or neuroendocrine in nature. Abeler et al (1988) suggested that two types of small cell carcinoma exist; those in young women being of germ cell origin, similar to ovarian carcinoid tumours, and the rare cases in older patients which are undifferentiated non-neuroendocrine carcinomas. These tumours are usually large and unilateral. Microscopically, they are composed of small, closely packed cells with little cytoplasm and deeply haematoxyphilic nuclei. Mitoses are numerous. 'Follicle-like' structures resembling the macrofollicles of granulosa cell tumours are a typical feature. Approximately one-quarter of cases show areas with larger eosinophilic cells which, when dominant, make up the large cell variant of the tumour. Hyaline globules may be evident. AFP is not produced and positive staining for both vimentin and cytokeratin is typical. There is no argyrophilia but some tumours stain for NSE and electron dense granules may be present.

Mural nodules in mucinous tumours

Mural nodules in cyst walls are most commonly seen in mucinous tumours and they may represent anaplastic carcinoma (Prat et al 1982b, Czernobilsky et al 1983), leiomyoma (Lifschitz-Mercer et al 1990) or sarcoma (Prat & Scully 1979). The most intriguing occurrence, however, is of highly pleomorphic nodules in association with benign, borderline and malignant mucinous tumours, which contain a mixed population of osteoclast-like cells, mononuclear inflammatory cells and pleomorphic giant cells (Russell et al 1981). These nodules, described as 'sarcoma-like', do not modify the prognosis of the tumour. Occasional cases of sarcoma-like nodules have been reported in serous cystadenocarcinomas (Clarke 1987) and are associated with a poor prognosis; they may represent anaplastic carcinomas or carcinosarcomas.

Ovarian lymphomas

Bilateral ovarian involvement is seen in 75% of patients with Burkitt's lymphoma and 20% present with ovarian tumours; other than that, only 1 in 300 lymphomas present in this way (Osborne & Robboy 1983). Hodgkin's disease presenting as an ovarian lesion is rare (Rotmensch & Woodruff 1982) and almost all ovarian lymphomas are non-Hodgkin's types (Fox et al 1988). Major differential diagnoses are granulosa cell tumour, dysgerminoma, metastatic carcinoma and undifferentiated small cell carcinoma.

Metastatic sarcomas

Sarcoma metastatic to the ovaries is far less common than metastatic carcinoma. Young & Scully (1990) have studied 21 examples. Eleven of these originated in the uterus; eight were stromal sarcomas and three leiomyosarcomas. The other metastases were a varied collection but the largest single group were leiomyosarcomas.

Great difficulty was experienced in differentiating metastatic uterine stromal sarcomas from ovarian sex cord-stromal tumours and in determining whether the tumours were primary endometrioid stromal sarcomas of the ovary or metastases. The major feature allowing differentiation from sex cord-stromal tumours was felt by Young & Scully (1990) to be the characteristic and prominent network of small arteries within the stromal sarcoma. The metastatic stromal sarcomas were bilateral in most cases and there were other, extra-ovarian, deposits. No case showed coexistent endometriosis which would support a primary ovarian origin (Young et al 1984b).

SEX CORD STROMAL TUMOURS

Granulosa cell tumour (GCT) variants

Juvenile granulosa cell tumour

The majority of GCT occurring in young women and girls have a distinctive microscopic pattern (Young et al 1984a) and in prepubertal girls 80% are associated with isosexual pseudoprecocity. The gross appearance of these tumours is variable, they may be solid or predominantly composed of multiple cysts, or even a single cyst. Necrosis and haemorrhage may be seen. Microscopically, there are sheets or aggregates of granulosa cells with variable numbers of follicles, often irregularly shaped. These follicles are intermediate in size between those of a macrofollicular adult GCT and a Call-Exner body. The lining cells may superficially resemble the 'hobnail' cells of a clear cell carcinoma. Theca cells are often present between the granulosa cell sheets and the two cell types may intermingle; a reticulin stain is helpful in differentiating these components. Broad intersecting fibrous bands may produce a pattern similar to a sclerosing stromal tumour. The granulosa and theca cells are typically luteinized with moderate to large amounts of eosinophilic cytoplasm. Mitoses are more numerous than in the adult and some cases show marked nuclear atypia.

The major danger is misdiagnosis as anaplastic carcinoma or small cell carcinoma. The prognosis for juvenile GCT is good, with a 5-year survival of more than 90%. Stage is the most important prognostic factor.

Granulosa cell tumour with bizarre cells

This variant makes up only 2% or so of GCT (Young & Scully 1983a). Histologically, there are foci of mono- or multinucleate cells with large, bizarre, hyperchromatic nuclei. These changes do not affect prognosis and have been likened to 'symplastic' change in leiomyomas.

Calcified thecomas

Ovarian thecomas typically occur in peri- or post-menopausal women. Focal calcification is not rare, but is hardly ever extensive. This contrasts with fibromas where approximately 10% are calcified to varying degrees.

Young et al (1988) have described a variant pattern in thecomas with extensive calcification which involved at least a quarter of the tumour mass. All patients were below 30 years of age.

Stromal tumours with minor sex cord elements

Tumours in the granulosa-theca group which contain a significant granulosa cell component behave as GCT and should be diagnosed as such. A minor component (perhaps up to 10% of the volume) may show granulosa cell, Sertoli cell or indifferent sex cord cell differentiation in a variety of stromal tumours, e.g. in fibromas, thecomas, stromal-Leydig cell tumours and even fibromatosis, without modifying the outcome (Young & Scully 1983b). The sex cord stromal elements occur in small groups, often at the periphery of the main tumour mass.

Variants of Sertoli Leydig cell tumours (SLCT)

SLCT with heterologous elements

Approximately 20% of SLCT contain heterologous elements (Prat et al 1982c, Young et al 1982a), usually mucinous epithelium of hindgut type with cyst and gland formation. Argyrophilic cells are seen in 30% of these cases and small foci of carcinoid tumour are commonly present. The mucinous component is usually benign but borderline or malignant tumours have been described. Sometimes the mucinous component may predominate with the SLCT represented only by a mural nodule. Rarely, hepatocyte-like cells and neuroectodermal elements have been described but the second commonest heterologous components, in approximately 25% of cases, are immature cartilage or skeletal muscle. These 'mesenchymal' elements tend to be associated with poorly differentiated SLCT and, when extensive, the prognosis is poor (Prat et al 1982c). The true nature of these tumours, i.e. whether teratomatous or metaplastic, is not clear.

A much commoner practical difficulty is the distinction between a well-differentiated SLCT and a well-differentiated endometrioid ovarian carcinoma, especially the Sertoliform variant (Roth et al 1982). Both tumours may have small, hollow and solid, tubular or cord-like structures and an interlacing cell pattern. The luteinized stromal cells in an endometrioid carcinoma can also be confused with Leydig cells. The most useful differentiating features are the presence in endometrioid carcinomas of foci of confluent cell growth, mucin production, squamous metaplasia, the presence of ciliated cells and an adenofibromatous component (Young et al 1982a). Immunohistochemical staining for EMA may also be useful and is positive in almost all endometrioid adenocarcinomas but negative in the great majority of SLCT (Aguirre et al 1989).

Retiform variant of SLCT

A pattern resembling the rete testis is seen in approximately 10% of SLCT, always of intermediate or poor differentiation. This component varies from small foci to an almost pure retiform pattern (Young & Scully 1983c, Roth et al 1985b). Microscopically, these tumours show irregular slit-like tubules and cysts. Some tubules may resemble thyroid acini and papillae, and oedematous polyps projecting into the cysts are common. The pattern may mimic a borderline serous tumour and atypia in the lining cells can lead to a close similarity to serous or endometrioid adenocarcinoma. Heterologous elements are seen in 17% to 40% of cases.

It has been suggested that this pattern of differentiation reflects the close embryological origins of Sertoli cells and the rete testis. It should be noted that true rete ovarii cysts, adenomas and carcinomas do occur, albeit rarely (Rutgers & Scully 1988c).

Sex cord tumour with annular tubules (SCTAT)

These tumours are too well described to merit extensive discussion (Young et al 1982b, Russell & Bannatyne 1989a). Almost all female patients with Peutz-Jegher's syndrome will develop SCTAT. They are characteristically small, bilateral, multifocal and calcified. They present at a slightly younger age than those in patients without Peutz-Jegher's syndrome (mean age 27 vs 34 years) and are benign. They may on rare occasions be associated with minimal deviation adenocarcinoma of the cervix or other genital tract malignancies. They should perhaps be regarded as hamartomas rather than true tumours. This suggestion is supported by recent studies on the ovaries of normal infants (Safneck & DeSa 1986) where structures mimicking gonadoblastoma and SCTAT were seen in approximately one-third of the infants, usually in association with follicle cysts. SCTAT unassociated with Peutz-Jegher's syndrome are different: they are large and unilateral, more than half produce hyperoestrinism and 20% are malignant.

Histologically, SCTAT in both groups show the same pattern of ovoid or rounded epithelial islands with solid tubules consisting of a double row of nuclei and encircling acidophilic, PAS-positive areas. There is typically a dense fibrous stroma condensed at the margins of the epithelial structures and a thick basement membrane is evident. In cases without Peutz-Jegher's syndrome there are commonly areas of differentiation either to micro-follicular GCT or SLCT and these areas may become dominant.

OVARIAN STROMAL PROLIFERATIONS, HYPERPLASIAS AND RELATED TUMOURS

Stromal hyperplasia, hyperthecosis, stromal luteoma and pregnancy luteoma

A minor degree of stromal hyperplasia is common around and after the menopause. Recently Snowden et al (1989) have described a simple morphometric method for its assessment. Excess androgen production by the stroma may lead to masculinization or, by peripheral conversion to oestrone, to hyperoestrinism. There is also some evidence of direct production of oestradiol (Lucisano et al 1986).

In hyperthecosis there are luteinized stromal cells at a distance from the follicles, either in clusters or scattered singly in the stroma. It is usually accompanied by stromal hyperplasia of at least moderate severity and, in its more florid forms, by virilization due to androgen production by the luteinized cells (Sasano et al 1989). An increased risk of endometrial hyperplasia and carcinoma is reported. Clinically evident hyperthecosis tends to occur in the reproductive age group and may present during pregnancy, but minor degrees are common in post-menopausal women when occasional luteinized stromal cells might be considered a normal finding (Boss et al 1965). Both stromal hyperplasia and hyperthecosis are almost invariably bilateral. In both conditions, the ovaries are usually enlarged, measuring up to 7 cm diameter, but cases with normal sized ovaries are described. The cut surface is firm, pale and white to yellow. Microscopically, there is nodular or diffuse cortical and medullary proliferation of stromal cells. Cystic follicles, when present, show theca luteinization. Small nodules of metaplastic smooth muscle may be seen.

There are close similarities between hyperthecosis in the reproductive age group and the polycystic ovary syndrome, where there is always theca cell hyperplasia (Greenblatt & Mahesh 1976), and often luteinization. Persistence of these cells after disappearance of other follicle remnants leads to clusters similar to those seen in hyperthecosis. Stromal hyperthecosis shows little or no response to clomiphene and often only a temporary response to wedge resection. A further differentiating feature is that most premenopausal patients with hyperthecosis have normal gonadotrophin levels (Judd et al 1973, Karam & Hajj 1979). A small proportion of patients with hyperthecosis have insulin resistance and acanthosis nigricans. It has been suggested that the basic defect in these women is insulin resistance and all other features are secondary (Barbieri & Ryan 1983).

Hyperthecosis also shows a continuum from prominent nodular aggregates of luteinized theca cells (nodular hyperthecosis) to the appearance of a 'dominant' nodule, composed of large rounded lutein cells without Reinke crystalloids (allowing distinction from a stromal Leydig cell tumour) and without a non-luteinized component or the hyaline plaques typical of a luteinized thecoma. Most regard such nodules as stromal luteomas (Sternberg & Dhurandar 1977, Hayes & Scully 1987a), but others reserve that term for tumours of identical appearance which occur, extremely rarely, in the absence of stromal hyperthecosis (Russell & Bannatyne 1989b). Stromal luteomas tend to occur in postmenopausal women and produce oestrogenic effects.

Other conditions associated with hyperthecosis include Leydig cell hyperplasia, Leydig cell tumour, massive ovarian oedema and thecoma (Clement 1987).

'Pregnancy luteoma' is usually diagnosed at or near term; it is bilateral in 30% of cases and multiple in 50% and should be regarded as a non-neoplastic proliferation of lutein cells under the stimulus of HCG. It presents as a soft fleshy mass with a median diameter of 6 cm. Masses of polygonal, eosinophilic, luteinized cells are seen with abundant cytoplasm and little or no lipid, showing mitotic activity and growing in trabecular, follicular or diffuse arrays (Clement 1987). Regressive changes are seen during the puerperium including infarction, cellular degeneration and fibrosis and removal is not necessary.

The majority of patients with pregnancy luteomas have been black and multiparous. There is virilization in approximately 25% of cases, which may affect the infant.

Leydig cell hyperplasia and tumours

Leydig cells may be found in the hilus of virtually all adult ovaries and are closely related to non-myelinated nerves. Hyperplasia may be confined to the hilar region or be diffuse throughout the ovary and may occur in pregnancy. Hilar region hyperplasia is characterized by a nodular or diffuse increase in Leydig cells with nuclear pleomorphism, mitotic figures and multinucleation. Occasional cells containing Reinke crystalloids are seen in the stroma in diffuse hyperplasia. The two patterns are not clearly separate and often coexist. Stromal proliferation with hyperthecosis or changes of polycystic ovary syndrome are usually present. Stromal luteomas, 'pure' Leydig cell tumours or stromal-Leydig cell tumours may coexist.

'Pure' Leydig cell tumours, which are almost always benign, may be hilar or non-hilar (Roth & Sternberg 1973). The hilar variant (hilus cell tumour) is more common and occurs after the menopause, producing virilization in most cases. The tumour is small and red-brown or yellow in colour. The cells have large amounts of eosinophilic cytoplasm and often contain lipochrome pigment. Reinke crystalloids are seen in 50% of cases but the overall appearances and hilar site allow diagnosis even in their absence. The presence of nuclear clustering with adjacent cytoplasmic pools is a very characteristic feature. One case with minor sex-cord elements has been described (Young & Scully 1983b). The non-hilar variant is extremely rare and can only be differentiated from stromal luteoma by the presence of Reinke crystalloids (Fig. 10.5).

Stromal-Leydig cell tumours are also rare (Sternberg & Roth 1973). They are composed of nondescript, spindled stromal cells, but include groups of lutein-like cells containing Reinke crystalloids. If stromal luteoma and 'pure' non-hilar Leydig cell tumours may be considered analogous 'female and male' tumours, then the 'female' equivalent of the stromal-Leydig cell tumour is the partly luteinized thecoma.

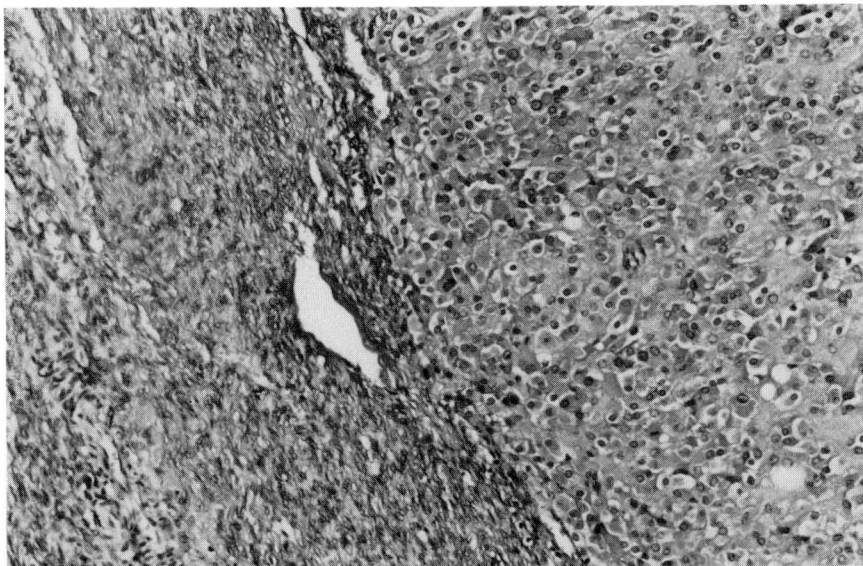

Fig. 10.5   This tumour (to right of photograph) was completely invested by ovarian stroma and is composed entirely of large pale lutein-type cells. Reinke crystalloids were seen indicating that this is a non-hilar Leydig cell tumours rather than a stromal luteoma. H & E × 95.

Steroid cell (lipid cell) tumours

Stromal luteomas and Leydig cell tumours fall into the category of steroid cell tumours which also includes a group which, although the commonest, cannot be further classified. All stromal luteomas and most Leydig cell tumours are benign but between 25% and 45% of the unclassifiable group behave in a malignant fashion (Hayes & Scully 1987b). These tumours may occur at any age and more than 40% are virilizing. They vary in colour, from yellow to black, depending on their lipid and lipochrome content. All the malignant tumours have been more than 7 cm in diameter and most show a mitotic count of more than 2 per 10 high power fields (Hayes & Scully 1987b). Nuclear atypia, necrosis and haemorrhage also suggest malignancy. Tumour cells are arranged diffusely or in cords with numerous intervening small vessels, and little fibrous stroma. They may be pale, vacuolated and lipid rich or small and eosinophilic.

Ovarian steroid cell tumours occurring in association with Cushing's disease may form a separate adrenal cortical type and carry a poor prognosis (Young & Scully 1987b).

Massive oedema and fibromatosis

These two conditions appear to be closely related (Young & Scully 1984).

Massive oedema occurs usually in young women (mean age 21) who present with abdominal pain or swelling and menstrual disturbances. Meigs' syndrome and virilization have been noted occasionally. Partial or intermittent ovarian torsion occurs in approximately half of cases. There is distinct right-sided dominance in the condition and only 10% of cases are bilateral. Ovarian enlargement is due to diffuse stromal oedema; vascular and lymphatic channels are prominent and haemorrhage may be seen; 40% of cases show foci of luteinized cells.

Ovarian fibromatosis also occurs predominantly in young women (mean age 25) and its manifestations are similar. It is usually unilateral but bilateral cases are documented. The ovary is enlarged up to 10 cm in diameter by a dense proliferation of collagen-producing spindle cells surrounding the normal ovarian structures. Foci of oedema and occasionally luteinization of the stroma are seen. Occasional cases have shown sex-cord elements in the stroma. A single case associated with intra-abdominal fibromatosis has been reported (Roche & DuBoulay 1989).

ASPECTS OF OVARIAN PATHOLOGY IN INFERTILITY AND PREGNANCY

Hyperreactio luteinalis and hyperstimulation syndrome

These two conditions are, histologically, virtually identical. Both show

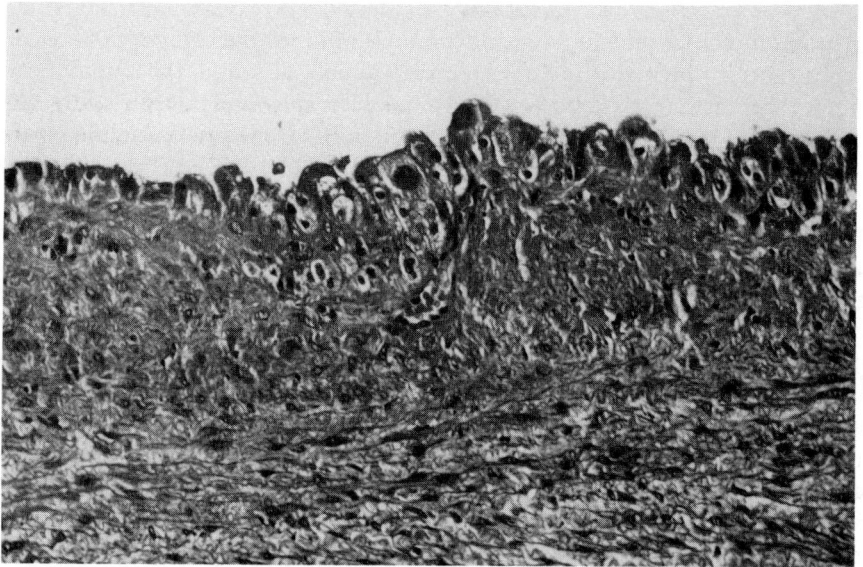

Fig. 10.6   The lining of this solitary luteinized follicle cyst is composed of large, pale, finely vacuolated cells, a few of which show pleomorphic, giant nuclei. The lining varies from one to several cells thick. H & E × 130.

numerous follicle cysts with luteinization of theca interna, and often of granulosa layers with ovarian enlargement, sometimes to more than 20 cm. Stromal oedema and luteinization are marked.

Hyperreactio luteinalis is related to gestational conditions causing high levels of HCG such as hydatidiform mole, choriocarcinoma, fetal hydrops and multiple gestations. It rarely occurs in normal pregnancies. The disease regresses post-partum or after removal of abnormal trophoblastic tissue. Ovarian hyperstimulation syndrome in its severe form is life threatening and may lead to acute fluid shift with ascites, pleural effusions, electrolyte imbalance, haemoconcentration, oliguria and thromboembolism. It is a complication of ovulation induction therapy (Friedman et al 1984, Haning et al 1985, Golan et al 1989).

Solitary luteinized follicle cyst of pregnancy and the puerperium

Another possible cause of ovarian enlargement related to pregnancy is the solitary luteinized follicle cyst of pregnancy and the puerperium (Clement & Scully 1980). The median diameter of these cysts is 25 cm and they are unilateral. They are lined by a single, or several, layers of luteinized cells which show marked nuclear atypia (Fig. 10.6). No separation into granulosa and theca cell layers is seen, though a granulosa cell origin for the lining is likeliest. These cysts are HCG dependent. There is nothing to suggest an origin in the corpus luteum of pregnancy.

Premature ovarian failure

This may be defined as the onset of secondary amenorrhoea and infertility before the age of 35–40 years, though it may develop prior to puberty with incomplete development of secondary sexual characteristics. Most patients have a normal female karyotype, though exceptions have been described (e.g. 47XXX, 45X0/46XX). Oestrogen levels are low and gonadotrophin levels are markedly elevated (hypergonadotrophic ovarian failure). Three major histological types have been described.

(a) Resistant ovary (gonadotrophin insensitivity) syndrome

This occurs in approximately 15% to 20% of cases. Its cause is not understood but deficiency of FSH and LH receptors in the ovary or an antibody response to these receptors have been postulated. Some patients with coexistent myasthenia gravis have been described with an antibody that impairs binding of FSH (Escobar et al 1982). The presence of normal menstruation prior to the onset of symptoms argues against any abnormality of FSH itself. Others have suggested that the disease is the early stage of premature menopause (Maxson & Wentz 1983). Menses have returned in some patients after therapy with oestrogen, high dose FSH, steroids or plasmapheresis.

The ovaries are of normal size but show a dense and superficially sclerotic stroma with variable numbers of primordial follicles. Follicle development varies and may be completely absent, as in hypogonadotrophic hypo-gonadism. 'Dysplastic' follicles may be seen, which are enlarged with irregular outlines and thickened basement membranes. Granulosa cells may be present in clusters and ribbons with intervening hyaline material and Call-Exner bodies may be frequent (Russell & Bannatyne 1989c).

(b) True premature menopause

This condition has multiple aetiologies. Leaving aside irradiation and chemotherapy, they include mumps oophoritis, genetic abnormalities, anti-ovarian antibodies, ataxia telangiectasia and galactosaemia. Some cases with auto-antibodies appear to represent end-stage auto-immune oophoritis and considerable overlap in the two conditions occurs. However, in the majority of women with true premature menopause, no cause is detectable. The ovaries are typically small and histologically there is complete or almost complete absence of follicles (Russell et al 1982). The stroma has a dense postmenopausal appearance. Stigmata of previous ovulation may be seen in the form of corpora albicantes or, less commonly, corpora lutea, and occasional atretic follicles are often present.

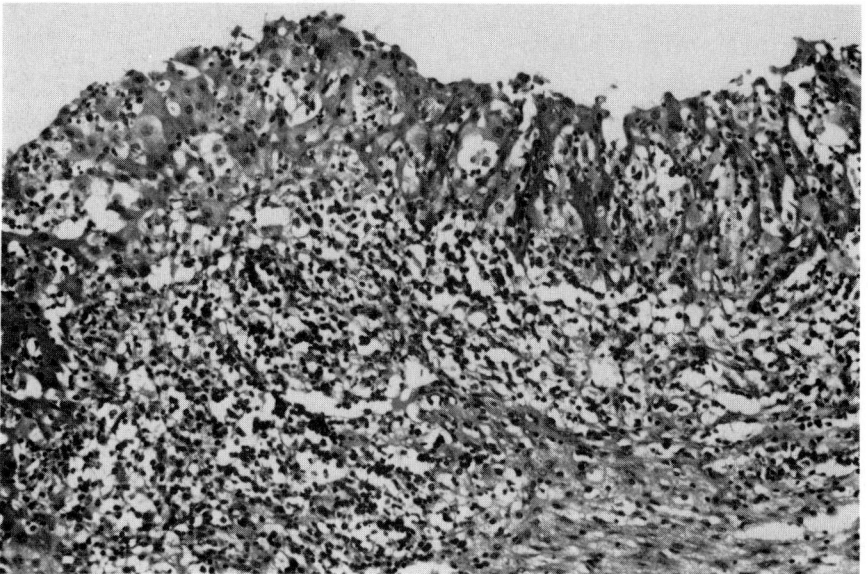

Fig. 10.7   Auto-immune oophoritis. The wall of a cystic follicle showing intense inflammation of the theca interna with extension into the luteinized granulosa. H & E × 105.

(c) Auto-immune oophoritis

This is a rare but probably under-reported condition. Patients present with primary or secondary amenorrhoea. The histological appearances are characterized by lymphoplasmacytic infiltration in relation to developing follicles, atretic follicles and corpora lutea, but most marked around cystic follicles. Eosinophils may also be seen in the infiltrate. Granulomas have been described (Russell et al 1982) but it is debatable whether this pattern of inflammation represents the same disease process. Inflammation tends to be concentrated in the theca interna layer of the follicles (Fig. 10.7). Perivascular and hilar inflammation is also well described. Primordial and pre-antral follicles are usually preserved and are not inflamed. Dysplastic follicles are occasionally seen and theca interna luteinization may make differentiation of antral follicles from corpora lutea difficult (Bannatyne et al 1990).

Despite the apparent rarity of this condition its recognition is important as therapy may occasionally allow ovulation and possibly prevent disease progression (Sedmak et al 1987, Bannatyne et al 1990). Many of these patients have other auto-immune diseases.

REFERENCES

Abeler V, Kjørstad K E, Nesland J M 1988 Small cell carcinoma of the ovary. International Journal of Gynecological Pathology 7: 315–329
Adcock L L, Dehner L P 1989 Surgical staging of ovarian tumours: the individual and integrative roles of the oncologist and pathologist. In: Nogales F (ed) Current topics in pathology. Vol 78. Springer-Verlag, Berlin, pp 41–68
Addis B J, Fox H 1983 Papillary mesothelioma of the ovary. Histopathology 7: 287–298
Aguirre P, Thor A D, Scully R E 1989 Ovarian endometrioid carcinomas resembling sex-cord stromal tumors. An immunohistochemical study. International Journal of Gynecological Pathology 8: 364–373
Aslani M, Ahn G-H, Scully R E 1988 Serous papillary cystadenoma of borderline malignancy of broad ligament. A report of 25 cases. International Journal of Gynecological Pathology 7: 131–138
Austin R M, Norris H J 1987 Malignant Brenner tumor and transitional cell carcinoma of the ovary: a comparison. International Journal of Gynecological Pathology 6: 29–39
Baak J P A, Fox H, Langley F A et al 1985 The prognostic value of morphometry in ovarian epithelial tumors of borderline malignancy. International Journal of Gynecological Pathology 4: 186–191
Baak J P A, Langley F A, Talerman A et al 1986 Interpathologist disagreement in ovarian tumour grading and typing. Annals of Quantitative Cytology and Histology 8: 354–357
Baak J P A, Wisse-Brekelmans E C M, Uyterlinde A M et al 1987 Evaluation of the prognostic value of morphometric features and cellular DNA content in FIGO I ovarian cancer patients. Annals of Quantitative Cytology and Histology 9: 287–290
Baak J P A, Schipper N W, Wisse-Brekelmans E C M et al 1988 The prognostic value of morphometrical features and cellular DNA content in cis-platin treated late ovarian cancer patients. British Journal of Cancer 57: 503–508
Bannatyne P, Russell P, Shearman R P 1990 Autoimmune oophoritis: a clinicopathologic assessment of 12 cases. International Journal of Gynecological Pathology 9: 191–207
Barbieri R L, Ryan K J 1983 Hyperandrogenism, insulin resistance, and acanthosis nigricans syndrome: A common endocrinopathy with distinct pathophysiologic features. American Journal of Obstetrics and Gynecology 147: 90–101

Barnabei V M, Scott Miller D, Bauer K D et al 1990 Flow cytometric evaluation of epithelial ovarian cancer. American Journal of Obstetrics and Gynecology 162: 1584–1592

Bell D A, Scully R E 1985 Atypical and borderline endometrioid adenofibromas of the ovary: a report of 27 cases. American Journal of Surgical Pathology 9: 205–214

Bell D A, Scully R E 1990a Serous borderline tumours of the peritoneum. American Journal of Surgical Pathology 14: 230–239

Bell D A, Scully R E 1990b Ovarian serous borderline tumours with stromal microinvasion: A report of 21 cases. Human Pathology 21: 397–403

Bell D A, Weinstock M A, Scully R E 1988 Peritoneal implants of ovarian serous borderline tumours: histologic features and prognosis. Cancer 62: 2212–2222

Bichel P, Jakobsen A 1989 A new histologic grading index in ovarian carcinoma. International Journal of Gynecological Pathology 8: 147–155

Bjorkholm E, Pettersson F, Einhorn N et al 1982 Long term follow up and prognostic factors in ovarian carcinoma: the Radiumhemmet series 1958 to 1973. Acta Radiologica Oncology (Fasc 6): 413–419

Blaustein A 1984 Peritoneal mesothelium and ovarian surface cells—shared characteristics. International Journal of Gynecological Pathology 3: 361–375

Boss J H, Scully R E, Wegner K H et al 1965 Structural variation in the adult ovary—clinical significance. Obstetrics and Gynecology 25: 747–763

Clarke T J 1987 Sarcoma-like mural nodules in cystic serous ovarian tumours. Journal of Clinical Pathology 40: 1443–1448

Clement P B 1987 Non-neoplastic lesions of the ovary. In: Kurman R J (ed) Blaustein's pathology of the female genital tract. 3rd edn. Springer-Verlag, New York, pp 471–515

Clement P B, Scully R E 1980 Large solitary luteinized follicle cyst of pregnancy and the puerperium. A clinicopathological analysis of eight cases. American Journal of Surgical Pathology 4: 431–438

Clement P B, Young R H, Scully R E 1987 Endometrioid-like variant of ovarian yolk sac tumour. American Journal of Surgical Pathology 11: 767–778

Colgan T, Norris H J 1983 Ovarian epithelial tumors of low malignant potential: a review. International Journal of Gynecological Pathology 1: 367–382

Cramer S F, Roth L M, Ulbright T M et al 1987 Evaluation of the reproducibility of the World Health Organization classification of common ovarian cancers. Archives of Pathology and Laboratory Medicine 111: 819–829

Czernobilsky B, Morris W J 1979 A histologic study of ovarian endometriosis with emphasis on hyperplastic and atypical changes. Obstetrics and Gynecology 53: 318–323

Czernobilsky B, Dgani R, Roth L M 1983 Ovarian mucinous cystadenocarcinoma with mural nodule of carcinomatous derivation. Cancer 51: 141–148

Dickersin G R, Kline I W, Scully R E 1982 Small cell carcinoma of the ovary with hypercalcaemia: a report of 11 cases. Cancer 49: 188–197

Dienemann D, Pickartz H 1987 So-called peritoneal implants of ovarian carcinomas. Problems in differential diagnosis. Pathology, Research and Practice 182: 195–201

Erhardt K, Auer G, Forsslund G et al 1984 Prognostic significance of nuclear DNA content in serous ovarian tumours. Cancer Research 44: 2198–2202

Escobar M E, Cigorraga S B, Chiauzzi V A et al 1982 Development of the gonadotrophin resistant ovary syndrome in myasthenia gravis; suggestion of similar autoimmune mechanisms. Acta Endocrinologica 99: 431–436

Feichter G E, Kuhn W, Czernobilsky B et al 1985 DNA flow cytometry of ovarian tumors with correlation to histopathology. International Journal of Gynecological Pathology 4: 336–345

Fox H 1989 The concept of borderline malignancy in ovarian tumours: a reappraisal. In: Nogales F (ed) Current topics in pathology. Vol 78. Springer-Verlag, Berlin, pp 111–134

Fox H, Langley F A, Govan A D T et al 1988 Malignant lymphoma presenting as an ovarian tumour: a clinicopathological analysis of 34 cases. British Journal of Obstetrics and Gynaecology 95: 386–390

Friedlander M L, Taylor I W, Russell P et al 1983 Ploidy as a prognostic factor in ovarian cancer. International Journal of Gynecological Pathology 2: 55–63

Friedlander M L, Russell P, Taylor I W et al 1984 Flow cytometric analysis of cellular DNA content as an adjunct to the diagnosis of tumours of borderline malignancy. Pathology 16: 301–306

Friedman C I, Schmidt G E, Chang F E et al 1984 Severe ovarian hyperstimulation following follicular aspiration. American Journal of Obstetrics and Gynecology 150: 436–437

Gershenson D M, Silva E G 1990 Serous ovarian tumours of low malignant potential with peritoneal implants. Cancer 65: 578–585

Goepel J R 1981 Benign papillary mesothelioma of peritoneum: a histological, histochemical and ultrastructural study of six cases. Histopathology 5: 21–30

Golan A, Ron-El R, Herman A et al 1989 Ovarian hyperstimulation syndrome: an update review. Obstetrical and Gynecological Survey 44: 430–440

Greenblatt R B, Mahesh V B 1976 The androgenic polycystic ovary. American Journal of Obstetrics and Gynecology 125: 712–726

Haapasalo H, Collan Y, Atkin N B et al 1989 Prognosis of ovarian carcinomas: prediction by histoquantitative methods. Histopathology 15: 167–178

Haning R V Jr, Strawn E Y, Notten W E 1985 Pathophysiology of the ovarian hyperstimulation syndrome. Obstretics and Gynecology 66: 220–224

Hayes M C, Scully R E 1987a Stromal luteoma of the ovary: a clinicopathological analysis of 25 cases. International Journal of Gynecological Pathology 6: 313–321

Hayes M C, Scully R E 1987b Ovarian steroid cell tumors (not otherwise specified). American Journal of Surgical Pathology 11: 835–845

Ishikura H, Scully R E 1987 Hepatoid carcinoma of the ovary. A newly described tumor. Cancer 60: 2775–2784

Judd H L, Scully R E, Herbst A L et al 1973 Familial hyperthecosis. Comparison of endocrinologic and histologic findings with polycystic ovarian disease. American Journal of Obstetrics and Gynecology 117: 976–982

Kallioniemi O-P, Mattila J, Punnonen R et al 1988a DNA ploidy level and cell cycle distribution in ovarian cancer: relation to histopathological features of the tumor. International Journal of Gynecological Pathology 7: 1–11

Kallioniemi O-P, Punnonen R, Mattila J et al 1988b Prognostic significance of DNA index, multiploidy, and S-phase fraction in ovarian cancer. Cancer 61: 334–339

Karam K, Hajj S 1979 Hyperthecosis syndrome. Acta Obstetrica Gynecologica Scandinavica 58: 73–79

Khoury N, Raju U, Crissman J D et al 1990 A comparative immunohistochemical study of peritoneal and ovarian serous tumors and mesotheliomas. Human Pathology 21: 811–819

Klemi P K, Joensuu H, Salmi T 1990 Prognostic value of flow cytometric DNA content analysis in granulosa cell tumor of the ovary. Cancer 65: 1189–1193

Kwang-Sun S, Silverberg S, Rhame J G et al 1990 Granulosa cell tumor of the ovary. Archives of Pathology and Laboratory Medicine 114: 496–501

Lauchlan S C 1990 Review article. Non-invasive ovarian carcinoma. International Journal of Gynecological Pathology 9: 158–169

Lifschitz-Mercer B, Dgani R, Jacob Z et al 1990 Ovarian mucinous cystadenoma with leiomyomatous mural nodule. International Journal of Gynecological Pathology 9: 80–85

Lucisano A, Russo N, Acampora M G et al 1986 Ovarian and peripheral androgen and oestrogen levels in post-menopausal women: correlation with ovarian histology. Maturitas 8: 57–65

Ludescher C, Weger A-R, Lindholm J et al 1990 Prognostic significance of tumor cell morphometry, histopathology and clinical parameters in advanced ovarian carcinoma. International Journal of Gynecological Pathology 9: 343–351

McCaughey W T E, Kirk M E, Lester W et al 1984 Peritoneal epithelial lesions associated with proliferative serous tumours of the ovary. Histopathology 8: 195–208

Mauri F, Barbareschi M, Scampini S et al 1990 Nucleolar organizer regions in mucinous tumours of the ovary. Histopathology 16: 396–398

Maxson W S, Wentz A C 1983 The gonadotrophin resistant ovary syndrome. Seminars in Reproductive Endocrinology 1: 147–160

Michael H, Sutton G, Roth L M 1987 Ovarian carcinoma with extracellular mucin production. Re-assessment of 'pseudomyxoma ovarii et peritonei'. International Journal of Gynecological Pathology 6: 298–312

Nakashima N, Fukatsu T, Nagasaki T et al 1987 The frequency and histology of hepatic tissue in germ cell tumours. American Journal of Surgical Pathology 11: 682–692

Osborne B M, Robboy S J 1983 Lymphomas or leukaemia presenting as ovarian tumors. An analysis of 42 cases. Cancer 52: 1933–1943

Oud P S, Soeters R P, Pahlplatz M M M et al 1988 DNA cytometry of pure dysgerminomas of the ovary. International Journal of Gynecological Pathology 7: 258–267

Ovarian Tumour Panel of the Royal College of Obstetricians and Gynaecologists 1983 Ovarian epithelial tumours of borderline malignancy: pathological features and current status. British Journal of Obstetrics and Gynecology 90: 743–750

Patsner B, Piver M S, Lele S B et al 1985 Small cell carcinoma of the ovary. A rapidly lethal tumor occurring in the young. Gynecologic Oncology 22: 233–239

Prat J, Scully R E 1979 Sarcomas in ovarian mucinous tumors. Cancer 44: 1327–1331

Prat J, Bhan A K, Dickerson G R et al 1982a Hepatoid yolk sac tumor of the ovary (endodermal sinus tumor with hepatoid differentiation). A light microscopic, ultrastructural and immunohistochemical study of seven cases. Cancer 50: 2355–2368

Prat J, Young R H, Scully R E 1982b Ovarian mucinous tumors with foci of anaplastic carcinoma. Cancer 50: 300–304

Prat J, Young R H, Scully R E 1982c Ovarian Sertoli-Leydig cell tumors with heterologous elements. II. Cartilage and skeletal muscle. A clinicopathologic analysis of twelve cases. Cancer 50: 2465–2475

Roche W R, DuBoulay C E H 1989 A case of ovarian fibromatosis with disseminated intra-abdominal fibromatosis. Histopathology 14: 101–107

Rodenburg C J, Cornelisse C J, Heintz P A M et al 1987 Tumour ploidy as a major prognostic factor in advanced ovarian cancer. Cancer 59: 317–323

Rose P G, Reale F R, Longcope C et al 1990 Prognostic significance of oestrogen and progesterone receptors in epithelial ovarian cancer. Obstetrics and Gynecology 76: 258–263

Roth L M, Sternberg W H 1973 Ovarian stromal tumors containing Leydig cells. II. Pure Leydig cell tumor, non hilar type. Cancer 32: 952–960

Roth L M, Liban E, Czernobilsky B 1982 Ovarian endometrioid tumors mimicking Sertoli and Sertoli-Leydig cell tumors. Sertoliform variant of endometrioid carcinoma. Cancer 50: 1322–1331

Roth L M, Langley F A, Fox H et al 1984 Ovarian clear cell adenofibromatous tumors. Benign, of low malignant potential, and associated with invasive clear cell carcinoma. Cancer 53: 1156–1163

Roth L M, Dallenbach-Hellweg G, Czernobilsky B 1985a Ovarian Brenner tumors. I. Metaplastic, proliferating, and of low malignant potential. Cancer 56: 582–591

Roth L M, Slayton R E, Brady L W et al 1985b Retiform differentiation in ovarian Sertoli-Leydig cell tumors. A clinicopathologic study of 6 cases from a gynecologic oncology group study. Cancer 55: 1093–1098

Rotmensch J, Woodruff J D 1982 Lymphoma of the ovary: report of twenty new cases and update of previous series. American Journal of Obstetrics and Gynecology 143: 870–875

Russell P 1979 The pathological assessment of ovarian neoplasms. II. The proliferating 'epithelial' tumours. Pathology 11: 251–282

Russell P 1984 Borderline epithelial tumours of the ovary: a conceptual dilemma. Clinical Obstetrics and Gynecology 1984 11: 259–277

Russell P, Bannatyne P 1989a Sex cord tumours with annular tubules. In: Russell P, Bannatyne P (eds) Surgical pathology of the ovaries. Churchill Livingstone, Edinburgh, pp 368–371

Russell P, Bannatyne P 1989b Stromal hyperplasia and hyperthecosis. In: Russell P, Bannatyne P (eds) Surgical pathology of the ovaries. Churchill Livingstone, Edinburgh, pp 113–118

Russell P, Bannatyne P 1989c Ovarian failure. In: Russell P, Bannatyne P (eds) Surgical pathology of the ovaries. Churchill Livingstone, Edinburgh, pp 57–67

Russell P, Wills E J, Schweitzer P et al 1981 Mucinous ovarian tumours with giant cell mural nodules. Diagnostic Gynaecology and Obstetrics 3: 233–249

Russell P, Bannatyne P, Shearman R P et al 1982 Premature hypergonadotrophic ovarian failure: clinicopathological study of 19 cases. International Journal of Gynecological Pathology 1: 185–201

Rutgers J L, Scully R E 1988a Ovarian Müllerian mucinous papillary cystadenomas of borderline malignancy. A clinicopathologic analysis. Cancer 61: 340–348

Rutgers J L, Scully R E 1988b Ovarian mixed-epithelial papillary cystadenomas of borderline malignancy of Müllerian type. A clinicopathologic analysis. Cancer 61: 546–554

Rutgers J L, Scully R E 1988c Cysts (cystadenomas) and tumors of the rete ovarii. International Journal of Gynecological Pathology 7: 330–342

Safneck J R, DeSa D J 1986 Structures mimicking sex-cord stromal tumours and gonadoblastomas in the ovaries of normal infants and children. Histopathology 10: 909–920

Sasano H, Fukunaga M, Rojas M et al 1989 Hyperthecosis of the ovary. Clinicopathologic study of 19 cases with immunohistochemical analysis of steroidogenic enzymes. International Journal of Gynecological Pathology 3: 311–320

Sedmak D D, Hart W R, Tubbs R R 1987 Autoimmune oophoritis: a histopathologic study of involved ovaries with immunologic characterization of the mononuclear cell infiltrate. International Journal of Gynecological Pathology 6: 73–81

Sevelda P, Vavra N, Schemper M et al 1990 Prognostic factors for survival in Stage I epithelial ovarian cancer. Cancer 65: 2349–2352

Silva E G, Robey-Cafferty S S, Smith T L et al 1990 Ovarian carcinomas with transitional cell carcinoma pattern. American Journal of Clinical Pathology 93: 457–465

Silverberg S 1989 Prognostic significance of pathologic features of ovarian carcinoma. In: Nogales F (ed) Current topics in pathology. Vol 78. Ovarian pathology. Springer-Verlag, Berlin, pp 85–109

Slotman B J, Nauta J J P, Rao B R 1990 Survival of patients with ovarian cancer. Apart from stage and grade, tumor progesterone receptor content is a prognostic indicator. Cancer 66: 740–744

Snowden J A, Harkin P J R, Thornton J G et al 1989 Morphometric assessment of ovarian stromal proliferation—a clinicopathological study. Histopathology 14: 369–379

Snyder R R, Norris H J, Tavassoli F 1988 Endometrioid proliferative and low malignant potential tumors of the ovary. American Journal of Surgical Pathology 12: 661–671

Sternberg W H, Dhurandhar H M 1977 Functional ovarian tumors of stromal and sex cord origin. Human Pathology 8: 565–582

Sternberg W H, Roth L M 1973 Ovarian stromal tumors containing Leydig cells. I: Stromal Leydig cell tumor and non-neoplastic transformation of ovarian stroma. Cancer 32: 940–951

Truong L D, Maccato M L, Awalt H et al 1990 Serous surface carcinoma of the peritoneum: a clinicopathologic study of 22 cases. Human Pathology 21: 99–110

Ulbright T M, Roth L M, Brodhecker C A 1986 Yolk sac differentiation in germ cell tumors. A morphologic study of 50 cases with emphasis on hepatic, enteric, and parietal yolk sac features. American Journal of Surgical Pathology 10: 151–164

Ulbright T M, Roth L M, Stehman F B et al 1987 Poorly differentiated (small cell) carcinoma of the ovary in young women: evidence supporting a germ cell origin. Human Pathology 18: 175–184

Young R H, Scully R E 1983a Ovarian sex cord-stromal tumors with bizarre nuclei. A clinicopathologic analysis of seventeen cases. International Journal of Gynecological Pathology 1: 325–335

Young R H, Scully R E 1983b Ovarian stromal tumors with minor sex cord elements. A report of seven cases. International Journal of Gynecological Pathology 2: 227–234

Young R H, Scully R E 1983c Ovarian Sertoli-Leydig cell tumors with a retiform pattern: a problem in histopathological diagnosis. A report of 25 cases. American Journal of Surgical Pathology 7: 755–771

Young R H, Scully R E 1984 Fibromatosis and massive edema of the ovary, possibly related entities: a report of 14 cases of fibromatosis and 11 cases of massive edema. International Journal of Gynecological Pathology 3: 153–178

Young R H, Scully R E 1987a Oxyphilic clear cell carcinoma of the ovary. A report of nine cases. American Journal of Surgical Pathology 11: 661–667

Young R H, Scully R E 1987b Ovarian steroid cell tumors associated with Cushing's syndrome. A report of 3 cases. International Journal of Gynecological Pathology 6: 40–48

Young R H, Scully R E 1988 Urothelial and ovarian carcinomas of identical cell types: problems in interpretation. A report of three cases and review of the literature. International Journal of Gynecological Pathology 7: 197–211

Young R H, Scully R E 1990 Sarcomas metastatic to the ovary: a report of 21 cases. International Journal of Gynecological Pathology 9: 231–252

Young R H, Prat J, Scully R E 1982a Ovarian Sertoli-Leydig cell tumors with heterologous elements. I. Gastrointestinal epithelium and carcinoid: a clinicopathologic analysis of thirty six cases. Cancer 50: 2448–2456

Young R H, Welch W R, Dickersin G R et al 1982b Ovarian sex-cord tumour with annular tubules: review of 74 cases including 27 with Peutz-Jegher's syndrome and 4 with adenoma malignum of the cervix. Cancer 50: 1384–1402

Young R H, Dickersin G R, Scully R E 1984a Juvenile granulosa cell tumor of the ovary. A clinicopathological analysis of 125 cases. American Journal of Surgical Pathology 8: 575–596

Young R H, Prat J, Scully R E 1984b Endometrioid stromal sarcomas of the ovary. A clinicopathologic analysis of 23 cases. Cancer 53: 1143–1155

Young R H, Dickersin G R, Scully R E 1987 Small cell carcinoma of the ovary. An analysis of 75 cases of a distinct ovarian tumor commonly associated with hypercalcaemia (Abstract). Laboratory Investigation 56: 89a

Young R H, Clement P B, Scully R E 1988 Calcified thecomas in young women. A report of four cases. International Journal of Gynecological Pathology 7: 343–350

11

Congenital heart disease

G. A. Russell

Cardiac malformations are the commonest group of life-threatening congenital anomalies. Histopathologists have a central role in the assessment of clinical diagnosis and management and in providing data on which to base counselling advice. Advances in the developmental biology, classification, epidemiology and the prediction of recurrence risks of congenital heart disease are highlighted in this chapter.

MECHANISMS OF CARDIAC MALFORMATIONS

Most cardiac malformations (90%) are thought to have a multifactorial aetiology whereby a genetic predisposition and environmental factors interact. Relatively few cases (8%) are due to Mendelian and chromosomal defects. Table 11.1 lists the chromosomal disorders which carry a high risk of cardiovascular defects. Purely environmental factors account for only 2% of cases (Nora & Nora 1978).

Table 11.1 Chromosomal disorders associated with congenital cardiovascular malformations (based on Bruyere et al 1987)

Syndrome	% of affected individuals who have cardiovascular defects	Commonest defect
trisomy 8	20	VSD, PDA
trisomy 9	>50	VSD, coarct, DORV
trisomy 13	80–90	VSD, PDA, ASD, DORV
trisomy 18	99	VSD, PDA, PS
trisomy 21	40–50	AVSD, ASD, VSD, PDA
trisomy 22	60–70	ASD, VSD, PDA
del(5p) cri-du-chat	20–25	VSD, PDA
del(13q)	10–25	VSD
del(14q)	>50	PDA, ASD, TF
del(18q)	<50	VSD
Turner (45X)	30–35	AS, PS, coarct, ASD
49 XXXXY	15	PDA

VSD = ventricular septal defect; ASD = atrial septal defect; AVSD = atrioventricular septal defect; PDA = patent ductus arteriosus; PS = pulmonary stenosis; DORV = double outlet right ventricle; coarct = coarctation of the aorta; TF = tetralogy of Fallot; AS = aortic stenosis; PVS = pulmonary valvular stenosis; TGA = transposition of great arteries; del = deletion.

Table 11.2   Environmental risk factors of human congenital heart disease (based on Bruyere et al 1987, Pexieder 1987)

Risk factor	Average relative risk	Common defects
Confirmed		
Alcohol	45.7 (high)	VSD, ASD, TF
Maternal rubella	67.4 (high)	PDA, PS, PVS
Thalidomide	40.7 (high)	VSD, TF, TA
Maternal diabetes	9.6 (moderate)	VSD, coarct, TGA
Anticonvulsants	5.5 (low)	VSD, ASD, TF
Probable		
Maternal hyperphe-		
nylalanemia or PKU	38.3 (high)	PDA, VSD, TF
Maternal *Toxoplasma*		
gondii infection	29.6 (high)	VSD
Valproic acid	11.8 (moderate)	?
Diphenylhydantoin	13.9 (moderate)	VSD
Isotretinoin	14.3 (moderate)	conotruncal and aortic arch defects
Lithium	10.6 (moderate)	?
Possible		
Anaesthetics	2.8 (low)	?
Barbiturates	2.2 (low)	?
Phenothiazines	3.7 (low)	?
Controversial		
Amphetamines	2.5 (low)	?
Insulin	6.3 (moderate)	?

For abbreviations see Table 11.1.

Between the 14th and 60th days of gestation the developing heart passes through a period of vulnerability to the effects of teratogens. The timing, intensity and duration of the environmental insult act together with a genetic predisposition to determine the type of malformation. An example of the latter is the cytochrome P450 enzyme system. This is inducible in embryonic cells and can generate reactive oxidized agents which are teratogenic. The conjugating enzymes necessary for detoxification are deficient in the embryo, and thus the reactive intermediates accumulate and injure cells (Bruyere et al 1987). A list of known and suspected cardiac teratogens is shown in Table 11.2.

Normal intracardiac patterns of blood flow seem to be essential for the proper development of cardiac chambers and valve orifices. This is supported by a variety of animal experiments which have demonstrated that altered blood flow may induce malformations in the developing heart (Clark & Rosenquist 1978). Congenital tumours of the heart which project into the lumina of the cardiac chambers and disturb blood flow are sometimes associated with cardiac malformations (Russell et al 1989). Early stages of cardiac development such as the looping of the primitive heart tube and the formation of the endocardial and conotruncal cushions are independent of blood flow and may be genetically determined. Elegant microangiographic studies in the embryonic chick heart suggest that patterns of intracardiac blood flow do not directly determine cardiac septation (Yoshida et al 1983). Thus the interaction of genetically determined events and haemodynamic forces seems to be essential for the normal development of the heart. Complex malformations may be the result of a 'deformation sequence' whereby an early anatomical anomaly alters the intracardiac blood flow which in turn induces a malformation which further disturbs the blood flow, and so on. Malformations with putative haemodynamic mechanisms include hypoplastic left and right heart syndromes and perimembranous ventricular septal defects (Clark 1987).

As well as the processes of cell proliferation, migration and differentiation, active cell death may also have a role in normal cardiac development. Pexieder (1975) has demonstrated that the normal patterns of cell death that occur in the embryonic heart may be altered by teratogens or abnormal intracardiac haemodynamic forces. The effects of these external influences may be to increase or occasionally to inhibit normal cell death in the embryonic heart; in some cases new foci of cell death may be induced.

THE ROLE OF THE NEURAL CREST IN CARDIAC DEVELOPMENT

Classical concepts of cardiac embryology describe how the definitive organ is entirely derived from the mesoderm. However, recent work has indicated that parts of the outflow tract of the heart are formed of ectoderm-derived mesenchymal cells ('ectomesenchyme') which migrate from the cranial neural crest between the mid-otic placode and the caudal limit of somite 3. This area has been designated the 'cardiac neural crest' because of the contribution it makes to the developing heart (Kirby & Waldo 1990). These observations first arose from attempts to create an aneural chick heart by removing portions of the cranial neural crest known to provide the heart with its postganglionic parasympathetic innervation. The experiments produced a high rate of outflow tract anomalies such as truncus arteriosus and double outflow right ventricle (Kirby et al 1983).

The quail–chick chimera has been used to study the migration of neural crest cells. This model relies on the presence of distinctive central heterochromatin condensation in the quail cells which allows their recognition by light microscopy. Microsurgical techniques allow equivalent segments of embryonic neural crest to be transplanted from a quail embryo to fill the excised segment in the chick. Following incubation, transplanted quail neural crest cells can be identified within the aorticopulmonary septum, truncal folds and the media of the aorta and pulmonary artery of the chick (Fig. 11.1) (Kirby et al 1983). When non-cardiac neural crest is transplanted, there is a high rate of cardiac malformations, indicating that the non-cardiac neural crest is unable to effect truncal septation (Kirby 1989).

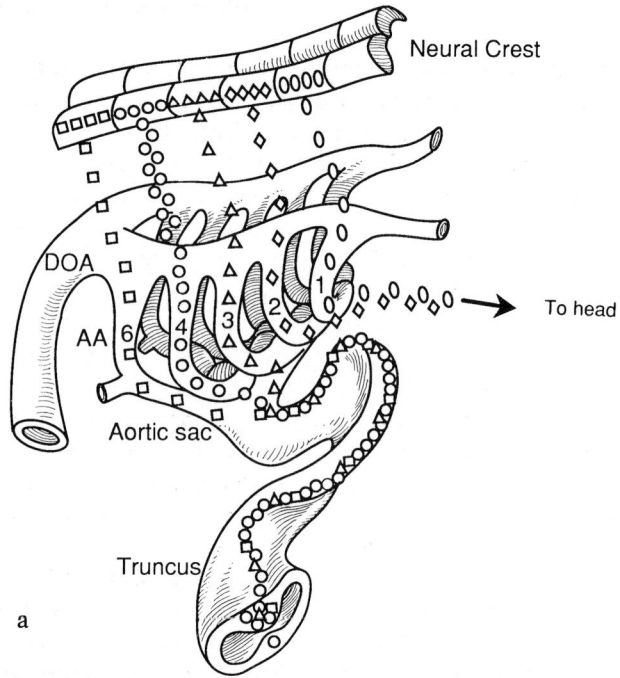

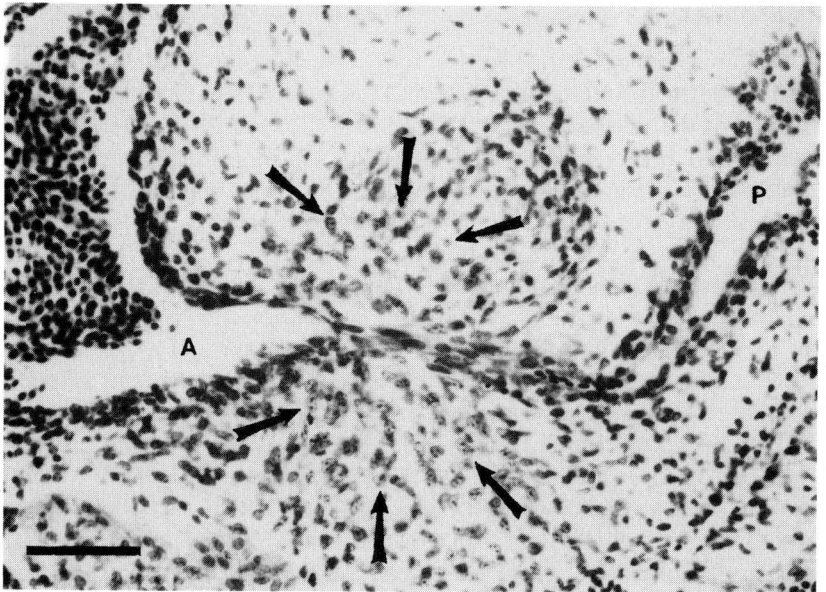

Fig. 11.1 **(a)** The migratory pathway of cranial neural crest cells through the pharyngeal region into the outflow tract of the developing heart AA, aortic arch; DOA, dorsal aorta. (Reproduced from Kirby & Waldo 1990, with kind permission of the authors, the Editor of *Circulation* and the American Heart Association.) **(b)** Truncal region during septation in a 6-day chick embryo with bilateral quail neural fold transplant at the level of somites 1 and 2 at stage 10. Typical quail cells (arrows) can be seen in the region of the developing septum. A, aorta; P, pulmonary trunk. Scale bar, 50 μm (reproduced from Kirby et al 1983, with kind permission of the authors and the Editor of *Science*).

Ablating portions of cardiac neural crest before the migration of the component cells results in various cardiac malformations in the chick. The size and the precise site of the ablation affects the type of malformation produced whereas the age of the embryo at the time of ablation influences the incidence. Lesions confined to the cardiac neural crest lead to a high rate of truncus arteriosus provided that the lesion exceeds two somite lengths, whilst lesions outside the cardiac neural crest never result in truncus arteriosus. This suggests that truncus arteriosus arises as a result of a decrease in the amount of ectomesenchyme derived from the cardiac neural crest (Kirby 1987). The nitrosurea derivative, nimustine hydrochloride, causes truncus arteriosus and ventricular septal defects in the chick. When quail–chick chimeras are treated with this agent and examined 24 h later there is extensive cell death in areas populated by quail neural crest cells. This suggests that truncus arteriosus induced by nimustine is caused by the loss of neural crest cells destined to participate in cardiac outflow tract septation (Miyagawa & Kirby 1989).

Excision of cardiac neural crest tissue also has complex effects on cardiac innervation and haemodynamics which may produce malformations by more indirect mechanisms. When ablation is confined to cardiac neural crest, but is less than one somite in length, the resultant cardiac malformation is one of a range of defects described as a 'dextroposed aorta' which include Fallot's tetralogy and double outlet right ventricle. However, the same anomalies can be produced by ablating cranial portions of the neural crest which do not contribute cells to the developing heart. Cells from all levels of the cranial neural crest contribute to the developing aortic arch arteries (Kirby 1988) and their ablation results in abnormal patency or closure of these vessels with resultant haemodynamic changes. Such changes have been measured in the chick embryo following cardiac neural crest ablation and shown to precede the development of the outflow tract (Stewart et al 1986). The implication is that some of the malformations which result from cardiac neural crest manipulation are secondary to haemodynamic alterations in the arch arteries, compounding the deficiencies of cellular migration to the heart.

Removal of cardiac neural crest also causes maldevelopment of structures derived from the pharyngeal pouches. These include the parathyroid and thymic connective tissue and the C cell component of the thyroid. The associations seen in the di George syndrome suggest that there may be a primary abnormality of the cardiac neural crest. Other putative cardiac neural crest syndromes include the CHARGE association (coloboma, heart disease, atresia choanae, retarded growth, genital hypoplasia, ear anomalies), retinoic acid embryopathy, neuroblastoma with congenital heart disease and the cardiac anomalies of the fetal alcohol syndrome (Kirby & Waldo 1990).

The chick embryo models are uniquely versatile in providing a high rate of predictable malformations whose precise type can be manipulated. They have shown the influences of abnormal cellular migration and haemo-dynamics to be central to the pathogenesis of cardiac malformation.

ANIMAL MODELS

Early work on the development of cardiac malformations relied on correlating observations made on the developing normal embryo with those made on the definitive malformation in the neonate. The discovery that cardiac anomalies occur spontaneously with a high frequency in inbred strains of animal has led to the development of new models for the examination of the evolving, rather than the definitive, malformation. Some of the genetically determined animal models of cardiac malformation are shown in Table 11.3 but only two of the canine models are discussed below.

Table 11.3 Genetically determined animal models of congenital heart disease (based on Patterson et al 1982)

Species and breed or strain	Defect
Chicken	
Light Sussex	Persistent fourth aortic arch
Brown leghorn	Ventricular septal defect
Mouse	
iv/iv	Situs inversus; variable intracardiac anomalies; heterotaxia of veins, lungs, liver, spleen
experimentally induced trisomies: 10	Ventricular septal defect
12	Ventricular septal defect
13	Pulmonary stenosis, VSD and overriding aorta
14	VSD and DORV
16	VSD and DORV
A/j and CL/Fr	Atrial septal defects and cleft lip
Rat	
Long Evans (Olson-Gross)	Ventricular septal defect
Rabbit	
III VO/J	Vestigial pulmonary artery
AX/J and AXBU/J	Retro-oesophageal right subclavian artery
Cat	
Siamese and Burmese	Endocardial fibroelastosis
Pig	
Minipig (Netherlands)	Hypoplastic left heart
Dog	
Poodle	Patent ductus arteriosus
Beagle	Pulmonary stenosis
Newfoundland	Discrete subaortic stenosis
German shepherd	Persistent right aortic arch
Keeshond	Conotruncal septum defects
Cow	
Hereford	Ventricular septal defect

For abbreviations see Table 11.1.

Congenital heart disease has the same incidence in dogs as in man although there are differences in the distribution of types that occur. Coarctation of the aorta is a common human malformation but is rare in the dog, whereas persistent fourth right aortic arch is a frequent canine anomaly but is uncommon in the human (Patterson et al 1982). Breeding studies using poodle and keeshond models support a mode of inheritance in which several genes act together to determine the degree and severity of the cardiac malformation.

In the embryos of poodles from predisposed litters, the normally muscular media of the ductus arteriosus is replaced by non-contractile elastic tissue which is in continuity with, and histologically resembles, the aortic media. The extent to which this 'aortification' of the ductus extends towards the pulmonary artery determines the length of ductus whose lumen remains patent in the definitive malformation. If sufficient normal ductal tissue remains at the pulmonary artery end to permit closure of the duct then a blind-ending 'ductus diverticulum' of the aorta results. Breeding experiments indicate that the capacity of the ductus to constrict is related to the proportion of the genome that is derived from dogs with patent ductus arteriosus (Patterson et al 1982). The changes in the human duct are more subtle but support the proposition that persistent patency is a primary abnormality of the duct and that the presence of abnormal elastic tissue in the media is a morphological correlate of disordered closure (Gittenberger-de Groot 1977).

Cardiac anomalies are present in over 50% of keeshond dogs at autopsy. The malformations found are a spectrum of outflow tract and pulmonary valve lesions ranging from subclinical absence of the medial papillary muscle to double outlet right ventricle with ventricular septal defect and pulmonary stenosis. Serial sectioning studies on keeshond embryos (Van Meirop & Patterson 1980) and scanning electron microscopy studies (Pexieder & Patterson 1984) have demonstrated an early and temporary hypoplasia of the embryonic right ventricle. A delay in fusion and hypoplasia of the atrioventricular cushions contribute to the development of the ventricular septal defect and hypoplasia of the conotruncal cushions is central to the pathogenesis of the outflow tract anomaly. Pexieder (1980) also described abnormal foci of intensive cell death in the myocardial mantle underlying the conal cushions in keeshond embryos at a stage prior to normal conotruncal fusion.

SCANNING ELECTRON MICROSCOPY

Many classical studies of cardiac development were based on three dimensional reconstructions from serial sections of the embryonic heart. Whilst these techniques have provided useful information about the embryology of the heart, the extrapolation to the three dimensional organ has a potential for error. Scanning electron microscopic examination of the prenatal heart offers many advantages over light microscopy. Standardized methods of specimen preparation are necessary in order to avoid artefacts and to allow comparisons to be made between the results obtained by different groups of workers (Pexieder 1988). The heart must be perfusion fixed at low pressure using buffered fixatives whose osmolarity is adjusted to reduce damage to the endocardial surface. Microdissection using standard-ized incisions with scissors creates fewer artefacts than fracture techniques. Orientation of the heart on the final photographs requires reference to extracardiac fixed points such as the neural tube.

Application of these techniques to the study of embryonic mouse hearts killed at 8 h intervals has contributed to an understanding of the mechanisms of outflow tract septation (Vuillemin & Pexieder 1989). Fewer scanning electron microscopy studies have been made on the developing human heart because of a paucity of well preserved material from early pregnancy. However, Pexieder & Janecek (1984) have used the technique successfully to study perfusion fixed hearts from therapeutic terminations between 6 and 20 weeks' gestation.

EXPRESSION OF CARDIAC PROTEINS IN DEVELOPMENT AND DISEASE

The function of membrane bound granules within the atrial myocardial cells had remained mysterious until the experiments of de Bold et al (1981) demonstrated that atrial extracts had a diuretic and natriuretic activity when injected into rats. The granules contain a 28 amino-acid peptide, atrial natriuretic factor and its precursor forms. Physiological studies indicate a central role for this cardiac hormone in the regulation of fluid balance, electrolytes and blood pressure. The most clearly defined stimulus for release of the hormone is increased atrial stretch. Elevated levels of atrial natriuretic factor have been found in adults with congestive cardiac failure, systemic hypertension and tachyarrythmias (Condorelli & Volpe 1989).

Atrial natriuretic factor is more widely distributed in the fetus than it is in adults. The fetal ventricular myocardium and the main conducting bundles also contain the hormone, whereas in adults it is confined to the atria. There is a change in gene expression so that synthesis of the hormone in the ventricles declines after birth. Plasma levels of the hormone are higher in the fetus than in extrauterine life and premature infants have elevated levels (Smith et al 1989). Fetuses with rhesus disease also have raised plasma levels which is probably due to the associated volume overload (Kingdom et al 1989).

Raised levels of atrial natriuretic factor are also found in children with some forms of congenital heart disease. The plasma level correlates with left atrial size and it may influence the regulation of circulatory volume in these cases (Matsuoka et al 1988). Adults with acquired heart disease may revert to the fetal pattern of expression of atrial natriuretic factor whereby ventricular conducting tissue and myocardium contain the hormone (Wharton et al 1988).

This phenomenon of changing patterns of protein expression at different sites in the heart during development and in disease has also been described for the family of cardiac myosin heavy chains (Swynghedauw 1986). Distribution of different forms of myosin heavy chain differ between the atria, ventricles and conducting system at different developmental stages (Kuro-o et al 1986, Bouvagnet et al 1987). In human mitral stenosis the myosin heavy chain in left atrial myocytes changes from atrial to ventricular type (Gorza et al 1984). Other transitions in myosin type can be induced in the ventricle of the rat heart when the aorta or pulmonary artery are banded. These changes in myosin gene expression seem to be a direct response to pressure overload within the heart although the mechanisms are obscure (Imamura et al 1990).

NOMENCLATURE AND CLASSIFICATION

Complex terminology and cumbersome systems of classification have impeded communications amongst workers from diverse fields who study congenital heart disease. The same lesion can be described depending on whether one favours an embryological, a mechanistic or a morphological approach. For example, the terms complete atrioventricularis communis, endocardial cushion defect, common atrioventricular canal and atrioventricular septal defect can all be used to describe the same anomaly. Systems of classification based on cardiac embryology or putative mechanisms of malformation (Clark 1987) are of limited value while our understanding of these processes remains so incomplete (Becker & Anderson 1984).

A descriptive approach allows the anomaly to be documented in an unambiguous way without making assumptions about cardiac development or the pathogenesis of the malformation. This method of 'sequential chamber analysis' has found favour amongst clinicians and histopathologists although it has made less impression in the fields of embryology and teratology. This approach to diagnosis is based on the orderly examination of atrial arrangement, the atrioventricular connection, the ventricles and the ventriculoarterial junction, after which a catalogue of malformations is made (Anderson 1987). A patent ductus arteriosus or an atrial septal defect may form the major anomaly in the heart and as such may be the main focus of attention. However, associated abnormalities of the arrangement of cardiac segments or abnormal connection of the junctions may be present in one third of autopsy cases (Hegerty et al 1985). Sequential chamber analysis is quick and simple to apply and it is the closest we have to a lingua franca in the field of cardiac malformations.

INCIDENCE AND RECURRENCE RISKS

The incidence of different forms of congenital heart malformation depends on the age of the patients studied. This reflects the natural loss of severe malformations in fetal and neonatal life which allows the milder anomalies to assume a greater numerical preponderance in later years. Some malformations such as patent ductus arteriosus cannot be manifest during fetal life when patency is the normal condition. Bicuspid aortic valve, the commonest cardiac malformation, affects 2% of the population but presents in adult life. Inconsistencies in nomenclature and classification as well as differences in emphasis as to what might be the dominant lesion in a complex anomaly makes it difficult to compare incidence figures meaningfully and they may be further distorted by referral practices and expertise. Nevertheless, the data support the observation that complex defects are more common in fetal echocardiographic and abortus series than in live births, due to a high rate of intrauterine death in these conditions (Allan et al 1985). Table 11.4 shows the distribution of different forms of congenital heart disease at different ages.

Table 11.4 Percentage distribution of types of congenital heart defects in fetuses, abortuses, stillbirths and livebirths

Dominant lesion	A	B	C	D
Ventricular septal defect	9.7	10.4	34.7	32.5
Complete transposition	5.5	2.7	9.1	5.0
Tetralogy of Fallot	8.3	15.6	3.4	5.9
Interrupted aortic arch	4.1	5.3	—	0
Coarctation of the aorta	6.8	5.3	9.4	6.3
Hypoplastic left heart	5.5	2.7	3.0	2.8
Atrioventricular septal defect	13.8	10.4	6.8	2.4
Absent left atrioventricular connection	5.5	7.9	0	0
Double inlet atrioventricular connection	2.7	0	6.4	1.7
Absent right atrioventricular connection	2.7	7.9	} 1.1	} 2.5
Pulmonary atresia with intact septum	6.8	0		
Ebstein's anomaly	5.5	0		
Pulmonary stenosis	0	0	1.1	7.6
Atrial septal defect	—	—	10.2	5.9
Total anomalous pulmonary venous return	0	2.7	0	0.8
Myocardial disease	11.1	0	0	0
Double outlet right ventricle	1.3	10.4	0.4	0
Truncus arteriosus	1.3	2.7	6.0	1.1
Tumours	4.1	0	0	0
Corrected transposition	1.3	5.3	0	0
Patent ductus arteriosus	—	—	—	11.9
Aortic stenosis	2.7	2.7	0	5.1
Misc	1.3	7.9	6.4	8.0

A = fetal echocardiography series (Allan et al 1985).
B = spontaneous abortions less than 24 weeks' gestation with congenital heart disease (Allan et al 1985).
C = stillbirth series (pooled data from Hoffman 1987).
D = livebirth series (Dickinson et al 1981).

Left to nature, 60% of liveborn children with congenital heart disease would die in infancy, 25% in the newborn period, and probably only 15% would survive to adolescence and adult life (MacMahon et al 1953). Surgeons and cardiologists have changed the pattern of cardiac malformation seen in the adolescent and adult by improving survival rates in childhood. Complex arrhythmias, chronic myocardial dysfunction, paradoxical emboli and compensatory polycythaemia present new clinical problems in the late survivors of corrective or palliative surgery; these are in addition to well-established complications such as pulmonary hypertension and infective endocarditis. Undoubtedly, advances in treatment e.g. cardiac transplantation will further modify the manifestations of congenital heart disease in adult life (Somerville 1986).

A couple who have had a child with a cardiac malformation will wish to know the risk to subsequent pregnancies. Improved survival has also meant that affected patients may reach a childbearing age themselves, and also wish to know the risks to their offspring. In a multifactorial model of inheritance the risk to a sibling or a child of an affected person is approximately equal in both and is calculated as the square root of the population incidence of the condition. This model accurately predicts some forms of congenital heart disease such as patent ductus arteriosus where the observed recurrence risks of 2.3% in siblings and 2.5% in offspring correspond closely to the 2.5% predicted recurrence risk (Burn 1983). However, there is wide variation in quoted recurrence risks for other cardiac malformations and some authors have questioned the validity of the method. Some of the discrepancies may be accounted for by inclusions of a few high risk families who may distort the data, whilst other series included children with clinically insignificant anomalies such as small, spontaneously closing, ventricular septal defects which would not have been detected had older children been studied (Nora & Nora 1984).

Lesions with a presumed haemodynamic pathogenesis affecting the left side of the heart were much more frequent in relatives of affected patients than predicted in the large Baltimore–Washington infant study (Boughman et al 1987). Thus 13.5% of older siblings of children with hypoplastic left heart, 8.1% of siblings of patients with coarctation, and 11.1% of siblings of those with bicuspid aortic valve suffered from a malformation which was generally the same as found in the index case. The figures for the hypoplastic left heart syndrome were closer to that expected for an autosomal recessive condition than for a multifactorial one.

The recurrence risk to the offspring of an affected parent with congenital heart disease is generally quoted at between 1 and 3%. However, higher recurrence risks are reported for some specific lesions; for example, atrioventricular septal defect had a 10–14% recurrence risk in the study of Emanuel et al (1983). A prospective study of mothers with congenital heart disease referred for fetal echocardiography showed surprisingly high recurrence rates of 1 in 52 if there was already one affected child and 1 in 10

Table 11.5   Recurrence risks in siblings and offspring for different
congenital heart defects (based on Burn 1987)

Cardiac defect	Recurrence risk counselling figure (%)	
	Siblings	Offspring
Oval window ASD	3	4
AVSD	2	5–10
Ebstein's anomaly	1	5
VSD	3	4
Pulmonary stenosis	2	6
Tetralogy of Fallot	2	4
Aortic stenosis	3	5–10
Coarctation	2	3
Patent arterial duct	2.3	2.5
Isomerism sequence	5	1
Double inlet ventricle	3	5
Absent right AV valve	1	5
Absent left AV valve	2	5
Complete transposition	2	5
Pulmonary atresia	1	5
Anomalous pulmonary venous connection	3	5

For abbreviations see Table 11.1.

if there were two affected children (Allan et al 1986). Recurrence rates of 1 in
28 for aortic valve atresia, 1 in 11 for complex congenital heart disease, 1 in
15 for coarctation and 1 in 13 for truncus arteriosus were reported in this
study. Results such as these must cast further doubt on the applicability of a
polygenic threshold model to all forms of cardiac malformation.

It will be appreciated from the above that genetic counselling for
congenital heart disease is a complex area. Histopathologists have an
important role in the accurate assessment of cardiac and extracardiac
anomalies which may allow the case to be assigned to a specific syndrome,
and detailed correlation with echocardiography is essential for audit. The
advice that the overall recurrence risk of an isolated cardiac malformation is
in the region of 2–5% is probably still valid. In any case, a family pedigree,
antenatal echocardiography and fetal karyotyping are valuable adjuncts to
counselling (Lin & Garver 1988). Table 11.5 shows quoted counselling
figures of recurrence risk for different cardiac defects.

FETAL ECHOCARDIOGRAPHY AND ANTENATAL DIAGNOSIS

The techniques of fetal ultrasound have so rapidly improved in the past
decade that they can now provide an effective means of screening for
malformations. When performed at 18 weeks gestation, two-thirds of
cardiac malformations are theoretically detectable on a routine 4-chamber
view performed in non-specialist centres (Allan 1988).

Fetal echocardiography allows the cardiologist to follow the progression of the malformation during gestation by performing multiple scans. Some anomalies become more severe, less amenable to surgery or change their morphology as pregnancy proceeds. For example, a contracted form of endocardial fibroelastosis has been documented as developing from a dilated form detected earlier in pregnancy (Carceller et al 1990).

Valuable new data about specific malformations and their associations have been obtained from echocardiography. Such studies have shown that in fetal life nearly half of the cases of atrioventricular septal defect are associated with Down's syndrome while the other half have atrial isomerism, usually left sided, but Down's syndrome and atrial isomerism are never detected together (Machado et al 1988). Haemodynamic measurements made by echocardiography can also quantify the degree of obstruction or incompetence of a cardiac valve.

MYOCARDIAL INFARCTION AND CONGENITAL HEART DISEASE

The observation that children with cardiac malformations may suffer ischaemic myocardial necrosis is well established (Esterly & Oppenheimer 1967) but it remains poorly understood and under-reported. In one postmortem series 30 out of 76 consecutive autopsies on children with congenital heart disease had myocardial necrosis (Russell & Berry 1989). Although the majority of these had undergone recent open heart surgery and myocardial necrosis could be ascribed to problems with preservation during cardiopulmonary bypass, other children had not been operated upon.

Infarcts have been found in hearts with a wide variety of malformations but seem to be most frequent in those with outflow obstructions due to valve stenosis or atresia (Esterly & Oppenheimer 1967). Early observations suggested that the distribution of infarction reflects the anatomical site of the underlying cardiac malformation. Franciosi & Blanc (1968) described left ventricular infarcts in cases of congenital aortic stenosis and right ventricular infarcts in pulmonary valve stenosis. However, other studies have demonstrated the frequent presence of ischaemic lesions in the unobstructed right ventricle in children with hypoplastic left heart syndrome (Lloyd et al 1986).

Attention has been drawn to the precarious myocardial perfusion in cases of aortic valve atresia where the blood reaches the coronary arteries via the patent ductus arteriosus and by retrograde flow down the hypoplastic aorta. In addition, abnormal communications between the ventricular chamber and the coronary arteries exist in both aortic atresia (O'Connor et al 1982) and pulmonary atresia when the ventricular septum is intact (Bull et al 1982). These ventriculocoronary connections may protect the heart from the development of ischaemic lesions and endocardial fibroelastosis in pulmonary atresia with intact ventricular septum. However, obstructive

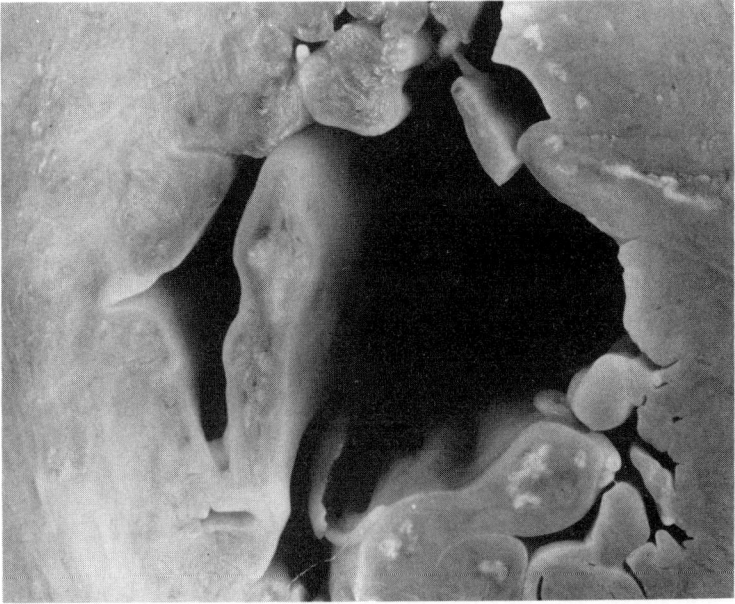

a

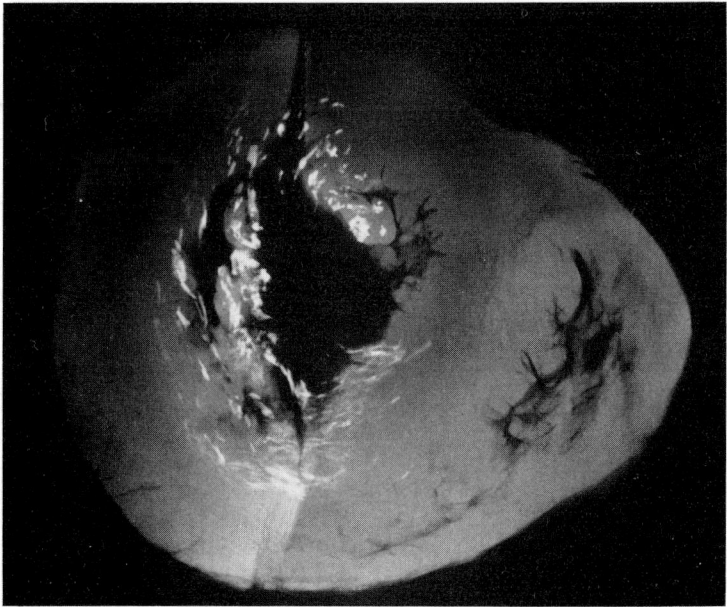

b

Fig. 11.2 (a) Calcified subendocardial necrosis from a child with severe congenital aortic stenosis. (b) Radiograph of same specimen (both figures from Russell & Berry 1989 with kind permission of the Editor of *The Journal of Clinical Pathology*).

lesions of the epicardial coronary arteries have been observed more frequently in children with ventriculocoronary connections and these may further impair the already disordered myocardial circulation (Gittenberger-de Groot et al 1988). The myocardium of malformed hearts may be rendered more vulnerable to ischaemia by extreme hypertrophy which increases the oxygen demand, and chamber dilatation which adversely affects the perfusion pressure.

Myocardial infarcts in children may be difficult to identify by naked eye examination at autopsy. The infarct will be visible in cases where the lesion has calcified or in jaundiced children when the areas of necrosis may take on a yellow-green appearance. Calcification is a rapid and common event in neonatal myocardial infarcts (Fig. 11.2) and a paucity of cellular reaction is typical. The vulnerable sites are the subendocardium and the papillary muscles although in severe cases the atrium may also be affected (Russell & Berry 1989). Random sections of heart from all four chambers should be examined histologically.

PULMONARY HYPERTENSION

The trend towards performing surgery in the first few months of life on children with cardiac malformations has highlighted some deficiencies in the classical concepts of pulmonary hypertension which were first elucidated in older children. Central to an understanding of the changes induced by increased pulmonary blood flow is an appreciation of the process of remodelling that the pulmonary vascular tree undergoes following birth and the onset of respiration. Extrauterine adaptation during the first 4 days of life involves an immediate reduction in pulmonary vascular resistance which is effected by dilatation of precapillary arterioles and recruitment of unopened muscular arteries into the circulation. Electron microscopy demonstrates a change in shape of the endothelial cells from a squat, cuboidal type with interdigitations to thinner, flatter cells with minimal overlap. The second stage of remodelling lasts until 3 to 4 weeks of age and involves the deposition of connective tissue around smooth muscle cells in small muscular arteries and the formation of definitive elastic laminae. During the growth stage from 3 weeks to 6 months of age the number of respiratory unit arteries increases with the formation of new alveoli and pericytes differentiate into smooth muscle cells in distal arteries (Howarth 1988).

The cardiac malformations that lead to pulmonary hypertension are typically post-tricuspid; these include ventricular and atrioventricular septal defects, patent ductus arteriosus, aorto-pulmonary window and truncus arteriosus. These anomalies lead to disturbance of the normal process of pulmonary vascular remodelling in the first weeks of life which may result in pulmonary vascular disease and altered vascular reactivity. Manifestations of abnormal remodelling include the premature differentiation of smooth muscle cells in more peripheral arteries than normal and the formation of excess type I collagen, both of which lead to medial hypertrophy. There is also an accumulation of myofilaments in the smooth muscle cells and a decrease in the number and size of arteries (Howarth 1987a).

The distribution and severity of the vascular changes as well as the predominance of different vascular lesions are related to the type of underlying cardiac malformation. Three forms of congenital heart disease have been shown to have different patterns of pulmonary vascular pathology. Isolated ventricular septal defect is associated with extension of muscle into intra-acinar arterial walls by 7 to 9 months of age but only mild, non-occlusive cellular intimal proliferation at the same age (Howarth 1987b). By contrast, children with atrioventricular septal defects show more severe cellular intimal proliferation (Howarth 1986). Children with transposition of the great vessels and ventricular septal defect have severe intimal cellular proliferation by 5 to 6 months of age which is accompanied by less pronounced muscularization of more peripheral arteries (Howarth et al 1987).

The interpretation of the early changes of pulmonary hypertension in lung biopsies from children with congenital heart disease requires the use of serial sectioning for the detection of focal abnormalities and for an appreciation of their microanatomy. In addition, these must be compared with age-matched controls to make allowance for the stage of remodelling expected in a normal child. A knowledge of the underlying anatomical malformation may help predict the pattern of abnormality. The biopsy must be sufficiently deep to include preacinar vessels which may show severe changes that are not reflected in the smaller distal vessels.

Ultrastructural studies on lungs from patients with plexogenic arteriopathy show early smooth muscle migration from the media to the intima followed by differentiation to a secretory myofibroblast (Smith et al 1990). The stimulus for this cellular migration may be a chemical one derived from the increased bronchial neuroendocrine cell population detected in this condition (Heath et al 1990). Rats injected with the toxin monocrotaline develop pulmonary hypertension with the early development of breaks in the internal elastic lamina of small pulmonary arteries possibly through abnormal elastase activity. These breaks may facilitate smooth muscle cell migration which can be diminished by inhibitors of elastase (Rabinovitch 1988).

Confusion has been generated by the tendency to equate the theoretical reversibility of the low grades of pulmonary hypertension with their operability. Although medial hypertrophy is potentially reversible it is by no means an insignificant lesion. Peri-operative mortality is high, when intra-acinar arteries have a medial thickness greater than 20% of their external diameter (Bush et al 1988). Pulmonary hypertensive crises immediately following successful repair of cardiac malformations are life-threatening and may not be predictable from the Heath-Edwards grading alone. It is not clear which of several factors is of most significance. Scanning electron microscopy has shown changes in the shape of pulmonary endothelial cells which may promote an abnormal interaction with platelets and leucocytes resulting in the release of vasoconstricting thromboxanes and leucotrienes. In addition, there are increased numbers of neuroendocrine cells containing the vasoconstrictors bombesin and serotonin in the lungs of children with pulmonary hypertension (Rabinovitch 1988). Immunohistochemical studies have demonstrated that the thick-walled pulmonary arteries in patients with congenital heart disease are prematurely innervated with tyrosinergic nerves which promote vasoconstriction. This abnormal innervation may be viewed as another example of disturbed pulmonary remodelling as it is an acceleration of the normal pattern of development (Allen et al 1989).

COARCTATION OF THE AORTA

It has been proposed that coarctation is due to a haemodynamic abnormality where there is an exaggeration of the normal aortic arch anatomy and low blood flow through the fetal isthmus (Rudolph et al 1972). The association of coarctation with malformations that reduce aortic blood flow supports this theory. An alternative hypothesis suggests that coarctation is primarily a malformation of the duct whereby an extension of the ductal media forms a circumferential sling around the lumen of the aorta (Wielenga & Dankmeijer 1968). Rosenberg (1990) suggests that the two hypotheses are not mutually exclusive if the abnormal ductal extension is regarded as a deformation secondary to altered haemodynamics. The ductal tissue in a coarctation is easy to identify microscopically in young children but it is increasingly difficult to recognize with age. Elzenga & Gittenberger-de Groot (1983) propose that all forms of coarctation result from abnormal ductal extension into the aorta. Severe stenoses present early, at the preductal site. Differential growth in the aorta and the tendency of the ductal tissue to undergo fibrosis lead to a relative 'migration' of the coarctation to paraductal and postductal positions. In less severe cases, secondary intimal thickening may present later as postductal ('adult type') obstruction. The suggestion that ductal tissue in coarctation is subject to similar changes as those occurring in the closing duct is borne out by the histological similarity between the two, including the presence of medial necrosis.

The implication of these observations for clinical management is not clear. The development of aneurysms at the site of balloon dilatation of coarctation has been attributed by some authors to the presence of 'cystic' medial necrosis (Isner et al 1987). The circumferential sling remains intact following balloon dilatation which may account for the high rate of restenosis observed in neonates following this procedure (Redington et al 1990). Surgical treatment in infants is associated with significant rates of recurrence whether the coarctation is excised and the ends anastomosed or whether the obstruction is incised and expanded by subclavian flap aortoplasty. Both techniques leave residual ductal tissue in the aorta and this tissue may have the potential for contraction as it matures (Russell et al 1991).

RHABDOMYOMAS AND TUBEROUS SCLEROSIS

Rhabdomyoma is the commonest cardiac tumour of infancy. The tumour is usually located within the ventricles where it forms a waxy, yellow nodule. Histologically it is composed of swollen, vacuolated, glycogen containing cells, interspersed with bands of normal myocardium. The tumour is usually asymptomatic but may present as an obstructive lesion or rhythm disturbance.

The association between cardiac rhabdomyoma and tuberous sclerosis is long established. Echocardiographic studies detect rhabdomyomas in 58% of children and 18% of adults with tuberous sclerosis, and in infancy the figure is probably even higher. These data suggest that a high proportion of these tumours regress or fail to enlarge as the patient grows. The tendency for regression suggests that conservative management should be considered in asymptomatic cases (Smith et al 1989).

Patients with multiple tumours nearly always have tuberous sclerosis. Those with a solitary rhabdomyoma clinically have a greater than 50% chance of having tuberous sclerosis, and autopsy frequently demonstrates microscopic rhabdomyomas too small for echocardiographic detection. A rhabdomyoma may be the earliest sign of tuberous sclerosis, preceding the development of the other classical stigmata. Non-invasive echocardiography is a recommended investigation for children with idiopathic infantile spasms, as 25% of these will subsequently prove to have tuberous sclerosis (Pampiglione & Pugh 1975). Attempts to identify and locate the tuberous sclerosis gene have suggested that two or more loci may be responsible and a genetic means of antenatal diagnosis by chorionic villus biopsy is not yet available (Lancet 1990). Selective fetal echocardiography in high risk pregnancies may also provide an effective, non-invasive means of screening for rhabdomyomas and hence tuberous sclerosis.

REFERENCES

Allan L D, Crawford D C, Anderson R H et al 1985 Spectrum of congenital heart disease detected echocardiographically in prenatal life. British Heart Journal 54: 523–526
Allan L D, Crawford D C, Chita S et al 1986 Familial recurrence of congenital heart disease in a prospective series of mothers referred for fetal echocardiography. American Journal of Cardiology 58: 334–337
Allan L D 1988 The diagnosis of fetal cardiac abnormality. British Journal of Hospital Medicine 40: 290–293
Allen K M, Wharton J, Polak J M et al 1989 A study of nerves containing peptides in the

pulmonary vasculature of healthy infants and children and of those with pulmonary hypertension. British Heart Journal 62: 353–360

Anderson R H, 1987 Terminology. In: Anderson R H, Macartney F J, Shinebourne E A, Tynan M (eds) Paediatric cardiology. Churchill Livingstone, Edinburgh, pp 65–70

Becker A E, Anderson R H 1984 Cardiac embryology: a help or a hindrance in understanding congenital heart disease. In: Nora J J, Takao A (eds) Congenital heart disease: causes and processes. Futura, New York, pp 339–358

Boughman J A, Berg K A, Astemborski J A et al 1987 Familial risks of congenital heart defect assessed in a population-based epidemiologic study. American Journal of Medical Genetics 26: 839–849

Bouvagnet P, Neveu S, Montoya M et al 1987 Developmental changes in the human cardiac isomyosin distribution: an immunohistochemical study using monoclonal antibodies. Circulation Research 61: 329–336

Bruyere H J, Kargas S A, Levy J M 1987 The causes and underlying developmental mechanisms of congenital cardiovascular malformations. American Journal of Medical Genetics (suppl) 3: 411–431

Bull C, de Leval M, Mercanti C 1982 Pulmonary atresia and intact ventricular septum: a revised classification. Circulation 66: 266–271

Burn J 1983 Congenital heart defects—the risks to offspring. Archives of Disease in Childhood 58: 947–948

Burn J 1987 The aetiology of congenital heart disease. In: Anderson R H, Macartney F J, Shinebourne E A, Tynan M (eds) Paediatric cardiology. Churchill Livingstone, Edinburgh, pp 33–37

Bush A, Busst C M, Howarth S G 1988 Correlations of lung morphology, pulmonary vascular resistance and outcome in children with congenital heart disease. British Heart Journal 59: 480–485

Carceller A M, Maroto E, Fouron J-C 1990 Dilated and contracted forms of primary endocardial fibroelastosis: a single fetal disease with two stages of development. British Heart Journal 63: 311–313

Clark E B, Rosenquist G C 1978 Spectrum of cardiovascular anomalies following cardiac loop constriction in the chick embryo. Birth Defects 14: 431–442

Clark E B 1987 Mechanisms in the pathogenesis of congenital cardiac malformations. In: Pierpont M E, Moller J H (eds) Genetics of cardiovascular disease. Martinus Nijhoff, Boston, pp 3–11

Condorelli M, Volpe M 1989 Endocrine function of the heart in cardiac disease. Acta Cardiologica 3: 203–219

de Bold A J, Borenstein H B, Veress A T et al 1981 A rapid and potent natriuretic response to intravenous injection of atrial myocardial extract in rats. Life Science 28: 89–94

Dickinson D F, Arnold R, Wilkinson J L 1981 Congenital heart disease among 160,480 liveborn children in Liverpool 1960 to 1969. British Heart Journal 46: 55–62

Elzenga N J, Gittenberger-de Groot A C 1983 Localised coarctation of the aorta, an age dependent spectrum. British Heart Journal 49: 317–323

Emanuel R, Somerville J, Inns A et al 1983 Evidence of congenital heart disease in the offspring of parents with atrioventricular septal defects. British Heart Journal 49: 144–147

Esterly J R, Oppenheimer E H 1967 Some aspects of cardiac pathology in infancy and childhood. Myocardial and coronary lesions in cardiac malformations. Pediatrics 39: 896–903

Franciosi R A, Blanc W A 1968 Myocardial infarcts in infants and children. Journal of Pediatrics 73: 309–319

Gittenberger-de Groot A C 1977 Persistent ductus arteriosus: most probably a primary congenital malformation. British Heart Journal 39: 610–618

Gittenberger-de Groot A C, Sauer U et al 1988 Competition of the coronary arteries and ventriculo-coronary arterial communications in pulmonary atresia with intact ventricular septum. International Journal of Cardiology 18: 243–258

Gorza L, Mercadier J J, Schwartz K et al 1984 Myosin types in the human heart. Circulation Research 54: 694–702

Heath D, Yacoub M, Gosney J R 1990 Pulmonary endocrine cells in hypertensive pulmonary vascular disease. Histopathology 16: 21–28

Hegerty A S, Anderson R H, Ho S Y 1985 Congenital heart malformations in the first year of life—a necropsy study. British Heart Journal 54: 583–592

Hoffman J I E 1987 Incidence, mortality and natural history. In: Anderson R H, Macartney F, Shinebourne E, Tynan M (eds) Paediatric cardiology. Churchill Livingstone, Edinburgh, p 5

Howarth S G 1986 Pulmonary vascular bed in children with complete atrioventricular septal defect: relation between structure and hemodynamic abnormalities. American Journal of Cardiology 57: 833–839

Howarth S G 1987a Pulmonary vasculature. In: Anderson R H, Macartney F J, Shinebourne E A, Tynan M (eds) Paediatric cardiology. Churchill Livingstone, Edinburgh, pp 127–145

Howarth S G 1987b Pulmonary vascular disease in ventricular septal defect: structural and functional correlations in lung biopsies from 85 patients, with outcome of intracardiac repair. Journal of Pathology 152: 157–168

Howarth S G, Radley-Smith R, Yacoub M 1987 Lung biopsy findings in transposition of the great arteries with ventricular septal defect: potentially reversible pulmonary vascular disease is not always synonymous with operability. Journal of the American College of Cardiologists 9: 327–333

Howarth S G 1988 Pulmonary vascular remodelling in neonatal pulmonary hypertension. Chest 93 (suppl): 133–138

Imamura S, Matsuoka R, Hiratsuka E et al 1990 Local response to cardiac overload on myosin heavy chain gene expression and isozyme transition. Circulation Research 66: 1067–1073

Isner J M, Donaldson R F, Fulton D et al 1987 Cystic medial necrosis in coarctation of the aorta: a potential factor contributing to adverse consequences observed after balloon angioplasty at coarctation sites. Circulation 75: 689–695

Kingdom J C P, Jardine A G, Doyle J et al 1989 Atrial natriuretic peptide in the fetus. British Medical Journal 298: 1221–1222

Kirby M L, Gale T F, Stewart D E 1983 Neural crest cells contribute to normal aorticopulmonary septation. Science 220: 1059–1061

Kirby M L 1987 Cardiac morphogenesis—recent research advances. Pediatric Research 21: 219–224

Kirby M L 1988 Role of extracardiac factors in heart development. Experientia 44: 944–951

Kirby M L 1989 Plasticity and predetermination of mesencephalic and trunk neural crest transplanted into the region of the cardiac neural crest. Developmental Biology 134: 402–412

Kirby M L, Waldo K L 1990 Role of the neural crest in congenital heart disease. Circulation 82: 332–340

Kuro-o M, Tsuchimochi H, Ueda S et al 1986 Distribution of cardiac myosin isozymes in human conduction system. Journal of Clinical Investigation 77: 340–347

Lancet 1990 Progress in tuberous sclerosis. ii: 598–599

Lin A E, Garver K L 1988 Genetic counselling for congenital heart defects. Journal of Paediatrics 113: 1105–1109

Lloyd T R, Evans T C, Marvin W J 1986 Morphologic determinants of coronary blood flow in the hypoplastic left heart syndrome. American Heart Journal 112: 666–671

Machado M V L, Crawford D C, Anderson R H et al 1988 Atrioventricular septal defect in prenatal life. British Heart Journal 59: 352–355

MacMahon B, McKeown T, Record R G 1953 The incidence and life expectations of children with congenital heart disease. British Heart Journal 15: 121–129

Matsuoka S, Kurashashi Y, Miki Y et al 1988 Plasma atrial natriuretic peptide in patients with congenital heart diseases. Pediatrics 82: 639–643

Miyagawa S, Kirby M L 1989 Pathogenesis of persistent truncus arteriosus induced by nimustine hydrochloride in chick embryos. Teratology 39: 287–294

Nora J J, Nora A H 1978 The evolution of specific genetic and environmental counselling in congenital heart diseases. Circulation 57: 205–213

Nora J J, Nora A H 1984 The genetic contribution to congenital heart disease. In: Nora J J, Takao A (eds) Congenital heart disease: causes and processes. Futura, New York, pp 3–13

O'Connor W N, Cash J B, Cottrill C M 1982 Ventriculocoronary connections in hypoplastic left hearts: an autopsy microscopic study. Circulation 66: 1078–1086

Pampiglione G, Pugh E 1975 Infantile spasms and subsequent appearance of tuberous sclerosis syndrome. Lancet ii: 1046

Patterson D F, Haskins M E, Jezik P F 1982 Models of human genetic disease in domestic animals. In: Harris H, Hirschhorn K (eds) Advances in human genetics, Vol 12, Plenum Press, New York, pp 263–340

Pexieder T 1975 Cell death in the morphogenesis and teratogenesis of the heart. Advances in Anatomy, Embryology and Cell Biology 51: 1–100

Pexieder T 1980 Cellular mechanisms underlying the normal and abnormal development of the heart. In: Van Praagh R, Takao A (eds) Etiology and morphogenesis of congenital heart disease. Futura, New York, pp 127–153

Pexieder T, Patterson D F 1984 Early pathogenesis of conotruncal malformations in the keeshond dog. In: Nora J J, Takao A (eds) Congenital heart disease: causes and processes. Futura, New York, pp 439–457

Pexieder T, Janecek P 1984 Organogenesis of the human embryonic and early fetal heart as studied by microdissection and SEM. In: Nora J J, Takao A (eds) Congenital heart disease: causes and processes. Futura, New York, pp 401–421

Pexieder T 1987 Teratogens. In: Pierpont M E, Muller J H (eds) Genetics of cardiovascular disease. Martinus Nijhoff, Boston, pp 25–68

Pexieder T 1988 SEM in studies on abnormal cardiac development. Teratology 37: 289–291

Rabinovitch M 1988 Problems of pulmonary hypertension in children with congenital heart defects. Chest 93 (suppl): 119–126

Redington A N, Booth D, Shore D F et al 1990 Primary balloon dilatation of coarctation of the aorta in neonates. British Heart Journal 64: 277–281

Rosenberg H S 1990 Coarctation as a deformation. Paediatric Pathology 10: 103–115

Rudolph A M, Heymann M A, Spitznas U 1972 Haemodynamic considerations in the development of narrowing of the aorta. American Journal of Cardiology 30: 514–525

Russell G A, Berry P J 1989 Postmortem audit in a paediatric cardiology unit. Journal of Clinical Pathology 42: 912–918

Russell G A, Berry P J, Dhasmana J P et al 1989 Coexistent cardiac tumours and malformations. International Journal of Cardiology 22: 89–98

Russell G A, Berry P J, Watterson K et al 1991 Patterns of ductal tissue in coarctation of the aorta in the first three months of life. Journal of Thoracic and Cardiovascular Surgery (in press)

Smith F G, Sato T, Varille V A et al 1989 Atrial natriuretic factor during fetal and postnatal life: a review. Journal of Developmental Physiology 12: 55–62

Smith H C, Watson G H, Patel R G et al 1989 Cardiac rhabdomyomata in tuberous sclerosis: their course and diagnostic value. Archives of Disease in Childhood 64: 196–200

Smith P, Heath D, Yacoub M et al 1990 The ultrastructure of plexogenic pulmonary arteriopathy. Journal of Pathology 160: 111–122

Somerville J 1986 Congenital heart disease in adults and adolescents. British Heart Journal 56: 395–397

Stewart D E, Kirby M L, Sulik K K 1986 Haemodynamic changes in chick embryos precede heart defects after cardiac neural crest ablation. Circulation Research 59: 545–550

Swynghedauw B 1986 Developmental and functional adaptation of contractile proteins in cardiac and skeletal muscles. Physiological Reviews 66: 710–771

Van Meirop L H S, Patterson D F 1980 Pathogenesis of conotruncal defects and some other cardiovascular anomalies in the keeshond dog. In: Van Praagh R, Takao A (eds) Etiology and morphogenesis of congenital heart disease. Futura, New York, pp 177–193

Vuillemin M, Pexieder T 1989 Normal stages of cardiac organogenesis in the mouse. II. Development of the internal relief of the heart. American Journal of Anatomy 184: 114–128

Wharton J, Anderson R H, Springall D et al 1988 Localisation of atrial natriuretic peptide immunoreactivity in the ventricular myocardium and conduction system of the human fetal and adult heart. British Heart Journal 60: 267–274

Wielenga G, Dankmeijer J 1968 Coarctation of the aorta. Journal of Pathology and Bacteriology 95: 265–274

Yoshida H, Manasek F, Arcilla R A 1983 Intracardiac flow patterns in early embryonic life. Circulation Research 53: 363–371

12

Technical advances in histopathology

P. Kirkpatrick   R. J. Marshall

Histopathology is the oldest branch of pathology and the one that remained technically unchanged for almost a century. Significant developments have occurred during the last 20 or 30 years with the advent of histochemistry, electron microscopy and immunohistochemistry, but the bulk of routine diagnostic work still relies on formalin-fixed, paraffin-wax-embedded tissue sections stained by empirical methods. This chapter deals with current advances and future prospects which are likely to affect basic technology in clinical laboratories.

TISSUE FIXATION, EMBEDDING AND PROCESSING

The major changes over the last few years concerned the refinement of block and section production. These include improved processing and embedding systems, new formula waxes, disposable blades and automated staining.

Different types of resin have been described as alternatives to wax. The choice of epoxy or acrylic compounds is determined by the requirement, e.g. the sectioning of hard tissues such as bone, or the production of semi-thin sections from lymphoid tissue where cytological, especially nuclear, detail is critical (Pallett et al 1986, Islam et al 1989). Resin embedding is of course required for electron microscopy and the attractions of having just one embedding medium for light and electron microscopy are obvious. In addition, the activity of most enzymes can be preserved in glycol methacrylate resin, if the increase in temperature at the polymerization stage is kept to a minimum (Murray 1988). Furthermore, many antigens can be demonstrated in resin-embedded material; the ease with which this can be done varies with the type of tissue and resin but standard immunohistochemical techniques can be used in some cases (Hogan & Smith 1982, Shires et al 1990).

Large paraffin sections are not new to histopathology but the national breast screening programme may make their routine use necessary, or at least desirable. In mastectomy specimens, the extent of the tumour is more reliably assessed if a whole cross-section is examined and, in addition, multiple carcinomas are detected which would have otherwise been missed (Gibbs 1982). Large blocks are particularly useful when dealing with impalpable mammographic lesions. Although a cross-section of a biopsy can be halved or quartered, this increases the risk of traumatizing the area of the specimen most in need of examination. In only a minority of cases are such difficulties encountered but large blocks are greatly recommended in all.

Fixation and processing of large blocks can be achieved routinely by limiting the thickness of tissue blocks to not more than 4 mm and by using modern, enclosed tissue processors. In order to minimize the technical disruption caused by the production of large blocks, they can be sectioned using disposable knives, which limit the width of the block to about 8 cm. The length can be much greater and a thickness of 4 µm can be achieved. This compares favourably with non-disposable blades, the maximum width of which is about 12 cm. The large slides produced are less easily examined and stored than standard slides, but are useful for teaching or demonstration purposes.

The localization of lesions detected by mammography can be difficult. Specimen radiography is recommended so that the surgeon can be assured that the abnormality has been removed; the radiograph can then be used as a guide for the histopathologist. Subsequent fixation may distort the specimen and it has been suggested that it remains attached to a perspex plate in which copper wires are inlayed to form a grid. The lines are printed over the specimen radiograph and allow accurate localization of the lesion for histology (Champ et al 1989).

Guide wires are often inserted into the breast to locate the lesion. However, the wire may be a poor guide as accurate placing of the tip is not easy to achieve. Moreover, the guide may move, cause haemorrhage or damage the tissue.

Further refinements and innovations have been made necessary by the mammography screening programme. Precise orientation of the excised specimen is important and different methods for marking excision margins have been suggested (Armstrong & Davies 1991). Traditionally, indian ink has been most commonly used for the purpose, but it is slow to dry and it tends to spread into the tissues; this may be prevented by suspension in acetone. Different artists' pigments have been recommended to distinguish the margins of excision (Paterson & Davies 1988). Six pigments were found which produced different colours under the microscope using ordinary illumination or polarized light. The main objection to this method is that the heavy metals present in some of these pigments are radiodense and therefore interfere with radiographic examination of specimen blocks, in which they can be confused with tissue microcalcification; they are also potentially toxic. Tipp-ex, a white solution used to erase typing errors, has also been recommended as a marker (Harris 1990). It is radiodense and is therefore unsuitable for mammography specimens, though convenient for visible or palpable lesions which do not require radiography. A method using coloured gelatins has also been advocated (Armstrong et al 1990).

These can provide several different colours and they are radiolucent. The application of six colours to the different margins of a specimen is time consuming, although gelatin dries as rapidly as other markers and much more rapidly if the tissue has been pre-cooled.

MICROWAVES

The first applications of microwave technology to histopathology were described 20 years ago and there is now a considerable literature on the subject. However, microwave ovens are still not in routine use. Microwave technology was reviewed recently by Leong (1988) and applications and methods were described in detail by Boon & Kok (1989).

There is virtually no aspect of histopathology where microwaves do not have a use. They fix tissue more effectively than conventional methods as the heat created, which coagulates protein, is evenly and consistently applied throughout. Reports differ as to whether additional formalin fixation is necessary. Good fixation can be achieved in normal saline (Leong et al 1985) or in Tris buffer (Kayser et al 1988). It might be considered safest to collect specimens in formalin, and good fixation is reported after $2\frac{1}{2}$ min irradiation of tissue placed for 1 h in formalin (Leong et al 1985). However, results are said to be more consistent when tissue is fixed for 4 h in formalin before irradiation (Boon et al 1988). The quality of such fixation is sufficient for conventional light microscopy, ultrastructural studies and immuno-histochemistry. Enzyme histochemistry can also be performed on tissue irradiated in saline (Marani et al 1988). It should be noted that tissue blocks less than 1.0 cm in their smallest dimension were used in all these studies. Large specimens can, however, be briefly irradiated for easy dissection, trimmed to block size and the blocks re-irradiated to complete the fixation process in a matter of minutes. This technique is applied with greatest advantage to brains removed at autopsy. Methods allowing the production of paraffin sections of mature and immature brains within one day were described by Boon et al (1989).

Microwave fixation of cryostat sections produces much better fixation and microscopic image than air drying (Kennedy & Foulis 1989). Adhesion of section to slide is enhanced by irradiation, though breast tissue may occasionally be difficult. Breast remains the tissue most likely to require cryostat sections and we have found it difficult to keep slide and section united following microwave fixation.

The procedures of dehydration and impregnation with paraffin wax, after formalin fixation, can also be accelerated by microwaves. For thicker tissue blocks (2–5 mm), this process can still take 3 h or so, but for small biopsy specimens it can be completed in 15 min (Kok et al 1988). In addition to accelerated diffusion, microwaves have been shown to speed up chemical linkages. This process can significantly reduce exposure times to solutions in a variety of staining techniques, particularly silver impregnation methods.

This applies not only to routinely processed tissues but also to frozen sections of fresh tissues (Kennedy & Foulis 1989).

Tissue antigens are well preserved following microwave irradiation. Leong found that some lymphocyte surface antigens, which were destroyed by formalin fixation, could be demonstrated following irradiation in saline (Leong 1988). The various incubation steps of a wide range of immuno-histochemical techniques can be shortened if these too are subjected to irradiation. Leong & Milios (1990) have described a streptavidin–biotin peroxidase method that requires only 20 min. Methods described by others take longer but still greatly reduce incubation time (Jackson et al 1988). Results are at least as good as those following routine methods and the demonstration of some substances, such as intermediate filaments, is actually enhanced. There are, however, some disadvantages. Increased concentrations of the primary antibodies are required by some methods, which adds to the cost of the technique and the number of slides that can be placed in an oven is limited, so that the time gained by a microwave method may be lost by having to do several consecutive runs. Microwave ovens are cheap, however, and there is no reason why a laboratory should be limited to one.

Microwaves have applications for electron microscopy also. Good ultrastructural preservation is obtained by seconds of irradiation in glutaraldehyde or a mixture of formaldehyde and glutaraldehyde (Leong et al 1985, Login & Dvorak 1985). Subsequent steps of resin impregnation and polymerization can be accelerated by microwaves and processing reduced to 1 to 2 h (McLay et al 1987).

Domestic microwave ovens can be used for these applications but some reservations have to be made. Heat distribution may not be uniform (McLay et al 1987) and there may be no facility for the extraction of fumes. Any method which requires the use of a volatile, inflammable liquid should not be attempted in such an oven. The H2500 Microwave Processor (Bio-Rad Microscience Ltd, Bio-Rad House, Maylands Road, Hemel Hempstead, Hertfordshire, HP2 7TD) is specifically designed for histopathology and provides accurate time and temperature controls and an extraction system for the removal of fumes. We use this machine in the routine laboratory for the rapid processing of urgent specimens and a domestic microwave in the mortuary for brain fixation. The laboratory oven is also used to improve the morphology of frozen sections, as described above. Rapid processing of urgent specimens is being developed. A small biopsy specimen can be fully processed and stained, ready for the microscope in 30 to 45 min.

LIGHT MICROSCOPY

Several refinements are now available for microscopy and many of these will find regular use in histopathology. Microscopes are widely available with built-in CCTV features, allowing microscopic features to be demonstrated to others and several manufacturers produce equipment capable of recording these on optical discs. These include the Eltime Video Image Archival System (Eltime Video Systems, 10/14 Hall Road, Heybridge, Maldon, Essex, CM9 7LA) which can store 800 high resolution colour pictures on a single optical disc, with an image recall time of 2 s. Each image can be individually referenced for recall from a directory and can carry up to seven major classification codes. A faster access time is obtained on the Laser Video Disc Recording System (Optivision (Yorkshire) Ltd, Ahed House, Dewsbury Road, Ossett, West Yorks, WF5 9ND). Both systems can also produce high quality colour prints for permanent record or display. The ability to transmit colour images via fax does not yet exist but is probably only a few years away.

If such optical disc storage proved to be cost-effective, it is possible that these systems could form part of an alternative long-term archive record for histopathology instead of the storage of heavy and bulky microscope slides. However, a complete change to disc recording is unlikely as it may not suit complex cases requiring numerous blocks or special stains and the transfer of suitable fields onto disc is time consuming on any scale.

Systems using video discs for undergraduate teaching have been described already (Mercer et al 1988, Kumar & Hodgins 1990). Further possibilities include the postgraduate teaching of trainee surgeons, physicians and histopathologists and the provision of educational updates for consultants. They may also prove to be a cost-effective method of training cytology screeners.

Other features which will become commonplace are motorized stages and autofocus microscopy systems, designed to take some of the fatigue out of prolonged and concentrated microscopy. Robotically controlled microscope stages have been developed, which allow remote control of the microscope. These make possible the microscopic examination of a specimen distant from the histopathologist—'telepathology' (Weinstein 1986). The need for this is greatest in hospitals where frozen section diagnosis is required but which are too small to justify a histopathologist on site and too remote for one to be summoned on demand. Such a system would also allow seeking an immediate expert opinion. The technology for telepathology, i.e. camera and monitors, already exists. The difficulty arises with the facilities necessary to transmit the image. Dedicated histopathology channels in a communications satellite are likely to be expensive and fibreoptic cable links are still being developed, but some are in use already.

A relatively new microscopy system, scanning laser confocal microscopy, bridges the gap between light and electron microscopy by combining a conventional light microscope with a laser light source and a beam scanning system. High resolution to about 0.2 µm can be achieved by point probing rather than field illumination and by excluding points not in the focal plane with a pinhole aperture. A specimen can be 'optically sectioned', images can be built up from different focal planes and used to provide a three-dimensional picture.

Such a system works particularly well with fluorescence microscopy, a disadvantage of which is unwanted signals from planes out of focus when using conventional microscopy. Astonishing detail of cellular organelles can be produced using appropriate antibodies in an immunofluorescence technique (White et al 1987). Scanning laser confocal microscopy has also been used to detect a diaminobenzidine reaction product with increased resolution (Robinson & Batten 1989). Because the laser beam can scan through a specimen, section thickness can be much greater than with conventional microscopy, with no loss of contrast, to a depth of 0.5 mm.

The uses of such a system are restricted to research applications at present. However, the possible quantitation of immunoperoxidase or immunofluorescence staining, the three-dimensional localization and increased resolution of cell organelles and the detailed imaging of chromosomes may well become part of routine investigations in the future.

ELECTRON MICROSCOPY

In recent years, electron microscopy has taken second place to immunohistochemistry in routine diagnostic practice. However, image enhancement and simplified image production should enable a revival of the service by reducing the time required of technician and histopathologist. High sensitivity TV camera systems are capable of enhancing EM images and provide optical disc storage and retrieval of selected areas. Accessories include a high resolution instant video printer which obviates the time-consuming and inconvenient steps of processing and printing conventional photographic film.

The techniques of cryoprocessing biological material for electron microscopy, for example in X-ray microanalysis and immuno-cryo-ultramicrotomy, are now firmly established research tools, but are unlikely to have an impact on routine diagnostic services for some considerable time.

IMMUNOHISTOCHEMISTRY

It is likely that the next major change in the provision of an immunohistochemical service will be the introduction of automation. This should increase through-put, improve standardization and minimize the time required of a skilled operator. Automatic immunostainers already are, or will shortly be, available. The Cadenza (Shandon Scientific Ltd, Astmoor, Runcorn, Cheshire WA7 1PR) uses a slide plus coverplate assembly into which reagents are pumped over the sections. The instrument can process up to 20 slides in a run and can perform two complete runs per day. About nine different primary antisera can be used in one run, if both monoclonal and polyclonal antisera are used. These antisera may have to be used at a higher concentration than with a manual technique, which increases reagent expense. Loading of slides into the machine requires expertise and cannot be left to junior or untrained staff. The Midas II (Midas II, BDH Ltd, Broom Road, Poole, Dorset, BH12 4NN) is a slide stainer which uses small submersion tanks, which can also be used for conventional staining techniques. It does not, however, automate the entire process, leaving primary antibody application to be carried out manually. The rest of the staining procedure can be automated but the cost of sufficient DAB chromogen to fill one tank may be prohibitive. Forty slides can be processed in one run and the automated part of the procedure takes 2 h. The AS Elite (Anglia Scientific, Broad Lane, Cottenham, Cambridge CB4 4SW) was developed from a prototype described by MaWhinney et al (1990). The basic concept is a heatable manifold with a series of individual chambers which are sealed with standard microscope slides (containing the dewaxed sections) against built-in seals. Reagents are then pumped from a carousel to chambers individually controlled by computer, where time and temperature can be set, monitored and recorded and a variety of fail-safe mechanisms automatically introduced: 96 slides can be stained in each run.

There is a temptation to regard immunohistochemistry as a highly skilled technical exercise requiring close attention to produce a good result. In fact, most steps lend themselves to automation and the results should be at least as good as those obtained by manual techniques. Primary antibodies are a problem as most departments use at least 15 routinely and may want to use more in a single run than a machine can handle. The primary antibodies are best changed between runs, which must cause some wastage. It may be better to keep this stage manual and automate the rest of the process. However, the cost of the reagents and antibodies is similar using automated or manual techniques. The capital and running costs of a machine must then be balanced against the considerable savings in skilled operator time. The rapid immunohistochemical staining, which can be achieved by microwave irradiation, may offer similar benefits (Leong & Milios 1990).

A further technique applicable to immunohistochemistry was described by Kraaz et al (1988). This used a skin punch biopsy instrument to remove 4 mm cores of tissue from wax blocks and re-embed them to form a 'multiblock' of tissues. This allows many different tissues to be examined in one section and is very economical when testing new antibodies, reagents or supernatants.

X-RAYS

The implementation of the mammography screening programme will make the presence of an X-ray cabinet in the histopathology department desirable if not essential. However, there are several other possible applications. Some of these may already be undertaken in the X-ray department, such as the examination of fetuses and infants, the assessment of specimen decalcification or radiography of thin sections of bony lesions. Others extend diagnostic accuracy; for instance, angiography of postmortem or surgical specimens can locate occluded vessels or the site of gastro-intestinal bleeding as in angiodysplasia and can increase the yield of lymph nodes from mastectomy, gastrectomy or colectomy specimens.

HEALTH AND SAFETY

With the advent of the Control of Substances Hazardous to Health Act (COSHH) in the United Kingdom, new safety issues emerge in a specialty such as histopathology where microbiological hazards have not been much of a problem. This legal requirement will affect matters as diverse as laboratory design and equipment choice as well as reagents and methods.

As an example, the continued use of formalin as the fixative of choice will require sophisticated ventilation systems to be installed, in order to comply with COSHH standards. This requirement can be met by installing a purpose built, ventilated histology work station. These are available from several companies and can be made out of stainless steel or Corian (CD (UK) Ltd, Whitehall Buildings, Whitehall Road, Leeds LS12 1BG). In future, such units will have to be specified as part of laboratory design and will require built-in, reagent-specific filters as well as airflow controls and alarms.

Histological equipment will also need to be designed and purchased with COSHH requirements in mind. Tissue processors using formalin or one of the conventional organic solvents should be one of the enclosed type, such as the VIP range (Miles Laboratories Ltd, Stoke Court, Stoke Poges, Slough SL2 4LY), the Hypercenter (Shandon Scientific Ltd) or the Concept (Clandon Scientific Ltd, Lysons Avenue, Ash Vale, Aldershot, Hampshire GU12 5QR), unless alternative reagents can be successfully used or a separate, ventilated room is available. Similarly, staining machines should be housed in fume extraction hoods either purpose made or separately provided, unless of the platen type, which present dry slides for mounting.

Automated coverslipping is another procedure which removes the user from exposure to harmful solvents and a choice of equipment is available for this. The technology already exists to coat slides with resin and, with some modification, it should be possible to produce a resin which would satisfy the mechanical and optical requirements of a final product without the need for glass coverslipping.

The AS650 Cryotome cryostat (Anglia Scientific, Broad Lane, Cottenham, Cambridge CB4 4SW) is designed with specific health and safety features, such as a separate specimen chamber for easy and efficient cleaning and disinfection. These features may also become a requirement in future.

COMPUTERS

If laboratories still exist without computerization, this will not be the case by the end of the century. Computers can perform many important laboratory functions. Practical uses include electronic requesting and reporting, bar-coded labelling of specimens, tissue blocks and sections and sophisticated statistical software for management and clinical purposes.

Bar-code labelling, combined with modern password-controlled computer links, will enable rapid access to a variety of hospital computer systems, allowing a complete review of relevant patient history prior to reporting. A currently available application is the Leitz Cy-Scan slide screening system (Leica (UK) Ltd, Davy Avenue, Knowlhill, Milton Keynes MK5 8LB). This produces bar-coded slide labels which record co-ordinate references and reporting data, subsequently available for immediate access. Similarly, the technology for automatic bar-coding of cassettes for filing and retrieval is likely to be available in the near future.

Computerization also permits detailed statistical analysis to be performed for both clinical and management purposes. The 1990s will see the introduction of a common workload measurement system in the United Kingdom, which will facilitate local management decisions by adding essential detail to Körner patient request figures.

Entirely automatic, computer-based systems requiring no analytical input for diagnosis from the histopathologist do not exist. They do exist, however, for the analysis of dispersed cells. It is possible to carry out a differential count of white blood cells for example and applications for urine analysis and karyotyping also exist (Kisner 1988). There are also systems for screening and diagnosis of cytology preparations but these are of limited usefulness. The cells must be automatically dispersed in a monolayer, rather than smeared by hand, which allows different properties, such as size, nuclear and cytoplasmic contours and nuclear-cytoplasmic ratio to be analysed. Such systems may allow the majority of normal cervical smears to be automatically 'screened out' but a full diagnostic service is still years away and may never be realized.

It is much more difficult for a computer to analyse a histological specimen, because it has to assess both overall architecture and cytological detail. Computerized interactive morphometry is concerned with the assessment of cells which are identified to the computer by a trained observer. This technique is already widely used for research purposes and its application to routine diagnostic pathology may not be far away. The equipment required is not expensive by the standards of general laboratory equipment. The system requires a computer with appropriate software, a video camera and monitor, some means, e.g. a mouse or light pen, for the observer to indicate the cells or areas of interest to the computer and a storage system. There have been many studies using computer-assisted technology and a few examples are described below.

The applications are generally geared to functions which a computer performs better than a human observer, e.g. the measurement of large numbers of features to minimize fatigue and statistical bias and the assessment of features beyond the resolution of the human eye. For example, differences in the staining properties and chromatin texture of intermediate cells in ectocervical squamous epithelium which were not apparent on routine examination, have been detected by a computer system (Wied et al 1989). Changes have also been detected in endocervical cells and related to prognosis. Non-Hodgkin's lymphomas have also been studied (Marchevsky et al 1986). About 100 nuclei per case were examined, the size being determined by comparison with superimposed concentric circles, the nuclear contour was assessed as cleaved or non-cleaved and a mitotic count was performed. The results were then applied to an algorithm to produce the diagnosis.

   With appropriate staining, it is quite simple to construct a ploidy profile of tumours and this may find many applications, for example in the assessment of malignant and borderline ovarian tumours. Computerized morphometry has also been used to assess the density of immunohisto-chemical staining to discriminate between malignant melanoma and benign melanocytic lesions (Williams et al 1986). However, if the histopathologist is to interact with a computer system, it is only worth it if the time spent is less than would normally be required to solve a difficult diagnostic problem. Some systems are still at the stage of discriminating between lesions which are easily separated by a trained observer and have yet to prove their value in difficult cases.

   A similar objection may be made to the use of expert systems in diagnosis. These prompt the user to assess various features in a specimen, such as pleomorphism or chromatin pattern; these are compared with a knowledge base and the computer then produces a diagnosis (Heathfield et al 1990). Nathwani et al (1990) discussed the reasoning behind the development of such systems and described their own experience. This was developed for lymph node pathology in particular but was so designed that it could be easily applied to other fields. The advantage is that the user has consciously to evaluate all the features required, a good practice not only for initial but also for on-going training. Few histopathologists, however, would allow a computer to offer a definite diagnosis where they were themselves in doubt and such automated systems are likely to remain limited in scope and in constant need of updating.

LIKELY FUTURE DEVELOPMENTS

How will histopathology have altered by the year 2000? Computerization will bring the greatest changes, some of which have been touched on in this chapter. Request forms may no longer be necessary, provided that the clinical information can be obtained automatically. Specimens will have bar-coded labels which follow them through the tissue block and slide stages into an optical disc archive.

   Small biopsy specimens will no longer be divided to provide material for immunohistochemistry, routine light microscopy and electron microscopy, as one embedding medium will serve for all. Tissue processing will be continuous throughout the day, since microwave processing will be built into automatic tissue processors. Most tissue samples will therefore be available for microscopy on the day they are removed. This will affect clinical practice since the availability of a biopsy report within an hour may render a second out-patient appointment unnecessary and should reduce the length of in-patient stay.

Straightforward histopathology reports will be entered into a hospital computer network, obviating the delay of a typed copy. Further histo-chemical and immunohistochemical stains will be requested by computer and be ready in minutes or hours. A final report on difficult and complex cases may still be available on the day of receipt of a biopsy.

The following scenario is extreme but not unlikely. There is a particularly difficult tumour; this is 'worked up' with special stains and combined light, scanning laser confocal and electron microscopy, allowing continuous magnification from $\times 10$ to $\times 100$ to $\times 100\,000$; a definite diagnosis is not reached. Representative areas are then recorded and faxed for the opinion of an expert who wishes to see more, and time is booked on PathSat 1. At the appointed hour, the histopathologists and clinicians concerned are linked to discuss the case. A diagnosis is agreed and the expert thanked. A sum of money is electronically switched between two accounts.

REFERENCES

Armstrong J S, Davies J D 1991 Laboratory handling of impalpable breast lesions: a review. Journal of Clinical Pathology 44: 89–93
Armstrong J S, Weinzwieg I P, Davies J D 1990 Differential marking of excision planes in screened breast lesions by organically coloured gelatins. Journal of Clinical Pathology 43: 604–607
Boon M E, Gerrits P O, Moorlag H E et al 1988 Formaldehyde fixation and microwave irradiation. Histochemical Journal 20: 313–322
Boon M E, Kok L P 1989 Microwave cookbook of pathology, 2nd ed. Coulomb Press, Leyden
Boon M E, Kok L P, Marani E 1989 Three strategies for microwave irradiation of human brains producing paraffin slides within one day. In: Bullock G R, Leathem A G, van Velzen D (eds) Techniques in diagnostic pathology, Vol I. Academic Press, London, pp 201–210
Champ C S, Mason C H, Coghill S B et al 1989 A perspex grid for localization of non-palpable mammographic lesions in breast biopsies. Histopathology 14: 311–315
Gibbs N M 1982 Large paraffin sections and chemical clearance of axillary tissues as a routine procedure in the pathological examination of the breast. Histopathology 6: 647–660
Harris M D 1990 Tipp-ex fluid: a convenient marker for surgical resection margins. Journal of Clinical Pathology 43: 346
Heathfield H A, Kirkham N, Ellis I O et al 1990 Computer assisted diagnosis of fine needle aspirate of the breast. Journal of Clinical Pathology 43: 168–170
Hogan D L, Smith G H 1982 Unconventional application of standard light and electron immunocytochemical analysis to aldehyde-fixed, araldite-embedded tissues. Journal of Histochemistry and Cytochemistry 30: 1301–1306
Islam A, Frisch B, Henderson E S 1989 Plastic embedded core biopsy: a complementary approach to bone marrow aspiration for diagnosing acute myeloid leukaemia. Journal of Clinical Pathology 42: 300–306

Jackson P, Lalani E N, Boutsen J 1988 Microwave-stimulated immunogold silver staining. Histochemical Journal 20: 353–358

Kayser K, Stute H, Lübcke J et al 1988 Rapid microwave fixation—a comparative morphometric study. Histochemical Journal 20: 347–352

Kennedy A, Foulis A K 1989 Use of microwave oven improves morphology and staining of cryostat sections. Journal of Clinical Pathology 42: 101–105

Kisner H J 1988 Principles and clinical applications of image analysis. Clinical Laboratory Medicine 8: 723–736

Kok L P, Visser P E, Boon M E 1988 Histoprocessing with the microwave oven: an update. Histochemical Journal 20: 323–328

Kraaz W, Risberg B, Hussein A 1988 Multiblock: an aid in diagnostic immunohistochemistry. Journal of Clinical Pathology 41: 1337–1339

Kumar K, Hodgins M 1990 Use of interactive videodisc for teaching of pathology laboratory cases. Journal of Pathology 160: 145–149

Leong A S-Y 1988 Microwave irradiation in histopathology. In: Rosen P P, Fechner R E (eds) Pathology annual. Appleton-Century-Crofts, New York, pp 213–234

Leong A S-Y, Milios J 1990 Accelerated immunohistochemical staining by microwaves. Journal of Pathology 161: 327–334

Leong A S-Y, Daymon M E, Milios J 1985 Microwave irradiation as a form of fixation for light and electron microscopy. Journal of Clinical Pathology 146: 313–321

Login G R, Dvorak A M 1985 Microwave energy fixation for electron microscopy. American Journal of Pathology 120: 230–243

Marani E, Bolhuis P, Boon M E 1988 Brain enzyme histochemistry following stabilization by microwave irradiation. Histochemical Journal 20: 397–404

Marchevsky A, Gil J, Silage D 1986 Computerized interactive morphometry as a potentially useful tool for the classification of non-Hodgkin's lymphomas. Cancer 57: 1544–1549

MaWhinney W H B, Warford A, Rae M J L et al 1990 Automated immunochemistry. Journal of Clinical Pathology 43: 591–596

McLay A L C, Anderson J D, McMeekin W 1987 Microwave polymerisation of epoxy resin: rapid processing technique in ultrastructural pathology. Journal of Clinical Pathology 40: 350–352

Mercer J, Pringle J H, Rae M J L et al 1988 The laser videodisc and computer-assisted learning. Journal of Pathology 156: 83–89

Murray G I 1988 Is wax on the wane? Journal of Pathology 156: 187–188

Nathwani B N, Heckerman D E, Horvitz E J et al 1990 Integrated expert systems and videodisc in surgical pathology: an overview. Human Pathology 21: 11–27

Pallett C D, MaWhinney W H B, Malcolm A J 1986 Plastic processing of cemented hip joint replacement specimens. Journal of Clinical Pathology 39: 339–342

Paterson D A, Davies J D 1988 Marking planes of surgical excision on breast biopsy specimens: use of artists' pigments suspended in acetone. Journal of Clinical Pathology 41: 1013–1016

Robinson J M, Batten B E 1989 Detection of diaminobenzidine reactions using scanning laster confocal reflectance microscopy. Journal of Histochemistry and Cytochemistry 37: 1761–1765

Shires M, Goode N P, Crellin D M et al 1990 Immunogold-silver staining of mesangial antigen in Lowicryl K4M- and LR gold-embedded renal tissue using epipolarization microscopy. Journal of Histochemistry and Cytochemistry 38: 287–289

Weinstein R S 1986 Prospects for telepathology. Human Pathology 17: 433–434

White J G, Amos W B, Fordham M 1987 An evaluation of confocal versus conventional imaging of biological structures by fluorescence light microscopy. Journal of Cell Biology 105: 41–48

Wied G L, Bartels P H, Bibbo M et al 1989 Image analysis in quantitative cytopathology and histopathology. Human Pathology 20: 549–571

Williams R A, Rode J, Dhillon A P et al 1986 Measuring S100 protein and neurone specific enolase in melanocytic tumours using video image analysis. Journal of Clinical Pathology 39: 1096–1098

Index